Running on Empty

In her award-winning book, Dr. Katrina H. Berne . . . gives a thorough and often poignant overview of this devastating yet poorly understood illness. Combining current medical knowledge of CFIDS with the results of patient interviews and entries from her personal journal, she discusses its physiological, psychological, and social aspects . . . .

Dr. Berne's personal and professional experience with CFIDS is evident throughout this book. The information she provides on CFIDS . . . is up-to-date, comprehensible, and complete. Interspersed with this information are insightful, sometimes intimate, statements about the psychological and sociological problems that persons with CFIDS experience at each stage of their illness . . . .

This book is more than a self-help book for CFIDS patients and a reference book for health-care professionals. It is insightful commentary on the devastating effects of chronic, debilitating illness.
— *American Medical Writers Association Journal*

RUNNING ON EMPTY provides the tools that patients and their families need to deal with this illness, from how to recognize the telling symptoms to how to choose and talk to doctors and apply for disability. With humor and sympathy, Berne also exposes the pain of her own experience, her low points and persistent hope. In her account readers will recognize a life being led as well as it can be. 'My illness can borrow my sanity but it can't have it,' writes Berne . . . . Her example, even more than the helpful information and advice, is what makes RUNNING ON EMPTY exceptional.
— *The CFIDS Chronicle*

The appendices are full of helpful information on CFIDS national organizations, consumer resources, books and other publications, sources of financial aid, and tips for organizing a support group.
— *Library Journal*

Extensive bibliographies and resource sections make this book invaluable for the growing number of CFIDS patients and the professionals who treat them. — *On The Bookshelf*
The Union Institute Bookstore

This comprehensive examination of CFIDS is up-to-date and gives excellent mechanisms for recognizing and coping with this debilitating syndrome. Dr. Berne's book is a current and well researched thesis on what is known about CFIDS, how it is diagnosed, and how one can learn to live with the deficits it causes. — David L. Payne, D.O.
CFIDS practitioner and researcher

Competing titles offer only a fraction of this information, often omitting surveys of field controversies in favor of exposing new research. — *The Bookwatch*

I highly recommend RUNNING ON EMPTY. As a physician who has been ill with CFIDS for four years, I find it highly accurate in terms of characteristics of the illness itself and regarding current research in progress. This book is written from the standpoint of both psychologist and patient and is written in a form that makes it readily understandable to the patient. I highly recommend this book to health care providers and patients.
— Sara S. Reynolds, M.D., AAFP
Executive Board Member, CFS Association of Arizona

CFIDS affects a surprising number of executives, and especially women executives. In facts, females who have been diagnosed with CFIDS outnumber male sufferers by a ratio as high as three to one.
... This book is the first to cover the disease from all angles and provide detailed explanations and advice on how to deal with it and its effects on career, family, and personal relationships.
— *Career Woman*

Running on Empty

The Complete Guide to Chronic Fatigue Syndrome (CFIDS)

Katrina H. Berne, Ph.D.

317175

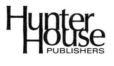

HUNTER HOUSE INC., PUBLISHERS
P.O. Box 2914
Alameda, CA 94501-0914

Library of Congress Cataloging-in-Publication Data
Berne, Katrina.
Running on empty : the complete guide to chronic fatigue syndrome (CFIDS) / Katrina H. Berne. — 2nd rev. ed.
p. cm.
Includes bibliographical references and index.
ISBN 0-89793-192-0 (hardcover). — 0-89793-191-2 (paper)
1. Chronic fatigue syndrome. I. Title.
RB150.F37R37   1995
616'.047—dc20   95-44914

Project Editor	*Production Manager*
LISA E. LEE	PAUL J. FRINDT
Copy Editor	*Sales & Marketing*
MARY LOU SUMBERG	CORRINE M. SAHLI
Proofreader	*Publicity & Promotion*
SUSAN BURCKHARD	DARCY COHAN
Index	*Scheduling & Administration*
MALI APPLE	MARÍA JESÚS AGUILÓ
Book Design	*Customer Support*
DIAN-AZIZA OOKA	SARAH BHATTACHARJEE, JOSHUA TABISAURA
Cover Design	*Order Fulfillment*
MIG DESIGN WORKS	A&A QUALITY SHIPPING SERVICES

Publisher
KIRAN S. RANA

Set in Goudy, Journal, and Zurich by 847 Communications, Alameda CA
Printed and bound by Publishers Press, Salt Lake City UT
Manufactured in the United States of America

9 8 7 6 5 4 3 2   Second edition

Table of Contents

To Mabel
who had stars in her eyes

Acknowledgments

Given my unpredictable and unrelenting health fluctuations, it's amazing I've completed this book, and I couldn't have done it without the support and encouragement of some very helpful and generous people.

My parents, Arthur and Claire Berne, who have seen me through my skinned-knees years and my I'll-never-get-through-college woes, have come through again on several fronts, supporting me in so many ways during my illness, doctoral studies, and the writing of this book.

My husband, Eldon, who married an unknown quantity (he married me post-onset but pre-diagnosis), has tolerated my mood swings, strange hours, and bizarre treatments (with their accompanying side effects and my complaints); listened to endless litanies on my various theories and ordeals; and weathered alternate declarations that I'll survive and triumph—and that I'll never make it. He has offered feedback, comfort, and consolation, and more love and encouragement than I thought humanly possible.

My kids, Karen and Jeffrey, who have continued to have needs of their own (as kids tend to do), have nonetheless tolerated a mother who spent most of her time at work, sick in bed, or writing and swearing at the computer.

The late Caroline Shrodes offered warmth, encouragement, and wisdom, not to mention help with punctuation. She pushed me to publish—to share my knowledge of CFIDS with others.

The wonderful folks at Hunter House offered encouragement, advice, and most importantly the opportunity to reach others with my work.

I am grateful to the dedicated physicians and other health professionals involved in CFIDS treatment and research who have risked the censure of a skeptical medical establishment to serve the needs of persons with CFIDS. I feel very close to other PWCs and wish to offer special thanks to those who filled out questionnaires, endured interviews that lasted hours, and urged me forward in my work.

I am endlessly grateful to these special people and to the others who have seen me through this far and who will probably stick around for more.

Important Notice

The material in this book is intended to provide a review of information regarding CFIDS. Every effort has been made to provide accurate and dependable information. The contents of this book have been carefully reviewed by medical doctors. The reader should be aware that health care professionals have differing opinions and ways of treating various problems, and advances in medical and scientific research are made quickly, so some of the information may become outdated.

Therefore, the publisher, author, editors, and reviewers cannot be held responsible for any error, omission, or dated material. Any treatments described should be undertaken only under the guidance of a licensed health care practitioner. The author and publisher assume no responsibility for any outcome of the use of any of these treatments in a program of self-care or under the care of a licensed practitioner.

If you have a question concerning your care or treatment, or about the appropriateness or application of the treatments described in this book, consult your health care professional.

Some of the therapies, treatments, or products mentioned in this book have been trademarked. When the author and publisher were aware of a trademark claim, the designations have been printed with initial capital letters.

Foreword

Through her own professional and personal experience with Chronic Fatigue Syndrome (CFS or CFIDS), Dr. Berne has developed an intimate and thorough knowledge of the disease. The horror, frustration, and anger produced by the disabling condition are graphically portrayed, yet balanced by the reality of palliative treatment and hope for future research.

Most Americans have heard of CFS, Chronic Epstein-Barr (CEBV), or "yuppie flu," or know someone suffering from the disease. However, the fledgling scientific literature of CFS has reached few patients and even fewer physicians. While patients are acutely aware of the potentially disabling power of the disease, most researchers and physicians continue to view CFS as a trivial anthill on the mountain of medicine.

While scientific research will ultimately yield answers to the many unknowns of CFS, this work is truly a landmark compendium of present knowledge in the field. For the physician, the book presents an historical summary, reviews theories of pathogenesis, and outlines current therapeutic strategies. Additionally, and perhaps more importantly, the author reifies the debilitating, disabling effects of the disease and contradicts the common perception that it is trivial or even nonexistent. Postulated etiologies of the disease challenge medical researchers to intensify their efforts.

Patients are presented with a complete, readable, and comprehensible self-study course in CFIDS. Chapters dedicated to self-help and adjustment to chronic disease are particularly critical for patients suffering from an incurable, long-lasting disease. Common pitfalls of self-diagnosis and self-treatment are clearly illustrated. Families and friends can find insight into the symptoms and reactions to symptoms which alter the physical functioning and personalities of their loved one. The author also suggests realistic and functional solutions to improve interpersonal relationships and to preserve the family structure. An extensive bibliography directs those interested in historic and current publications to scientific and lay literature on CFIDS. Physicians, patients, and their families are provided with a current list of support groups, research organizations, and governmental agencies serving the cause of CFIDS.

Finally, society at large is confronted with the desperate need for recognition of this worldwide health problem. Lack of research funding, lack of national interest on the part of federal and private research agencies, and physician misinformation and apathy combine to retard discovery into the pathogenesis and treatment of the disorder. Hopefully, this book will serve to unite and stimulate a broad base of support and research into CFIDS.

CFIDS is fraught with systematic difficulties including diagnostic and therapeutic confusion due in large part to unknown or unproved etiology and pathogenesis. This creates frustration for the physician as well as the patient and often leads to a dysfunctional and unsatisfactory patient/physician relationship. Dr. Berne strives to look beyond knowledge gaps and expose the poorly defined disease process in terms of its functional impact on the physical and mental health of the patient. Numerous real-life examples compel the physician to accept the seriousness of CFIDS; patients are reassured that they are not alone in the morass of signs and symptoms. The author has intertwined experiential data with hard science to produce the most complete overview of CFIDS to date. It will undoubtedly serve as a catalyst for future research and as a ready reference for patients and families of those suffering from CFIDS.

Daniel L. Peterson, M.D.
Incline Village, Nevada, 1992

Preface

A series of astonishing breakthroughs in medical research is gradually bringing the stark realities of CFIDS to the attention of the media, the general public, and the medical establishment. CFIDS is a devastating and elusive illness that afflicts millions and poses a major public health threat. It is a serious disease of immune dysfunction and neurological impairment that is finally being taken seriously.

The tremendous progress being made by a handful of dedicated CFIDS researchers inspires PWCs (persons with CFIDS) as nothing else can. It validates our disease as a distinct clinical entity and gives us hope that the cause(s) and cure(s) will soon be found. These advances also fill us with deep gratitude and pride. We will be forever grateful to the pioneering CFIDS physicians and researchers who have persevered despite the skepticism and derision of their "peers." And we are very proud that PWCs, their families, and friends are largely responsible for this success. We funded much of the research that is legitimizing CFIDS.

These accomplishments at the cutting edge are encouraging and impressive. But the translation of laboratory and clinical findings into diagnostic tools and effective treatments is painfully slow. CFIDS remains. Much of the medical profession continues to ignore, trivialize, or even "psychologize" CFIDS. And, running on empty, PWCs still have a long way to go.

This book is a comprehensive close-up study of CFIDS written by a true CFIDS insider. Without flinching, Katrina Berne, Ph.D., describes the emotional, physical, and cognitive onslaught of this disease, sharing the knowledge of a seasoned PWC and a trained psychologist who counsels and lectures on that which she knows much about. She explains both the science and the impact of CFIDS, making a mysterious, invisible disease visible and understandable.

Dr. Berne employs an array of devices to depict life with CFIDS: descriptive metaphors, excerpts from her own personal journal, and compassionate vignettes that tell the tales of other PWCs and their feelings. Her insights into the experience and trauma of CFIDS will touch many chords in people with the disease and those who care for them. And her exploration of what PWCs have lost is riveting and frightening.

There is almost nothing you cherish that CFIDS cannot take away. Your health, your mind, your job, your family, your home, your friends, your identity . . . . Inevitably, CFIDS disrupts or shreds the script for your life and those sharing it.

Fortunately, Dr. Berne pursues the difficult issue of "How do I live with CFIDS?" with the same vigor, wisdom, sympathy, and humor that she uses to explain the nature of the disease. She catalogues the many methods PWCs have devised to grapple with, endure, and grow from the experience of having CFIDS. Her advice on "what to do" includes an analysis of the medical profession and various approaches to healing, identification of treatment programs and lifestyle adjustments, extensive discussion of coping techniques and changes in life philosophy, open letters between PWCs and significant others, guidance on how to form and facilitate a support group, and lists of other resources.

The tools are here for PWCs, their families, their friends, and even their physicians to develop new scripts.

After reading *Running on Empty* you walk away feeling full. It is authoritative but friendly, personal, and easily accessible. It is a resource for everybody and anybody who has an interest in CFIDS. It is the single most useful book on CFIDS to date.

Marc M. Iverson
President, The CFIDS Association, Inc.
Publisher of *The CFIDS Chronicle*

Author's Preface
to the Second Edition

On May 12, 1995, International Chronic Fatigue Syndrome (CFS or CFIDS) Awareness Day, Mark Loveless, M.D., an infectious disease specialist who heads an AIDS and CFS clinic at Oregon Health Sciences University, testified at a U.S. congressional briefing. He stated that *every day* a CFIDS patient feels significantly the same as an AIDS patient feels two months before death.

Dr. William Reeves, chief of Viral Exanthems and Herpesvirus Branch at the Centers for Disease Control and Prevention (CDC), stated that between 76 and 220 per 100,000 Americans have a CFIDS-like illness, revising the earlier underestimate of 4 to 9 cases per 100,000.

CDC officials have recently added CFIDS to the list of Priority One New and Reemerging Infectious Diseases.

Anthony Komaroff, M.D., a CFIDS researcher, clinician, and head of a research/treatment center funded by the National Institutes of Health (NIH), reports serious brain damage in persons with CFIDS, and this has been corroborated by extensive research.

CFIDS is one of the most common illnesses of our time, and its symptoms overlap with those of numerous other possibly related illnesses. Compounding the already confusing picture is the emergence of other CFIDS-like illnesses, such as Gulf War Syndrome, fibromyalgia, post-polio syndrome, environmental illness, and symptoms suffered by women with breast implants. The connections among these illnesses are not well understood. Among private insurers, CFIDS is the fastest rising cause of disability for men and women.

The impact of chronic fatigue syndrome has been significantly underestimated. Government officials will have to start paying attention to researchers, practitioners, and patients (i.e., constituents) regarding the devastation that has been caused by a disease that was once dismissed as "yuppie flu" or as a nonexistent "fad" illness. (Who would follow such a fad? Who wants this disease?) While we are running on empty, our elected officials are asleep at the wheel. Our insurance companies, to whom we have paid substantial premiums over the years, are cutting us off at every opportunity.

We now know that the illness is severely debilitating and often disabling, that it robs people of their lives as they knew them, and that the socioeconomic impact alone is devastating to our nation. What is it going to take?

Ten years plus after the documented outbreak in Incline Village, Nevada, we are still begging for recognition and for research money. We are the vocal minority—those with CFIDS who spend what little time, energy, and money we have fighting for our interests while battling an illness that is unpopular in the extreme. CFIDS, the disease, is unpopular with us too, but the issue is not. And we represent the tip of the iceberg. There are many more who are silent, and many who remain undiagnosed.

This illness will not go away; in fact, its numbers are increasing. We need help. We need research funding to discover causes, treatments, and perhaps a cure. We need the support of everyone, from government officials to our immediate families and friends. We need some relief. We need information. We need to feel like valuable, valued individuals again.

My place in the struggle is to help restore a sense of self-worth for persons with CFIDS (PWCs), to educate them and their significant others, and to provide support and help with problem solving. Readers and patients often ask me how I chose this specialty. The answer is simple: it chose me. I have been ill with CFIDS for 11 years. I am still dumbfounded and baffled that I have spent that period of time living with the illness, helping others who have it, researching and writing about it, and coming up with so little that is concrete. It keeps me humble. And I am one of the lucky ones. I have been able to continue my work in a modified fashion. My family and friends do understand my situation and limitations as best they can. My life abounds with love and support—but also with symptoms and limitations. The ultimate dilemma, the world's worst irony: being too ill to be the activist and advocate I'd like to be.

My goals in writing the second edition of *Running on Empty* are to provide support and education, to present current theories and treatment options, and to suggest ways to cope with the illness and lead a meaningful life. As in the first edition, I have no answers, but in the years that have passed, causal theories, treatment options, and attention to the illness have begun to flourish. Still, the answer to many specific questions is, "I don't know." There is so much we don't know, but we have leads to follow and exciting work ahead. There is still much room for hope.

Katrina Berne
Winter 1995

Part I

Chronic Fatigue Immune Dysfunction Syndrome (CFIDS): What It Is

Chapter 1

An Overview of CFIDS

Jane awoke one morning feeling flu-ish and decided to stay in bed. An active, energetic, "Type A" woman, Jane knew she might feel ill for a few days before returning to her normal responsibilities and activity level, as had always been the case with minor illnesses. She'd either keep going despite the illness, or at most take a few days off before resuming her busy schedule. This time didn't feel any different; she felt a bit off-balance and spacey, as if her head were filled with cotton, and had aching joints, a sore throat, tender lymph nodes, and fatigue. "It's just the flu," she told herself. "A week or so of this and then I'll be fine."

Two years later Jane is still in bed most of the time, knowing now that it wasn't just the flu but a lingering illness that has left her debilitated. Her responsibilities—work and family—aren't being fulfilled as well as she'd like, and her former leisure time activities—jogging, hiking, racquetball, lunches with friends, dinner parties—have dwindled to almost nothing. She is often depressed and wonders if she'll ever feel any better. She's feeling crazy and lazy, since no doctor has been able to diagnose her illness. It has been implied and sometimes suggested outright that what she is experiencing is merely the blues, depression, or an anxiety problem; and Jane is beginning to believe what several doctors have told her: that it is "all in her head."

Logically she knows that she would never voluntarily have given up her previous lifestyle—the income, the work she enjoyed, her many leisure activities—just to stay in bed and feel awful. She has to drag herself out of bed even to do the basics, such as minor household chores and personal grooming. She feels guilty for neglecting many of her responsibilities but has found that if she pushes herself to be active and to "take care of business" her symptoms flare. "I don't understand what's happening to me. I'm just not myself anymore. I used to be able to do *everything*—and do it well. I always took care of everything and everyone, and I'm not able to do that anymore."

Jane wonders whether her life will ever return to normal and fights the possibility that she may have to adapt to this debilitated state and modify her lifestyle significantly in order to cope. And worse, she doesn't understand why she feels so awful all the time. Jane says, "I can handle anything as long as I understand it and know what I'm up against. This feeling, this illness . . . I just can't make sense out of it. I don't know if it's something I'm doing to myself or something from 'out there' I can't control." She wonders how much "legitimacy" her illness has and how it could have happened to her.

Robert has always regarded himself as a low-energy person, reporting frequent illnesses as a child and even as an adult. "I get everything that's going around," he laments. "Whatever flu bug everyone is getting, I always get it too. I've had measles, flu, chicken pox, mono . . . . I've just gotten used to it." His previous allergies are now worse, as is his already-low energy level. Over a period of time, Robert has felt more and more fatigued. Unable to work even part time, he is fighting the maze of paperwork that accompanies his attempt to obtain disability benefits. His self-esteem, as a hard worker and a good provider, has plummeted along with his ability to live a "normal" life. "I don't get it. I've been sick a lot—but never this sick, and never for so long." Robert has been to a number of doctors and has finally found one who is familiar with his illness, which is called Chronic Fatigue Syndrome (CFS), or Chronic Fatigue Immune Dysfunction Syndrome (CFIDS).

CFIDS may be a new problem or a modern version of an illness that has occurred in outbreaks for well over a century. However, it remains a poorly understood illness. It is a disease of immunological and neurological dysfunction, and its cause may be viral. At one time it was called "Chronic Epstein-Barr Virus Syndrome," but this name is no longer used since the Epstein-Barr virus is no longer believed to be the causative agent.

Patients and practitioners alike have complained about the name chronic fatigue syndrome, suggesting that the "f" word be dropped, since fatigue is only one of a myriad of debilitating symptoms associated with the illness. Many physicians and patients feel that the name chronic fatigue syndrome trivializes the illness, making it seem like a "crazy and lazy" phenomenon. Walter Gunn, Ph.D., former chief CFIDS researcher for the Centers for Disease Control and Prevention (CDC), said, "The term Chronic Fatigue Syndrome is demeaning to the people who have it," adding that at present we have no basis for giving the disease a more accurate name.

Other names have been suggested: myalgic encephalomyelitis (ME), the term used in some other countries, or myalgic encephalomyelopathy. Other suggested names include major acquired brain dysfunction, postviral fatigue syndrome, chronic viral syndrome (or postviral syndrome), Gilliam Ramsay's syndrome, Florence Nightingale syndrome, and chronic multiple systemic dysfunction. The term chronic fatigue immune dysfunction syndrome (CFIDS) has come into common usage since it includes the immune abnormalities that have been found in many PWCs (Persons With Chronic fatigue immune dysfunction syndrome). According to an article in The CFIDS Chronicle (Spring 1995), the name CFIDS "represents a transitional term until research progresses to the point at which a name that accurately describes the etiology (cause), pathogenesis (mode in which the disease develops), or pathophysiology (mechanism of the disease) can be determined."

Suspects for the causative agent(s)—there may be more than one—include retroviruses, herpesviruses, adenoviruses, and other infectious agents. But not everyone exposed to the causative agent(s) will necessarily develop the disease. Current research suggests that the onset of CFIDS is a multicausal event, including not only a triggering agent (viral or otherwise), but other factors including age, sex, exposure to environmental toxins, a stressful lifestyle and/or a period of intense stress or work, prior surgery or illness, and genetic predisposition.

CFIDS is believed to be both an endemic and an epidemic phenomenon; that is, isolated cases are believed to exist in the general population at all times, with epidemic outbreaks occurring periodically. Although such outbreaks have occurred for more than a hundred years, it is not known if the current epidemic is identical to past outbreaks. Descriptions of earlier outbreaks match the current illness definition quite well but have been poorly documented. Because each outbreak was given a name, noted briefly in the medical literature, and then dismissed, we lack sufficient information to draw solid conclusions. And to further complicate the matter, in examining the illness we may be looking at a number of similar illnesses that fall under one "umbrella."

There have been pockets of CFIDS outbreaks across the United States and in other countries as well—CFIDS is literally all over the map. CFIDS crosses all barriers—age, nationality, gender, income, lifestyle, and occupation—although certain predisposing factors make some people more susceptible than others.

The onset of CFIDS is abrupt in about 75% of cases: most patients can pinpoint exactly when they became ill. "I was sitting in the airport the day before Thanksgiving when I suddenly started to feel awful," says Tom. "My flight was fine, but I wasn't; I don't even remember the time I spent with my relatives. I slept through the entire visit." However, the onset may not be as abrupt as it seems. Often, patients note in retrospect that they experienced a number of CFIDS-like symptoms over a period of years, often throughout their lifetimes: easy fatigability, allergies, frequent infections, unexplained body pain, and such. These symptoms were mild or intermittent and did not cause significant distress until an infectious agent, toxic exposure, and/or major life changes initiated the onset of full-blown CFIDS. The distinction between gradual and abrupt onset of CFIDS is blurry.

Female PWCs are believed to outnumber males by a 2:1 or 3:1 ratio. This phenomenon is not uncommon in autoimmune diseases, which CFIDS may indeed prove to be. "What are *you* doing with a *woman's* disease?" asked one insensitive doctor of a male PWC. In fact, CFIDS may be less frequently diagnosed among males because men often do not seek medical attention when they are ill. If the "sex bias" does exist, it may be explained by hormonal differences and/or occupational differences. The majority of known cases have occurred among professionals, health care workers, airline personnel, and businesspeople, while blue-collar workers and those in solitary professions seem to be less affected. It has been hypothesized that Type A personalities may be more susceptible to developing CFIDS.

However, the notion that CFIDS and occupation or personality type are linked may prove to be false. "CFS is an Equal Opportunity Attacker," wrote Dennis Jackson, Ph.D. (*The CFIDS Chronicle*, Spring 1991). Several studies comparing healthy individuals and PWCs indicate that their socioeconomic status and educational levels were about the same. No one is exempt from the possibility of developing CFIDS.

The average age at onset is 37, and most patients are in their middle or "prime" years, in the 25–50 age range. Numerous studies indicate that about 75% of patients are aged 20–49; 50–60% are 30–49. The preponderance of cases in these middle, normally productive years is potentially devastating to our work force. However, the age range may be skewed because the illness is probably underdiagnosed in children and in the elderly. CFIDS is found in every age group.

Symptoms vary widely among patients and will vary in severity and change over time in each PWC. Many CFIDS symptoms have been experienced by healthy individuals from time to time, but in PWCs the symptoms are more continuous, severe, and pronounced. A college professor who was forced by CFIDS into early retirement calls it "the disease of jumping symptoms." Another PWC notes, "The fatigue, disequilibrium, and frequent illnesses that plagued me in the first year of my illness aren't such a problem anymore. But I now have more difficulty with allergies, digestive problems, and sometimes muscle pain. I'm ill all the time, but the severity and the symptoms keep changing. It's really hard to plan anything or live any kind of predictable life with this crazy stuff going on. I'm getting really angry and fed up, and so is my family. We never know what to expect."

For the sake of convenience, we may describe CFIDS symptoms as falling into three general categories.

General or **physical symptoms** include: debilitating fatigue; sore throat; swollen or tender lymph nodes; frequent infections; unusual and often severe headaches; allergies (worsening of previous allergies and/or new allergies); sensitivities to foods, odors, or chemicals; weight change, usually a gain unaccompanied by a change in eating habits; muscle and joint aches; gastrointestinal problems such as gas, diarrhea, nausea, and abdominal pain; rashes; low-grade fevers; night sweats; shortness of breath with minimal or no exertion; heart palpitations; chest pain; cough; urinary tract problems; decreased sex drive.

Neurological symptoms include: sensitivity to bright light; disequilibrium (balance problems, "spaceyness," and disorienta-

tion); difficulty with concentration and memory; impaired calculation and word-finding abilities; numbness or tingling feelings; sleep
disturbance; visual problems; seizure-like episodes or "blackouts";
unusual and disturbing nightmares; and altered spatial perception,
which is often most evident when driving a vehicle. These neurological symptoms are a hallmark of CFIDS.

Emotional problems associated with CFIDS include: depression, which may be accompanied by suicidal ideation or attempts;
anxiety with or without panic attacks; mood swings; irritability
and/or "rage attacks." The depression may be both endogenous
(chemically caused) and exogenous (caused by external events—in
this case, being chronically ill). Although patients often *feel* crazy,
many of the emotional changes they experience are directly caused
by the illness. Most did not experience such problems prior to the
onset of CFIDS.

PWCs generally feel poorly understood by others, experiencing self-doubt as well as relationship conflicts. It is impossible for
those without CFIDS to understand the true impact of the illness
and the havoc it can wreak. Because patients invariably appear
healthier than they feel, those with whom they come into contact
are not immediately aware of CFIDS-related limitations and often
expect the PWC to behave "normally"—that is, to be active and
to handle the same responsibilities as in the past. It is difficult for
PWCs to communicate the degree of their physical impairment
and emotional pain to others, and as a result many relationships
are disrupted. In addition, the PWC copes daily with lowered self-
esteem, a very restricted activity level, an inability to predict
health fluctuations, and feelings of powerlessness and worthlessness
due to the inability to function as in the past. Many have based
their self-esteem on *what they were able to do* rather than on *who
they were and are*, leading to changing roles and identity problems
that must be addressed. The emotional fallout of CFIDS can be as
devastating as the symptoms themselves.

There is no laboratory test to diagnose CFIDS. Diagnosis is
based on symptoms, length of the illness, degree of impairment,
and by ruling out other illnesses with similar symptoms. In the past
an Epstein-Barr antibody panel was used, but this should no longer
be regarded as a diagnostic tool since the elevation of Epstein-Barr
virus antibodies found in most patients is now viewed as an

epiphenomenon—a secondary phenomenon accompanying another and caused by it—rather than a cause of CFIDS. Many PWCs see numerous doctors before being diagnosed. CFIDS is both underdiagnosed (when patients' symptoms are not understood or taken seriously by their doctors) and overdiagnosed (when fatigue is caused by other factors, including anemia, sleep disorders, psychological/psychiatric disorders, effects of drugs, metabolic disorders, and other chronic illnesses).

The severity of the illness varies considerably among patients as well as in individual patients across time. Some are mildly affected and can carry on a modified activity schedule, others are extremely debilitated, and many are completely disabled. Those in the latter group are unable to work and may be bedbound or housebound. Most cases fall between these extremes, with the illness following a waxing and waning cycle.

The Centers for Disease Control and Prevention, initially resistant to acknowledging the existence of this illness, issued a definition and symptom criteria for the diagnosis of Chronic Fatigue Syndrome (the term they prefer) in March 1988. Revised diagnostic criteria were published in December 1994. Although the criteria were developed for research purposes, they are often used as a diagnostic tool by physicians and the Social Security Administration. CFIDS researchers, medical practitioners, and patients agree that their definition is quite narrow in scope and needs to be updated.

The mode of transmission is unknown. Multiple cases of CFIDS in families are common, and those afflicted are usually genetically related (blood relatives) rather than nonblood relatives such as spouses. Some researchers suspect that the risk for partners of PWCs of developing the disease increases over time due to increased viral "load" or repeated exposure, while others believe that the risk of contagion is high only in the early stages of the disease. However, there is *no* evidence that CFIDS is contagious or transmissible. If CFIDS is found not to be highly contagious, then genetic predisposition and/or exposure to environmental agents may explain the route by which the disease is contracted.

Spouses and others close to the PWC may develop subclinical cases of CFIDS, although the incidence of this is unknown. In about 10% of cases in an outbreak in Lake Tahoe, both spouses became ill, and the risk of contagion to a spouse was highest in the first year of the illness. A parent and a child or children may fall ill at the same time. A study of patients with pets in Charlotte, North Carolina, indicated that 50% of these pets were ill; this study has not been replicated and its significance is unknown (Cheney 1991).

Because of the uncertainties regarding contagion, PWCs are advised not to be blood or organ donors. Some experts believe that PWCs should not obtain immunizations as these may challenge an already-disrupted immune process; others assert that flu shots pose no danger and are advisable. Because the transmissibility of the illness has not been determined, some physicians advise against anything that would cause contact with the saliva of the PWC, such as sharing eating utensils and drinking glasses or kissing on the mouth, and recommend the use of condoms for those who are sexually active with more than one partner. Other physicians feel that such precautions are unnecessary, so it is up to the individual to decide whether precautions are appropriate.

Although there is no known cure, CFIDS is treatable. Rest and lifestyle modification are the most helpful treatments. PWCs who are used to being active achievers find that moderating their activity levels falls somewhere between inconvenient and impossible. However, it is absolutely necessary to adapt by altering one's activity level. The worst thing PWCs can do is push themselves too hard, thereby inviting relapses and possibly prolonging the course of the illness.

In addition to rest and moderation of activity, general and symptomatic treatments are available. It is essential to work with a physician who is knowledgeable about CFIDS and current treatment regimens. Individual or group psychotherapy is helpful for dealing with the emotional devastation that invariably accompanies CFIDS: illness-imposed limitations, anger, losses, depression, relationship and family issues, and lifestyle alterations. Instruction in relaxation and stress-reduction techniques can also be helpful. Most support groups provide referral lists of recommended professionals.

Is there life after CFIDS? *Do* people recover? Many PWCs have been told by their physicians that they will get well in a specified amount of time, such as three to five years. However, it is impossible to predict how long an individual will remain ill or whether full or significant recovery will take place. Although the prognosis is uncertain in individual cases, various clinicians have noted trends in the course of the illness. Daniel Peterson, M.D., has noted that 75% of patients improve gradually, 20% reach a plateau at a certain level of dysfunction, and 3% remain severely disabled and may continue to deteriorate. Paul Cheney, M.D., has reported that about 12% of patients recover fully, usually during the first one to two years or during the fourth to fifth year. Another expert finds that 30% of patients experience significant remission, although full recovery is unlikely. Degree of recovery seems to be associated not with how severe the illness is, but with how long it has lasted. Several experts observe that those who remain ill for longer than three years have a low incidence of complete recovery, although many improve. Those who have become fully disabled often remain disabled for many years. The majority of patients continue to have chronic moderate-to-severe symptoms. Although most continue to have symptoms, a small subgroup recovers and most patients do improve—often substantially—over time.

PWCs are encouraged to play an active role in treatment and to obtain current, accurate information. Appendix C contains numerous sources of information: publications and organizations that offer information about CFIDS treatment, research, patient advocacy, coping tips, and emotional support.

PWCs have cause for hope. The medical community is becoming increasingly sensitive to CFIDS and those it afflicts; researchers are searching for causes, treatments, and cures; and a significant number of patients do recover—fully, or to some degree. Meanwhile, self-care, education, medical treatment, and emotional support remain the most precious resources of persons with CFIDS.

Chapter 2

Definition and History of CFIDS

Some doctors still dismiss its existence, but chronic
fatigue syndrome could be the next crippling, global epidemic.

Maggie Strong, *Mainstay: For the Well Spouse of the
Chronically Ill*

WHAT CFIDS IS...

"CFIDS is a mystery waiting for a miracle," wrote one PWC.
"CFIDS changes your priorities and puts you firmly in the *now*.
You can't remember yesterday, and you can't predict tomorrow.
When your *now* is full of pain and frustration, it's the end of the
world. When your *now* improves, there's hope in your heart."

CFIDS has been defined and described by many experts. Paul
Cheney, M.D., noted that although we lack a specific definition of
this syndrome, "we know it when we see it" (February 1990). He
described the common denominators of PWCs as immune system
dysregulation and neurocognitive dysfunction. Noting both similarities and differences among PWCs, Mark Loveless, M.D., calls
CFIDS a "spectrum of disease."

Jay Goldstein, M.D., has referred to CFIDS as "the most
complex disease I have ever studied." He defined CFIDS in March
1991: "I regard CFIDS as the final common pathway of a multifac-
torial psychoneuroimmunologic disorder with a limbic encephalopathy causing autonomic dysfunction and subtle neuroendocrine
derangements." Although this definition is the most specific to date,
it is difficult for those outside the medical profession to understand.
Its essence is that disruption in normal brain functioning is the
cause of most or all CFIDS symptoms, although the causes of the
brain abnormalities are not currently known. Defining CFIDS as a
psychoneuroimmunologic disorder addresses the interactions among

behavior, the immune system, and the central nervous system. These interactions are quite complex and form the basis for understanding illness and wellness in an appropriate and meaningful way.

Various community-based studies indicate that the prevalence of CFIDS is between 76 and 267 cases per 100,000 people in the United States. Some estimates indicate 2 to 10 million cases in this country alone, and millions more in other countries around the world. Because systematic studies have not been done and many cases remain undiagnosed, we can only guess at the actual number of PWCs. One reason for the underdiagnosis of the syndrome is the resistance or unwillingness of many physicians to diagnose a poorly understood illness whose name reflects only one symptom: fatigue—the most common complaint among all medical patients. CFIDS is an illness that is easy to diagnose if the physician has experience with it; however, it is difficult and expensive to treat, making it especially unpopular with HMOs (health maintenance organizations). Pocket outbreaks of the illness have occurred in many areas, including Incline Village, Nevada; Lyndonville, New York; and parts of North Carolina and northern and southern California. The CDC, the CFIDS Association of America, local support groups, and health practitioners are continually deluged with requests for information about CFIDS. Clearly this is an epidemic of huge proportions.

...AND WHAT CFIDS ISN'T

CFIDS isn't just chronic fatigue. The medical profession and general public have tended to confuse chronic fatigue and chronic fatigue *syndrome,* an unfortunate result of the terminology used for this illness. The name CFIDS is often preferred because it includes the "immune dysfunction" aspect of the illness, but the term "CFS" remains more widely used. The CDC insists on using this name, a point of contention for many researchers, practitioners, and PWCs.

CFIDS isn't "just" depression. Because fatigue is a symptom of depression, and because depression is a part of the CFIDS symptom complex, the distinction frequently becomes blurred. In most cases the onset of depression in PWCs occurs after the onset of CFIDS and is an effect rather than a cause of the syndrome. Chapter 4 contains a more detailed discussion of the clinical differences between CFIDS and depression.

CFIDS isn't AIDS. Viral involvement is common to both illnesses (evidence of activation or reactivation of such viruses as Epstein-Barr virus, cytomegalovirus, and human herpesvirus type 6). Although the causal agent of AIDS is the human immunodeficiency virus (HIV), the causal role of a virus in CFIDS is suspected but has not been established.

In HIV disease the immune system is down-regulated, resulting in an immunocompromised state in which one is susceptible to opportunistic illnesses and infections. AIDS is fatal in most or all cases, whereas CFIDS tends to improve over time. Although some CFIDS-related deaths have been reported, this is a fairly unusual occurrence, and most have been suicides. As several PWCs have said, "The difference between AIDS and CFIDS is that AIDS kills you and CFIDS makes you wish you were dead."

In contrast to HIV disease, certain aspects of immune functioning in CFIDS are inappropriately "up-regulated"—as if an *on* switch had been pushed mistakenly—alternating with periods of "down-regulation." During the periods of down-regulation PWCs develop various infections such as upper respiratory infections and reactivation of other viruses, especially early in the course of the illness.

Other distinctions between the two diseases exist. Weight loss is associated with HIV disease, whereas weight gain is more common in CFIDS. Although the mode of transmission of CFIDS is unknown, we know HIV to be transmitted by bodily fluids such as blood, semen, and vaginal secretions. We currently have no evidence that CFIDS is transmitted in these ways.

Still, similarities exist. Certain symptoms are common to both illnesses, and both follow a waxing and waning pattern. Incidence of activation or reactivation of other viruses is common to both. Both are currently considered epidemics posing serious health threats worldwide, and both have been insulted and ignored by the press, the medical profession, and government agencies.

The prejudices attached to both illnesses are based on myths—AIDS is no more a "gay disease" than CFIDS is "yuppie flu" or "crazy and lazy disease"—but such stigmas are widespread. However, HIV research may ultimately be of great benefit to PWCs in that some HIV treatments may help PWCs as well.

A BRIEF HISTORY OF CFIDS

Outbreaks of CFIDS-like illnesses have been occurring in numerous countries, including the United States, for hundreds of years. The documented outbreaks have generally appeared in cooler countries rather than those with tropical climates: England, Scotland, Canada, Switzerland, Japan, Iceland, Australia, New Zealand, Germany, and South Africa. Outbreaks were given various names, including postviral fatigue syndrome, the English sweats, muscular rheumatism, neurasthenia, chronic active Epstein-Barr syndrome, chronic mononucleosis-like syndrome, Royal Free disease, Icelandic disease, postinfectious (or epidemic) neuromyasthenia, Addington's disease, vegetative neuritis, Akureyri disease, chronic hyperfatigability syndrome, low natural killer cell disease, and benign myalgic encephalomyelitis.

Unfortunately, most of these outbreaks were only briefly noted in the medical literature and later forgotten. The similarities and possible connections among them had not been fully explored until relatively recently, when the incidence of numerous pocket epidemics began to receive serious attention from the medical profession, government agencies, and the media. This attention was generated in large part by a grassroots movement among patients who were sick and tired . . . and sick and tired of not being taken seriously.

The current outbreak in the U.S. was first noted in Incline Village, Nevada, where a large portion of the population was stricken with an unusual illness in about 1984. Drs. Daniel Peterson and Paul Cheney treated many of these patients and in 1985 called upon the Centers for Disease Control and Prevention (CDC) to investigate the outbreak, which occurred in surrounding areas as well. The CDC (Gary P. Holmes, M.D., and colleagues) initially denied the existence of an epidemic, but later claimed they had indeed taken it seriously and they suspected it to be an Epstein-Barr-virus-related illness. Later the CDC retracted this stance, taking the position that the illness was real but was not likely caused by the Epstein-Barr virus, since tests indicated the presence of various other viruses as well that may or may not have played a causal role. The CDC, obviously uncomfortable and/or uninterested in this difficult syndrome, essentially turned its back on the devastation that was occurring not only in Incline Village but elsewhere.

Stephen E. Straus, M.D., of the National Institute of Allergy and Infectious Diseases investigated the outbreak of CFIDS as well, taking the approach that since an etiologic agent (cause) hadn't been found, the illness may be a psychoneurotic disorder. Speaking and writing in double messages, Straus has acted both sympathetically and dubiously toward the CFIDS population, apparently concluding that psychopathology precedes the illness and is its primary cause. This concept does not fit with the majority of findings regarding CFIDS as a primarily organic disease. After consistent prodding, the CDC has become involved in researching CFIDS, but its efforts to date have been woefully inadequate—certainly disproportionate to the high incidence and devastation of CFIDS.

THE CFIDS PHENOMENON: STILL A MYSTERY

CFIDS has significantly affected us individually and collectively. By afflicting those in their most productive years, CFIDS is a serious threat to the nation's work force. The loss of workers, the mounting medical and research expenses, and the increasing number of disability cases and cumulative disability payments from Social Security and private insurers are potentially devastating to our national economy.

Also devastating are the divorce rate and suicide rate of PWCs. The divorce rate for chronically ill persons is an astounding 75%. The suicide rate is unknown but believed to be much higher than that of the general population. Because many PWCs (including children and adolescents) feel overwhelmed, misunderstood, depressed, and hopeless, suicide is often contemplated and sometimes attempted by PWCs as an alternative to a life of desperation and pain.

Anthony Komaroff, M.D., wrote, "Chronic fatigue syndrome and its related conditions represent an illness distinct from other known physical and psychological illnesses" (1988). Other researchers concur and remain baffled by this illness, which resembles other illnesses but is a phenomenon all its own. CFIDS is a disease like no other.

Chapter 3

The Onset of CFIDS

S udden onset of a chronic illness is unusual, but CFIDS is an exception. As many formerly active and healthy PWCs have said, "One day I got sick with what I assumed was the flu, but I never recovered." Abrupt onset of CFIDS in adults occurs in 75–90% of cases, often following a physically and/or emotionally traumatic event such as surgery, another illness, an accident or injury, vaccination, or a series of stressful incidents. Most common is onset with a flu-like illness, with neurological symptoms developing over time.

Others who develop CFIDS have a lifetime history of various illnesses, such as allergies, asthma, viral illnesses, PMS, irritable bowel syndrome, endometriosis, and bacterial infections. They become considerably sicker and begin to develop the markers of CFIDS, often over a period of time. Those in this category are often unable to pinpoint the onset of CFIDS because they have been ill so frequently. These individuals initially believe that they had been healthy all their lives, but realize in retrospect that they had long harbored the precursors of CFIDS. Those individuals, however, who experienced low-level or subclinical symptoms (such as frequent illnesses, fatigue, malaise, and allergies) and went on to develop full-blown CFIDS following triggering events did not typically experience such symptoms as sleep disorders, emotional problems (anxiety, depression, and mood swings), and various other neurological complaints prior to the onset of CFIDS.

Kyle describes retrospective confusion about her illness. "I may have been sick for five years and not really known it. I [had been] sick with pneumonia, depression, inability to concentrate. [Later on] I had every kind of blood test in the world and x-rays. I still didn't know what was wrong with me."

Patients who experience an abrupt onset of symptoms generally assume they have a "normal" or self-limiting illness that will last a week or two. Very few expect that this is the beginning of a long-term illness whose symptoms will wax and wane over time, and for which adequate treatment is difficult to obtain.

Typically, patients begin to seek medical attention because their symptoms linger and because the symptom combinations and changes are so unusual. Unless the symptoms have persisted for longer than a few weeks or months, a diagnosis of CFIDS is not usually made. Patients may be given appropriate medical treatment, including recommendations for rest, symptomatic treatment, and encouragement to obtain follow-up treatment if symptoms are not resolved within a given time frame. Patients who receive inappropriate medical attention do not feel their complaints are taken seriously and are generally told such things as "This is all in your head. You've just worn yourself out. Relax. Get a little rest and go back to work." Such reactions have been described repeatedly by patients who were frustrated with how awful they felt and how insensitively their physicians responded.

Increasingly, patients are fortunate enough to see physicians who take their complaints seriously, believing that the symptoms are real although the diagnosis is elusive. These physicians may say, "I don't know what you have, but let's find out," or "You have CFS/CFIDS, but I really don't know much about it," followed by an appropriate referral.

As the symptoms linger for weeks and months, patients often experience a sense of unreality. Certain phrases are typical among prediagnosed PWCs: "What could be wrong with me? Why don't I get better? Why can't someone tell me what I have and just cure me? This can't be happening to me." Describing the onset of CFIDS, one PWC commented, "For no apparent reason, my life fell flat on its face."

I was not alarmed when I initially became ill—just tired, wiped out. This state of being was "not okay" for an active psychotherapist, college instructor, single mother, and exercise nut. I fought *it* hard, and *it* fought back harder. I experienced uncharacteristic mood swings, disequilibrium, and other bizarre symptoms. As additional symptoms developed, I sought medical advice and was told such nonsense as "You're too stressed. You need to exercise." (I had been a three-mile-a-day jogger, having stopped only because jogging made me sicker—much, much sicker. When I explained this to my doctor, he didn't seem to hear me.) "You're dehydrated. You're anxious." I was living in the Twilight Zone: my body had been hijacked by aliens and was doing mysterious things, not behaving like *my* body at all. And was I dehydrated? Anxious? Stressed? Maybe—but mainly I was vulnerable and confused. I couldn't trust my own perceptions and desperately needed information and understanding. At that time, I didn't get either.

Many PWCs formerly thrived on hectic lifestyles, striving for lives of perfection: the perfect student, employee, spouse, friend, parent. When CFIDS struck, these illusions crumbled as their optimism was replaced with a chaotic state of uncertainty, confusion, and fear.

Paula, a PWC, describes her experience:

> When I first came down with it, I couldn't cope with anything. I wasn't working that hard at the time; I babysat and watched ten kids, all preschoolers, and I was taking a few classes. I couldn't function, I couldn't think clearly, and I was having a hard time with my studies, [with] understanding the few simple courses I was taking. They weren't even difficult. I couldn't keep track of the bills to pay them. Little things . . . I'd go into a room and forget what I was going in there for and turn around and walk out again. I'd forget to call people back. I was snapping at everyone. Real dramatic. I couldn't cope. I'd cry very easily. I had physical and mental symptoms, and the confusion and frustration of trying to figure out what was wrong. At first I thought it was the flu and it would go away, but it didn't go away. I was fine one day and not fine the next—just that quick.

Notice Paula's comment: "I *wasn't working that hard* at the time"—a prime example of the self-imposed, perfectionistic standards of performance common to many PWCs. Attending school and providing daycare for ten children *is* hard work, but such a high activity level was normal for Paula. Several patients and doctors have commented that even PWCs who cut back considerably on their activities are still busier than many of their healthy counterparts.

Bill, another PWC, describes the abrupt onset of CFIDS at the airport one Thanksgiving Day.

I was eating breakfast and I felt sick, like the flu came on. I can remember it very distinctly: it was as if a switch had been turned on. The onset was abrupt. The ride was a little tough; I felt weak—an "I need to get to bed" type of feeling, like a bad flu. The next thing I can remember was the pictures that were taken of me at the Thanksgiving dinner when I was bent over and my head was supported by one of my arms and I was really wiped out and sick. During that ten-day stay at my in-laws' house, I spent 40–60% of the time in bed trying to sleep it off. I never really got better.

Yolanda, a recently remarried mother of three children, was attending law school when unusual symptoms began to appear. Her fatigue interfered with schooling and parenting, but she persevered and her symptoms increased in severity. She found that anything requiring mental activity made her sicker. She reported a "whole breakdown of my physical system," beginning with an ear infection and developing into "equilibrium and anxiety symptoms, numbness, shakiness, exhaustion, insomnia, allergic and viral-type problems." These problems developed and worsened over a period of several years, but Yolanda chose not to take the leave of absence from law school suggested by her doctor. Then, as she began a review course for the bar exam . . .

I totally fell apart. My mind had to focus on a whole lot of material crammed into a short period of time. After a few weeks, I couldn't even stay alert. I felt paralyzed and would completely collapse. I would fall asleep and be in another zone; it was almost like passing out. I was just in a fog. I got really concerned, like maybe I had AIDS or something. It was really scary. Sometimes I'd feel fine, but within forty minutes of going to class, that was it; it was over. I thought maybe this was a psychological thing; "I don't want to do this" or something. It wasn't a fun thing to do, but I'd done a lot of other things that weren't fun, and I didn't pass out doing them.

Lack of family support made the ordeal worse. No one could believe that "Superwoman" was having serious health problems. Now, many years later, Yolanda reports that she has failed the bar exam repeatedly and remains discouraged and unable to work.

In cases of acute onset, occasionally so severe as to require hospitalization, the illness is regarded as more "real" and is easier to diagnose. When the onset is gradual, bizarre symptoms take turns driving us crazy, although we're not "ill enough" to be taken seriously by others. Then the diagnostic process may take weeks, months, or years as the symptoms fluctuate unpredictably.

In her book *Living with Chronic Illness*, Cheri Register writes about the features of the initial phase of chronic illness, noting the waxing and waning of symptoms, attempts to attribute these symptoms to a psychological cause, difficulty obtaining a diagnosis, and determination to chase the illness away by changing habits and behavior. She describes numerous frustrating contacts with medical professionals as she sought to obtain a specific diagnosis, compounded by strained relationships with others, continuous stress, and changes in mood and personality.

Fear often accompanies the onset of strange, unexplained symptoms. People wonder if they're going crazy, and not uncommonly fear they will die of whatever it is that has drastically altered their lives. One patient comments: "I wondered if this is a terminal thing, because I felt so tired and drained and burned out and couldn't manage to keep going like that. I figured it was going to kill me, whatever it was." And another: "I just couldn't go any more. That wasn't like me. I could always say, 'I'm going to do this,' and do whatever was necessary. My body didn't work right; I was scared, and I burst into tears. I was crying because I was scared; I didn't know what was going on." A common thread is the feeling of being out of control, captive of an unknown, invisible force that seemed to come out of nowhere.

Experiencing such symptoms is a frightening experience for anyone, especially when a diagnosis is not easily found. It is terribly unfair that something alien, something beyond one's control, can simply appear and change one's entire life. The onset of symptoms is accompanied by a reaction that generally includes disbelief, sorrow, and fear. The symptoms and accompanying emotional devastation continue interminably as the illness lingers.

Chapter 4

Diagnosis: The Search for a Label

Patient: Doc, I sure hope I'm sick!
Doctor: Why on earth would you wish that?
Patient: I'd sure hate to feel this awful if I were well!

We all know what it's like to feel well and what it's like to feel sick, but the distinction is difficult to put into words. I know I'm sick when I don't want to do the things that are normally pleasurable; not only do I feel physically unable, I don't even have the energy or interest to want to do those things. Such feelings are often likely to be dismissed as merely "emotional" (i.e., as signs of depression). To make matters worse, the symptoms are often not observable or measurable, for example, joint pain, nausea, headache, light-headedness. And the symptoms come and go on their own schedule, inconveniencing and torturing PWCs without permission or warning. Others have difficulty understanding how sick (how absolutely rotten) we feel, in part because our numerous symptoms are invisible. "You look fine," they tell us. A PWC at the 1994 American Association for Chronic Fatigue Syndrome convention wore a button proclaiming "I look better than I feel."

Our society has many unwritten rules about being ill. People who become ill are expected to do one of two things: recover or die. It's okay to break a limb—as long as it heals in a timely manner and one does not complain excessively. Even an occasional headache, which is invisible, is acceptable and easily remedied. But to have symptoms that cannot be seen or understood by others is not okay. Anything that cannot be fixed or denied makes trouble.

PWCs have an especially hard time "legitimizing" their illness. Sometimes a diagnosis is made fairly quickly, but other times months or years may elapse between onset and diagnosis. Often the individual symptoms are not cause for alarm, but the number of symptoms experienced and the length of time they persist are problematic. The symptoms vary so much that it can take some time before it becomes apparent that they are all part of one syndrome. Patients experiencing light sensitivity or facial numbness, for example, may not mention such a trivial, seemingly irrelevant symptom to their doctors but will respond positively if asked whether they have experienced such a symptom. Often patients feel they can ignore the minor symptoms, assuming them to be transient.

Many patients have seen doctors who did not take their complaints seriously, and so have given up the pursuit of a diagnosis. Still others feel crazy reporting the numbers of varied symptoms they are experiencing; to visit a doctor complaining of depression, fatigue, equilibrium problems, brain fog, sore joints, shortness of breath, headache, ringing in the ears, and on and on . . . . Sounds pretty crazy, doesn't it? An approach-avoidance issue emerges: "I want a diagnosis, but I don't want to have to recite that crazy list of symptoms again and risk being told what I am secretly beginning to suspect—that I'm bonkers. I'm not handling my life right; I'm not coping; I'm copping out; I'm crazy and lazy. I'm afraid it might be true, even though I *know* this is organic, a virus or something . . . . There's something chewing on my wiring, sabotaging the controls. I'm not making this up—I'm really ill, really I am. You've got to believe me, doctor, even though if I were you, I probably wouldn't believe me, either. What is *happening* to me?"

The patient needs to be listened to and taken seriously. PWCs do not enjoy being ill, nor do they have anything to gain by pretending they are. It's easier, however, for society to dismiss those who have chronic complaints as people who just don't want to participate. We don't follow the rules. We slip through the cracks. We may not be well enough to go to work but may not be ill enough to spend all our time in bed. Some days we can accomplish a lot, other days mere survival needs require all of our limited energy. We are not an easy lot to deal with. Ask any doctor or family member of a PWC. For no apparent reason, our bodies and minds are not behaving right. We want—*need*—some sort of explanation. We want to know why and what to do about it. In the beginning we'll settle for a label, anything that validates our experience and reassures us we're not crazy.

Step one in the diagnostic process is to schedule an appointment with a doctor. The receptionist generally wants to know what the problem is, but usually the description of one's malady is so lengthy it will be interrupted several times by other incoming calls. The appointment may be granted as if it were a special favor rather than a two-way business transaction, and the preparation begins. "What can I say so the doctor will understand the seriousness of this; how can I describe what is happening to me? If I bring a list, the doc will think I'm neurotic. If I don't, I'm likely to forget a lot of important information. How healthy should I look? If I look okay, I won't be taken seriously. But what can I do? Paint circles under my eyes? Draw red dots on my body? I know I'm sick, so why should it be so difficult to convince someone else? And why should I have to convince anyone?"

As Sefra Pitzele wrote, we are in a "well until proven sick" situation. Although she is afflicted with lupus rather than CFIDS, her experiences will sound familiar to PWCs. She describes the unexpected rush of exhaustion that defies any standard definition of fatigue, the accompanying feelings of helplessness, and the search for a diagnosis. During this time we continually hear that our doctors cannot find any specific problem, and self-doubt flourishes as we wonder if our symptoms are imagined or fabricated. "As our confidence in our own judgment erodes still further, we depend more and more on the judgment of those people who seem to have grown numb to our complaints. Before long, we don't know what to believe" (Pitzele 1985). And we can even forget what it felt like to be well.

At our wits' end and with self-esteem at low ebb, we are surrounded by others who cannot understand how we feel. Armchair advice and diagnoses from concerned others may do more harm than good, and the same is true of the reactions of many of the doctors we approach with desperation and fear. Still we pursue a diagnosis: proof that we are really ill, that our symptoms—and we ourselves—are legitimate.

DEALING WITH DOCTORS

There is some argument as to whether diagnosis is an art or a science; ideally, it is a skilled combination of both. The expertise and intuition of the diagnostician supplemented with diagnostic tests are likely to yield the most useful information.

I wonder, if I didn't have this illness but were a doctor listening to someone who did, what would I think? I'd like to think that I'd take a patient-oriented, caring approach. That I'd listen, taking the patient's words seriously, and be willing to say "I don't know" if I didn't know. I'd like to think I wouldn't cop out and that I'd keep an open mind.

Humorist Dave Barry describes the "two most popular doctor options: to tell you to come back in a week, or to send you to the hospital for tests. Another option would be to say, 'It sure beats the heck out of me why your tongue is swollen,' but that could be a violation of the Hippocratic Oath." Barry suggests that perhaps only conditions involving "say, an icepick protruding from your skull" are likely to elicit a conclusive diagnosis, and that in the case of subtler problems, "you may never find out what's wrong" (1988). His statements are humorous and exaggerated, but his point is valid: diagnosing an elusive illness can be exceptionally difficult, especially when the cause is unknown and no specific diagnostic tests have been developed. The process is perplexing for the medical profession as well as patients and their families.

Most patients see several doctors before a correct diagnosis of CFIDS is made. Many patients see five, ten, or fifteen doctors; an astounding number see even more. It takes determination to continue the search, and doubtless many give up along the way. Although awareness within the medical profession has improved, many doctors still don't "believe in" chronic fatigue syndrome. But we're not talking about believing in ghosts or believing in God; we're talking about doctors believing their patients, their educated colleagues, and the medical literature. We are dealing with a serious problem and we need to work at finding out more about it rather than doubting those who have it.

Those who have had lengthy diagnostic searches have horror stories to tell about the process. Unfortunately, the fields of psychiatry and psychology become dumping grounds for those with elusive illnesses. When nothing "turns up" on lab tests, the patient is often presumed physically healthy but psychologically suspect.

Despite the psychological aspects of CFIDS, to assume that psychological factors cause the syndrome is to confuse correlation with causation. CFIDS generally occurs out of the blue, with a sudden onset and a host of physical symptoms that do not ordinarily accompany depression or anxiety syndromes—a fact often conveniently overlooked by those unwilling to delve into the unknown. The physician's personal feelings and judgment about the perceived mental status of the patient—as well as over-reliance on technology to provide definitive answers—can result in incorrect, often damaging, conclusions.

I saw a family practitioner, an otolaryngologist, a neurologist, a gynecologist, a gastroenterologist, an allergist, a cardiologist, and a host of other -ologists before finding out what might be wrong. I could write pages about the expense, self-doubt, emotional turmoil, degradation, and confusion I experienced. I got angry alternately at the doctors and at myself. Many of them took my complaints seriously—those who had known me prior to the onset of my symptoms and didn't consider me a garden-variety "hysterical female." The doctors who hadn't known me B.C. (before CFIDS) more often treated me like a "crock," a neurotic woman with multisystem complaints who probably enjoyed being attended to by the medical profession. The process was agonizing. The illness itself was crazy-making; insensitive, disbelieving physicians made the ordeal worse.

The anxiety of waiting for test results was more traumatic than the tests themselves. Like a teenager waiting to be asked to the prom, I sat near the telephone waiting to hear whether I had a brain tumor, hypoglycemia, heart problems, multiple sclerosis, an ulcer. . . . Initially I was relieved to know that I didn't have the dread disease of the week, then I became frightened again not to know what I *did* have. I assumed that if the right test were run, I'd have a diagnosis, followed by curative treatment that would make me well. With each negative test result I became *more* rather than less concerned because of the implied conclusion that I didn't "have" anything at all. I had been taught to believe in the wisdom of doctors and medical tests, but felt misunderstood, mistreated, and mislabeled. I look back and shudder. Two incredibly long years went by before I was properly diagnosed by a competent and thorough physician.

Bill described the diagnostic crazies he experienced during all the testing and doctor visits:

I got more and more depressed and finally got to the point where I was totally devastated. I'd been through heart tests and neurological tests, I'd been to an infectious disease doctor, I'd been through blood tests time and time again. My family doctor thought I might have E-B virus . . . . Although some doctors don't believe in it, she says too many people are having those symptoms. She believes it exists; she's more into calling an apple an apple. So I got into thinking that's what I've got, and the infectious disease specialist says, "I don't think you've got a viral problem, but I don't know what it is." Everything else is ruled out, but this is one thing you can't rule out. That doesn't mean you can rule it in. It's another vague diagnosis.

I saw another doctor and told him half the doctors don't take me seriously. He said, "I'm taking you very seriously. We need to look at several areas, including allergy and immunology." He thinks what I've been through is a travesty.

Sometimes the doctor does everything she or he can think of and finds no cause. That is understandable; we are dealing with an elusive and ill-defined phenomenon. To be told, as Bill later was, "The truth of it, quite honestly, is that I don't know what the hell you have. I don't know what else to check. I don't think it's going to kill you," is at least an honest statement. But to be told, "I can't find anything, so it must be a psychological problem. Go see a shrink" is not a constructive or fair statement to make. An honest "I don't know" is acceptable, but placing blame on the patient is totally inappropriate. To do so reinforces the irrational notion that we are responsible for being ill. Bill later said, "A smart doctor . . . will tell you that he can't find what's wrong with you, not that you have a psychological problem. People can be really damaged by that kind of a physician."

In his recent book, *What Your Doctor Didn't Learn in Medical School*, Stuart Berger wrote that many patients, particularly women, get stamped with the label "hypochondriac" or "hysteric" when it's unclear what is ailing them. Berger discussed the attitude of most doctors confronted with patients who report vague symptoms and just don't feel like themselves anymore. Doctors often become annoyed and skeptical because they are not well-acquainted with some of the more elusive illnesses. Many times the symptoms are diverse and vague, the clues are subtle, and the search is frustrating.

However, when a physician has seen a number of CFIDS patients, the picture becomes clearer. Byron Hyde, M.D., said, "This is a simple disease to diagnose despite what you've heard to the contrary. There is no disease even vaguely like it" (February 1990).

THE PROCESS OF DIAGNOSIS

The following discussion of diagnostic criteria and testing contains a lot of detailed medical terminology that may be difficult to follow. Readers may prefer to skim these sections now and come back and review them as they need and want to after reading the rest of the book.

Diagnostic criteria for chronic fatigue syndrome were first defined in a landmark article that appeared in the March 1988 *Annals of Internal Medicine;* these criteria were updated in a December 1994 article in the same journal. The strict criteria were developed for research purposes so that uniform groups of patients could be studied; thus, some PWCs do not fall exactly into the scope of the criteria. Many CFIDS symptoms not included in this definition are listed and described in Chapter 5.

The criteria include the following:

I. Clinical evaluation of cases of prolonged or chronic fatigue by:

A. History and physical examination

B. Mental status examination (psychiatric, psychological, or neurologic exam if appropriate)

C. Tests to exclude other illnesses with similar symptoms (screening tests: complete blood count with leukocyte differential [CBC]; erythrocyte sedimentation rate [ESR, or sed rate]; serum levels of alanine aminotransferase [ALT], total protein, albumin, globulin, alkaline phosphatase, calcium [Ca], phosphorus [PO4], glucose, blood urea nitrogen [BUN], electrolytes, creatinine, and thyroid-stimulating hormone [TSH]; urinalysis [UA]; plus additional tests as clinically indicated)

II. Classify as chronic fatigue syndrome if:
   A. Criteria for severity of fatigue are met (unexplained, per-
      sistent, or relapsing chronic fatigue that has not been life-
      long, is not the result of ongoing exertion, is not
      substantially alleviated by rest, and results in substantial
      reduction of activities), and
   B. Four or more of these symptoms are present for at least six
      months since the onset of the illness:
      1. Impaired short-term memory or concentration
      2. Sore throat
      3. Tender cervical or axillary lymph nodes
      4. Muscle pain
      5. Multijoint pain without joint swelling or redness
      6. Headaches of a new type, pattern, or severity
      7. Unrefreshing sleep
      8. Postexercise malaise lasting more than 24 hours

Patients are then divided into four subgroups depending on comor-
bid conditions, current level and duration of fatigue, and current
level of physical function as measured by an instrument.

The use of further tests may be indicated in individual patients, but there is no definitive test that rules in or rules out
CFIDS at this time. Many physicians order tests for viral antibodies and various immune parameters, and brain scans that may indicate abnormalities, but these tests are not considered diagnostic.
The criteria listed above are designed to separate CFIDS from
idiopathic chronic fatigue (that is, unexplained chronic fatigue
that does not meet the CFIDS criteria).

This case definition differs from that established in 1988 but
is still inadequate for diagnosis of the syndrome. There has been
much disagreement among researchers and practitioners as to what
would constitute a case definition for this illness. The article con-
cludes:

"We sympathize with those who are concerned that this
name [chronic fatigue syndrome] may trivialize this illness.
The impairments associated with chronic fatigue syndrome
are not trivial. However, we believe that changing the name
without adequate scientific justification will lead to confusion and will substantially undermine the progress that has

been made in focusing public, clinical, and research attention on this illness. We support changing the name when more is known about the underlying pathophysiologic process or processes associated with the chronic fatigue syndrome and chronic fatigue." (Fukuda et al. 1994)

Most physicians who are knowledgeable about CFIDS agree that the patient's history and description of symptoms are more helpful than the physical examination because many of the reported symptoms and sensations cannot be felt or measured in a physical exam. Because there is no definitive test for CFIDS, the diagnosis is based upon the exclusion of illnesses with similar symptoms. This process can be lengthy, stressful, and expensive, but if there is another illness present, particularly one that is curable or treatable, such information is essential. The tendency to self-diagnose is natural, especially when one's symptoms match those described by friends or in the media, but it is important to have one's suspicions confirmed by a professional who is experienced in diagnosing CFIDS.

Illnesses to be ruled out vary from case to case based upon the patient's signs and symptoms. Syndromes with similar symptoms that should be ruled out include the following:

Other viral illnesses, such as: cytomegalovirus (CMV); chronic mononucleosis (Epstein-Barr virus infection); toxoplasmosis; herpesviruses (simplex I and II, herpes zoster, HHV-6); mycoplasmal pneumonia; coxsackie-B; hepatitis A and B, chronic active hepatitis; rubella; HIV disease/AIDS.

Other infectious diseases, such as: localized infections; bacterial infections (e.g., tuberculosis, brucellosis, endocarditis, Lyme disease); collagen vascular diseases (e.g., systemic lupus erythematosus); rheumatoid arthritis; immune deficiency state (e.g., low Immunoglobin A, which helps fight infection); chronic inflammatory diseases (e.g., sarcoidosis, Wegener's granulomatosis); toxic agents (e.g., chemical solvents, heavy metals, and pesticides); allergies; malignancies, especially lymphoma; chronic psychiatric diseases (e.g., depression, anxiety, and/or panic disorder as the sole cause of symptoms); chronic systemic diseases (e.g., pulmonary, renal [kidney], cardiac, hepatic [liver], hematologic [blood]); anemia; neuromuscular diseases (e.g., multiple sclerosis and myasthenia gravis); fungal diseases, including candidiasis (which may be a separate illness or part of the CFIDS cluster); endocrine diseases such as hypothyroidism, Addison's disease, Cushing's syndrome, diabetes mellitus; parasitic infection (giardiasis, amoebiasis, or helminthic infection); drug side effects, dependency, or abuse (including alcohol); drug interactions

Note: Many of the above conditions may exist as the sole cause of symptoms or coexist as part of the CFIDS symptom spectrum.

THE OFFICE EXAM

Patients will often self-report symptoms found on the symptom checklist in Appendix A. If the patient is being seen early in the illness, sore throat, feverishness, lymphadenopathy, and flu-like malaise may be the major complaints. Those seen in the chronic stage of the illness usually describe easy fatigability, relapse after exertion or stress, and neurocognitive impairments as their primary symptoms.

Physical findings during an exam may reveal:

Abnormal oral pharynx (throat) exam, including buccal mucosal ulcerations (sores in the mouth); posterior cobblestoning or erythema (swelling or redness); blisters on tongue or coated tongue (sometimes thrush); and crimson crescents (purplish-red discoloration of both anterior pharyngeal pillars [areas behind the molars extending in symmetrical arcs from the uvula] which is not associated with pharyngitis [swelling or infection of the throat], found in about 80% of patients)

Difficulty with cognitive functioning: serial 7s (counting backwards from 100 by 7s); difficulty recalling the names of three items after intervening stimuli have been presented

Fever, or subnormal body temperature

Low blood pressure

Intermittent tachycardia (increased heartbeat)

End-gaze nystagmus (involuntary eye movements)

Intermittent aniscoria (unequal pupil size) in dim light

Photophobia (Light sensitivity)

Anterior and/or posterior cervical or axillary adenopathy or lymphadenia (swollen or inflamed glands in the neck or armpits), usually asymmetric

Rashes or sores

Brittle and/or thinning hair

Sallow complexion

Hyperreflexia (increased reflex reactions)

Intention tremor (quivering hand movements when attempting a task)

Mild tremor on drift testing (attempting to hold one's arm out in a stable position)

Mitral valve prolapse (an abnormality that causes a failure of this heart valve to close properly)

Tender points such as those found in fibromyalgia

Diffuse abdominal tenderness

Excessive titubation (staggering or stumbling) or inability to maintain Romberg or tandem stance and tandem walk (standing or walking with eyes closed)

Mild to severe skin atrophy of distal finger tips; loss of fingerprints

(Paul Cheney, M.D., Ph.D. and Charles Lapp, M.D., March/April 1993)

The above findings can be discovered through a careful examination. Harvey Moldofsky has said, "As I talked to these patients, I began to hear a recurrent theme. It was as though I was listening to the first four notes of Beethoven's Fifth Symphony. Once you've heard those notes, you know the rest of the music."

It is also important for the physician to ask questions about symptoms that the patient may have experienced but not associated with the more obvious ones, or which are difficult to describe without specific questioning:

Are you sensitive to bright light? To noise? Do certain fumes or strong odors such as cleaning products bother you? Do you have food intolerance? Do you feel cold or hot often, when others do not? Do you have difficulty following directions?

Do you get lost when driving? Do you frequently lose your train of thought in the middle of a sentence? Do you forget something you have just been told? Are you easily distracted from tasks? Is it difficult to get back on task once the distraction is over? Do you have difficulty recalling common everyday words or names? Do you lose your balance easily? Do you walk into doorjambs rather than through the doorway? Do you frequently feel "spacey" or disoriented? Do you have episodes when you feel as if you might faint? Do you have difficulty standing for long periods of time? Do you experience "brain fog"? Do you have difficulty doing more than one thing at a time? Do you have a difficult time engaging in conversation in the presence of such external stimuli as music or other conversations in the room? Do you have trouble hearing or understanding what is being said to you at times? Do you experience difficulty doing things you have done many times before (e.g., fastening your seat belt, following a recipe, remembering which light switch to use)? Do you have trouble balancing your checkbook or doing simple math in your head? Do you have difficulty understanding or recalling what you read? Do you feel worse following physical exertion or emotional stress? Do you feel worse at malls or crowded stores? Do you overreact to minor irritations? Do you become short of breath for no apparent reason?

Serial weight and temperature measures offer additional information. It is also immensely helpful for the physician when the patient keeps a daily log of symptoms, medications, and supplements taken, and uses a daily rating system to indicate fluctuations in the illness. These journals as well as periodically completed symptom checklists or rating scales may also be important in disability determination. In *The Doctor's Guide to Chronic Fatigue Syndrome*, Dr. David Bell presents the Disability Scale he developed as well as the Karnofsky Performance Scale, both of which are indicators of the individual's ability to function (1994).

LABORATORY TESTS

Medical practice is often quite reliant on laboratory tests for diagnostic purposes, which can be helpful as long as they are not misused. The emphasis on lab tests has been praised ("Incredible technology!") as well as damned ("Doctors treat test results instead of patients"). Sophisticated lab tests can be of great value, but some dangers are associated with their use. Lab tests should not replace the art of medicine, the practice of listening carefully to the patient, and open-mindedness on the part of the physician. Lab test results should not be regarded as the ultimate authorities about the patient's state of health. We should not value "scientific data" more than we do good judgment and intuition. Great variations exist among test results at different labs, since each sets its own standards for normalcy, and testing procedures vary from lab to lab. Errors are often made. Tests performed at a reliable lab are thus an adjunct to the artful practice of good medicine, representing only one part of the complex process of diagnosis.

The process of undergoing tests is emotionally and financially draining for patients, even though the procedures themselves may be relatively innocuous. Although the tests are routine for those who order and perform them, they are journeys into the unknown for already confused and ill patients, who often feel diminished by the process. The equipment and procedures can be intimidating; technology can cause panic in the uninitiated—as it probably should.

The cost of the test may present greater discomfort than the test itself. Waiting for test results is nerve-wracking; the prospect of coming up with nothing is frustrating, and the prospect of coming up with a serious disorder is frightening. The hours or days spent waiting for test results seem like months or years, and although we do not want to find out that we have, for example, a brain tumor, we are nonetheless disappointed to have gone through blood tests and brain scans and then be told we have "nothing."

Although no specific diagnostic test for CFIDS exists, certain laboratory tests should be performed as part of the diagnostic process. In the process of testing for other illnesses with similar symptoms, another illness may be correctly diagnosed as the cause of symptoms.

A basic workup should include the following:

Complete blood count
SMA-20 (chemistry panel)

Sedimentation rate (ESR)
Tuberculin skin test and/or chest x-ray
Urinalysis (qualitative and microscopic)
Thyroid profile, including free thyroxine index (thyroxine
    and T_3 takeup)
Thyroid stimulating hormone (TSH)
Antinuclear antibodies (ANA)
RPR or VDRL (syphilis test)

Additional tests that should be performed on a case-by-case basis, depending on the patient's symptomatology and in some cases to document abnormalities for disability determination include:

Allergy testing; skin test for anergy (lack of immune
    response)
Antithyroid antibodies
Tests as indicated for: cancer; hepatitis; HIV; lyme disease;
    lupus; myasthenia gravis; multiple sclerosis
Viral antibodies (HHV-6, CMV, EBV, etc.)
Stool specimen test for parasites
Fecal occult blood
Exercise testing with oxygen consumption measurements
Functional capacity evaluation
Toxic chemical analysis
Brain scans: CT, MRI, Topographic Computer EEG,
    NeuroSPECT and PET scans
Neuropsychological testing
Vestibular (balance) testing
Immune tests of the following: circulating immune com-
    plexes; IgA levels and IgG subclasses
Lumbar puncture (spinal tap)
Upper and lower gastrointestinal (GI) series
Liver and spleen scan
Bone marrow aspirate
Lymph node biopsy

It should be emphasized that most of the above tests are indicated only when other illnesses are suggested by particular (and usually severe) symptomatology to rule out specific disorders.

ABNORMALITIES

Various multisystem abnormalities have been detected in PWCs, but findings are not consistent and are a matter of ongoing research and debate. Until testing is standardized and consistent findings are identified, we will not have a diagnostic marker for CFIDS—that is, an abnormality or group of abnormalities that are present in all PWCs and absent in other people.

Immune Abnormalities

Some immune parameters fluctuate over time, making it difficult to establish a typical CFIDS immune profile. It is not known whether immune dysfunction is a cause or epiphenomenon or both.

In the 1980s, the Epstein-Barr virus (EBV) was erroneously assumed to be the cause of CFIDS since EBV antibody titers (concentrations in the blood) tend to be elevated in PWCs. However, since that time it has become apparent that elevated antibody titers to a number of viruses are common, but these viruses are unlikely to play a causal role in CFIDS. Therefore, testing EBV antibody titers is of no practical use in diagnosing CFIDS. Additionally, it is possible that antibodies are being produced due to immune system dysregulation rather than because of viral replication.

The CFS Advisory Council, governing body of the American Association for Chronic Fatigue Syndrome (AACFS), reached a consensus about certain abnormalities found in PWCs, which they have grouped into categories and described in their March 12, 1993, "Official Statement of the National Chronic Fatigue Syndrome Advisory Council Regarding Immunological and Virological Aspects of Chronic Fatigue Syndrome" as follows:

" . . . the most frequent abnormalities found include:
Chronic T-cell activation as determined by flow cytometric markers
Decreased natural killer (NK) cell activity (which seems to fluctuate with the severity of the illness)
Reduction of the CD8-suppression cell subset as determined by flow cytometry
Increased levels of the antibody to the Epstein-Barr virus early antigen (EBV-EA)

Other immune abnormalities that have not been consistently reported include:
Skin test anergy (lack of immune response)
Low proliferative responses to lectins (e.g., PHA, PWM)
    and antigens
IgG subclass deficiencies
Abnormal CD4 and CD8 numbers and ratios
Abnormal macrophage, B-cell, and neutrophil functions
Abnormalities in the complement cascade as demonstrated
    by C_3, C_4, $CH_{50,}$ and immune complex levels

Parameters currently under investigation include:
Increased levels of cytokines (e.g., interleukins, interferons,
    and tumor necrosis factor)
Differences in subsets of CD4+ cells

This report contains cautions about generalizing these findings. Since not all PWCs exhibit the same abnormalities, they cannot be used in the evaluation of individuals with CFIDS. That the research-ers involved were able to concur on these abnormalities indicates significant progress in our understanding of CFIDS-related immune abnormalities and provides fertile ground for continued research.

Immune abnormalities found by other researchers include:

Various lymphocyte abnormalities and depression of cell-
    mediated immunity
Elevated antibodies to herpes group viruses
Perturbations of the 2'–5'A synthetase/RNAse L pathway
    (intracellular antiviral cellular defense mechanism; an
    enzymatic pathway that is activated when defending
    against a virus)
Allergies
Recurrent illnesses and infections, including systemic
    candidiasis and parasitic infection, especially early in the
    disease (acute phase)
Low sedimentation rate (although in some cases it is
    slightly elevated)
Changes in white blood cells (mild leukocytosis, mild leuk-
    openia, moderate monocytosis, atypical lymphocytes,
    slightly elevated SGOT and SGPT)

Mild LFT (liver function test) elevations

Macrocytosis with elevated MCV (large red blood cells
with elevated mean corpuscular volume)

Presence of autoantibody production

Presence of antinuclear antibodies (usually at low levels
and variable)

Presence of antithyroid antibodies

Note: Many of these abnormalities suggest up-regulation of the immune system.

Neurocognitive Abnormalities

Impaired concentration

Attention deficit

Memory impairment as measured on Wechsler Memory
Scale, Revised (WMS-R), Mini-Mental Status Exam
(MMSE), Wisconsin Card Sort Test (WCST), Trail-
Making Test (TMT), Boston Naming Test (BNT), Visual-
Function Scale (subtest of the Luria Nebraska
Neuropsychological Battery) showing short-term memory
impairment: memory consolidation deficit; slowing of
mental but not motor scanning as information increases;
delayed decision making; vulnerability to interference;
inability to benefit from cuing and context; proactive inhibition; delay in mental scanning; forgetfulness; "weak
memory traces that were very easily perturbed." (Sandman et al. 1993)

Word-usage difficulties

Difficulties with math and using numbers

Deficits in auditory learning—more so than in visual learning: difficulty understanding the spoken word; difficulty
solving novel nonverbal problems

Concept formation deficit

Difficulty adapting behavior to current context

Impaired abilities to organize, consolidate, and retrieve
stored information

Use of simplistic and ineffective memory strategies that are
not in keeping with expected premorbid abilities

Difficulty synthesizing information and making decisions

Volitional problems: difficulty starting and/or stopping tasks

Abnormal Draw-a-Person tests, indicating organicity and possible relation to right parietal lobe dysfunction (sensory-perceptual abnormalities)

Elevated subscales on the MMPI-2 (Minnesota Multiphasic Personality Inventory) forming a profile unique to CFIDS patients

Abnormal results on subtests of the Halstead-Reitan Neuropsychological Test Battery

Decreased IQ as measured by the Wechsler Adult Intelligence Scale, Revised (WAIS-R): IQ scores (Full Scale IQ) lower than expected for this population, given educational level, in all subjects tested; greater decrease in Performance IQ scores than in Verbal IQ scores; most significant impairments found on the following subtests: Digit Span (especially repeating digits backwards), Arithmetic, Digit Symbol, Block Design, Picture Completion. This scatter (uneven performance) among subtest scores indicates attention-concentration, visual perception, and visual-motor speed impairments; problems with memory, sequencing, visual discrimination, abstract reasoning, and spatial organization; "IQ loss on repeated IQ measures over time . . . indicate definite shifts in intellectual functioning during the course of the illness." (Bastien and Peterson 1994, AACFS Conference proceedings)

Other Central Nervous System (CNS)-mediated Abnormalities

CNS dysfunction in CFIDS may be a primary phenomenon related to CNS damage, or it may be secondary to "undefined systemic factors" (Ichise 1992). Jay Goldstein, M.D., views virtually all of these abnormalities as stemming from "limbic system dysregulation in a neural network or an immunoneuroendocrine network that involves the brain and the entire body" (*The CFIDS Chronicle*, Summer 1993). CNS dysfunction can be evaluated using brain-scans, which fall into the two categories given below.

Structural brain scans
—MRI (magnetic resonance imaging—high resolution), which shows small high signal intensity lesions that

appear as small dots, primarily in the white matter of about 50–78% of PWCs, although the significance of these findings is unknown.

— MSI (magnetic source image—a scan which combines MRI with the SQUID [Superconducting QUantum Interference Device], which shows dysfunction primarily in the frontal, parietal, and temporal lobes. Integrative and learning difficulties are implicated by test results.

Functional brain scans:

— NeuroSPECT (Single-Photon Emission Computerized Tomography), or

— NeuroSPECT ^{99}Tc^m-HMPAO (this substance is administered prior to testing), which usually shows decreased perfusion, or blood flow, primarily to the temporal and frontal lobes in about 80% of PWCs; abnormalities seem to correlate with clinical status.

— PET (Positron Emission Tomography), which shows glucose metabolism, and hence brain activity.

— Topographic computerized EEG, which often shows increased slow-wave activity especially when the patient is engaged in certain cognitive tasks.

— Computer EEG topographical brain mapping. Results are generally consistent with hypoperfusion; may be normal during rest but abnormal during certain cognitive tasks (reading aloud, reading for comprehension, taking the Bender Gestalt test, or reciting digits forward and backward).

Neuroendocrine Dysfunction

Hypothalamic/metabolic dysregulation:

— Decreased corticotropin releasing hormone (CRH) and cortisol levels: "possibly a mild central adrenal insufficiency secondary to either a deficiency of CRH or some other central stimulus to the pituitary-adrenal axis" (Demitrack et al. 1991)

— Central endocrine dysfunction

— Thyroid abnormalities (often after the first few years of illness)

— Decreased libido

— Reduced growth hormone secretion
— Reduced prolactin response to 5-HT (a precursor to serotonin) challenges
— Increased cortisol response to 5-HT
— Reduced TSH (thyroid stimulating hormone) response to TRH (thyrotropin releasing hormone)
— Acylcarnitine, free carnitine, and serum total carnitine deficiency, possibly indicative of mitochondrial dysfunction
— Mitochondrial impairment (abnormality in the cells' ability to produce energy)
Altered sleep patterns and sleep-wave physiology—possibly due to alteration in immune functioning; decreased cellular ATP (adenosine triphosphate)
Gut permeability (leaky gut syndrome), presumed to be the basis of cellular energy deficiency
— Abnormalities in liver detoxification processes
— Decreased levels of certain amino acids
— Krebs cycle abnormalities
— Increased lactate
Sleep disorders:
— Acute phase: hypersomnia (sleeping many hours); chronic phase: hyposomnia (need for sleep but inability to fall asleep or obtain restful sleep; "tired and wired" feeling)
— Increased sleep latency (delayed onset of sleep)
— Shortened REM latency (delayed onset of rapid-eye-movement sleep)
— Increased REM activity and density
— Enhanced REM sleep latency response to cholinergic stimulation
— Reduced slow-wave sleep
— Increased sleep fragmentation
— Alpha-delta sleep: alpha wave (lighter) sleep intrusion into delta wave (deeper) sleep
— Early morning awakening
— Abnormal night temperature variations
— Night headaches, which may awaken patient
— Sleep paralysis: a state in which voluntary movement is

impossible, usually on awakening, despite clear consciousness. It may last for several minutes and may be accompanied by "vivid dreamlike hallucinations" (*Harvard Mental Health Letter*, September 1994).

— Thematic dreams, often vivid and disturbing; may be violent and intense
— Waking dreams: dreams continue into waking consciousness
— Increased incidence of nocturnal myoclonus (leg movement, restlessness, tingling—often helped by walking)
— Increased incidence of sleep apnea (frequent awakening due to breathing cessation)

Abnormal exercise ergometry:
— Defects in functional capacity, impaired VO2 utilization, irregular tidal volume rates (irregular breathing patterns)
— Quickly reaching anaerobic threshold (AT)—the point at which one becomes completely fatigued and cannot exercise any longer)
— Inefficient glucose usage
— Exaggerated increase in blood pressure
— Difficulty with regulation of breathing and erratic breathing patterns
— Lower-than-normal levels of cortisol, epinephrine, norepinephrine, and DHEA
— Decrease in body temperature
— Decreased cerebral perfusion (which increases in normals)
— Breathing abnormalities
— Dyspnea (shortness of breath) on minimal or no exertion

Vision-related abnormalities:
— Photophobia (light sensitivity)
— Blurred vision
— Latency in accommodation (changes in lens to focus)
— Eye sensitivity (dry, scratchy, gritty, burning)
— Nystagmus, usually primary horizontal nystagmus (eye cannot remain stable to fixate)
— Oscillopsia (bouncing, jiggling vision)
— Atypical blurring of vision at distance and up close
— Discomfort with fluorescent lighting

—Discomfort looking at complex patterns
—Less common: Diplopia (double vision)
Neuro-otologic abnormalities and balance problems:
—Dizziness and/or vertigo due to peripheral inner ear
  disorder and/or central vestibular sensory integration
  dysfunction. Tests include: routine audiometry, auditory
  brainstem response (ABR), electronystagmography
  (ENG), computerized dynamic posturography (CDP),
  and electrocochleography (EcOG). Most useful are the
  CDP and EcOG, which often detect endolymphatic
  hydrops.
—Disequilibrium
—Proprioceptive dysfunction: difficulty walking, frequent
  stumbling
—Neuromuscular abnormalities, including altered muscle
  metabolism
Psychological symptoms:
—Anxiety, with or without panic attacks
—Depression
—Sensory storms
—Irritability and overreaction to stimuli (especially when
  multiple stimuli are present); emotional lability (mood
  swings)
Short-term amnesia, often misdiagnosed as panic attack
"Spacing out" or blackouts, possibly related to subtle seizure
  activity
Seizure activity, often subclinical and often undiagnosed
Neurally mediated hypotension, also called vasodepressor
  syncope and neurocardiogenic syncope (misregulated
  blood flow and blood pressure that can lead to lightheadedness, fainting, or feeling an impending sense of fainting)—a recent finding whose relevance to CFIDS is not
  yet well demonstrated. This disorder involves miscommu-
  nication between the brain and the heart. A preliminary
  study has demonstrated this finding in a small number of
  patients on tilt-table testing, which revealed an abnormal blood pressure drop and failure of the restoration of
  normal circulation afterwards. No definite relationship
  between CFIDS and neurally mediated hypotension has

been found, but treating the latter has created symptom improvement in many PWCs. Modifications of this testing procedure are being made for further research studies. In the meantime, Florinef (fludrocortisone), atenolol (a beta-adrenergic blocker)—prescription medications for this condition—sometimes accompanied by increased salt and fluid intake, have been helpful to many PWCs. Research in this area continues.

OTHER ABNORMALITIES

Elevated red blood cell count
— Abnormal red blood cell membranes
Elevation of serum angiotensin-converting enzyme (ACE), a blood pressure regulating mechanism
Low levels of zinc and magnesium
Elevated blood lipids
Fever; low body temperature
Low blood pressure
Elevated liver enzymes
Alkaline urine
Fingertip abnormalities:
— Flattening of the dermal ridges, usually appearing first on the little (fifth) finger; may progress to other fingers and palm often resulting in loss of fingerprints (a phenomenon of aging that occurs at an accelerated rate in PWCs)
— Longitudinal creasing of the fingertips
CFSUM1, a urinary marker present in about 85% of PWCs and 45% of controls: a bacterial xenobiotic (substance foreign to the body) produced by aberrant gut bacteria whose base structure is methyloated proline (also the base of many pesticides), most likely an epiphenomenon of CFIDS related to gut bacteria exposed to pesticide residues that have mutated to produce this neurotoxin and metabolic toxin. This is a possible indicator of liver-gut dysfunction.
Oral health abnormalities:
— Oral infections, including abscesses
— Red, persistent sore throat

— Papules (elevated red bumps) and vesicles (resemble blisters) in the back of the throat and lining of the cheeks

— Aphthous stomatitis: inflammation of oral mucosa in back of throat, on tongue, gum tissue, buccal mucosa (inner cheeks and lips), similar in appearance to strep throat

— Cobblestone appearance of reddened spots in the back of the throat

— Crimson crescents

— Herpetiform lesions

— Candidiasis on tongue and cheeks

— Brown or black "hairy tongue"

— Burning sensations of tongue, gums, palate

— Xerostomia (dry mouth)

— Increased incidence of periodontal disease and gingivitis

— Altered taste buds

— Possible toxicity from dental restoration materials, primarily mercury (also tin, copper, nickel, silver, and zinc) in dental amalgam

— TMJ (temporomandibular joint) dysfunction (pain in and near the joint of the jawbone and the skull)

Assessment and comparison of these abnormalities are made more difficult by their fluctuation over time. Thus, despite patterns that have emerged in research, there are no standard abnormalities that lead to a definitive diagnosis of CFIDS. These lists of abnormalities are compiled from the work of Drs. Archard, Bastien, Behan, Caliguiri, Cheney, Daly, DeLuca, Demitrack, DuBois, Findley, Fudenberg, Goldstein, Grufferman, Gupta, Hamre, Handleman, Herberman, Hyde, Iger, Jessop, Jones, Klimas, Komaroff, Landay, Lapp, Levy, Lieberman, Lloyd, Loblay, Lottenberg, Loveless, Mena, Moldofsky, Nelson, Olson, Peterson, Pettibon, Rigden, Rozofsky, Sandman, Stern, Suhadolnik, Tosato, Wakefield, Whitaker, and others.

Note: It is suspected that many or all of these findings are related to central nervous system functioning.

OVERLAPPING AND/OR
RELATED DISORDERS

The following disorders share significant features with CFIDS, although it is not known in most cases whether a relationship between the disorders exists, or whether they are separate, associated, or overlapping illnesses.

• **Depression** is associated with CFIDS as a symptom but not a direct cause of the illness. The similarities and differences are explained later in this chapter.

• **Fibromyalgia (FM)** is diagnosed in the presence of pain in all four quadrants of the body and pain on palpation of 11 of 18 specified trigger points. Many PWCs fit these criteria. Overlapping symptoms between FM and CFIDS are fatigue, body pain, sudden onset, cognitive dysfunction, gastrointestinal symptoms, mood disorders, abnormal CRH (corticotropin releasing hormone), ataxia (problem with gait/balance), paresthesias (numbness or tingling sensations), sensitivity to cold, sleep disturbances, headache, anxiety, morning stiffness, normal results on routine lab tests, and numerous others. It is increasingly accepted in the research community that the two disorders are overlapping, if not identical, in almost all cases. The primary difference seems to be which symptoms are most severe; FM patients have greater musculoskeletal tenderness whereas PWCs have more severe cognitive problems. Often the specialty of the doctor diagnosing the disorder determines whether the illness receives the FM or the CFIDS label.

• **Gulf War syndrome** is the name given to the illness developed by many U.S. veterans of the Persian Gulf War. This syndrome strongly resembles CFIDS and multiple chemical sensitivity disorder. Many vets have become disabled as a result of this syndrome, and some spouses of veterans also have become ill. It has been estimated that between 2,000 and 8,000 veterans are afflicted. Numerous causative factors have been considered: immunizations, special suits worn, chemicals (pesticides; jet and diesel fuels; exhaust fumes; chemical warfare agents, although their use has been denied; a special paint containing cyanide; heavy metal exposure; decontamination solution; depleted uranium; petrochemicals;

fumes from kerosene heaters), primitive sanitation, rapid weather changes, and austere conditions.

• **Hypothyroidism** is common in the general population and afflicts some people in the chronic stages of CFIDS. Symptoms include fatigue, cognitive problems (impaired memory and concentration), depression, feeling cold often, constipation, muscle cramps, hair loss or damage, brittle fingernails, weight gain, unsteady gait, decreased exercise tolerance, joint pain, hoarseness, slow heart rate, tingling of fingers and toes, decreased sex drive, heavy or more frequent menstrual periods, puffy face, and elevated blood pressure and cholesterol levels. Blood tests are not always accurate in diagnosing hypothyroidism, but if it is suspected a full thyroid panel should be done. (See section on laboratory tests in this chapter.) Hashimoto's thyroiditis is the cause of most spontaneous hypothyroidism and may emerge after childbirth, administration of certain immune modulating drugs, or as a result of endocrine dysfunction.

• **Idiopathic CD4+ T-lymphocytopenia (ICL)** is an illness defined by low numbers of T4 cells (under 300 per cubic milliliter of blood volume) in the absence of HIV infection. The symptoms resemble those of CFIDS as well as HIV disease, although PWCs generally have T4 cell counts in the normal range (800–1200) and people with HIV do not. Only a small number of patients with this disorder have been identified to date.

• **Lyme disease** is caused by a tick bite around which a target-shaped reddened area develops. It is treated with antibiotics. However, Lyme disease may be falsely diagnosed, for example in cases where there is no response to antibiotic treatment and the illness becomes chronic. It is suspected that many diagnosed with Lyme disease actually have CFIDS or FM. Confusion among these disorders and lack of laboratory standardization suggest that differential diagnoses be made carefully.

• **Multiple chemical sensitivity syndrome (MCS) or environmental illness (EI)** may develop as the result of a single massive toxic exposure or repeated exposures to small amounts of toxins, with likely immune and endocrine dysregulation. Once sensitivity and symptoms develop, it takes less and less of any toxic substance to produce a strong reaction in the individual. Because multiple chemical sensitivities are common in CFIDS, there may be a strong link between the two disorders. Symptoms include fatigue, headaches, breathing problems, increased sensitivity to odors, flu-like symptoms, dizziness, confusion, vision problems, acquired alcohol intolerance, amenorrhea or dysmenorrhea, cold intolerance, arthralgia, skin rashes, digestive problems, cognitive problems, and depression. Food sensitivities are common, and those with this disorder often react to food additives and ingredients, including food colorings, flavorings, and preservatives. Not all people exposed to a given chemical will respond in the same ways, however. Triggering factors include genetic predisposition and toxic exposure (working in polluted environments outdoors or in closed buildings, or extreme sensitivity to certain chemicals, notably acetone, trichloroethylene, and chlorinated hydrocarbons).

• **Post-polio sequelae (PPS)** affects about 1.6 million American polio survivors. Fatigue (the major symptom), weakness in previously affected and unaffected muscles, joint pain, difficulty walking and climbing stairs, new breathing difficulties, attention deficit, word-finding difficulty, slowed information processing, difficulty with bladder function, headaches, sensory changes, brain lesions, and a blunted hormonal response to stress are symptoms of PPS. It is triggered by overexertion and/or emotional stress. It is known that polio causes spinal cord damage as well as damage to specific areas of the brain and brain chemicals. Polio epidemics and CFIDS/ME-like epidemics have often occurred in close conjunction with one another, and it is speculated that CFIDS/ME may be caused by an enterovirus, as is polio.

• **Sick building syndrome (SBS)** is a phenomenon that occurs in individuals in the same workplace, usually a "tight" building with little or no outside ventilation. Symptoms may be caused by common chemical exposure (including industrial cleaning solutions and office products, such as copier toner and typewriter correction fluid), molds and mildew in air conditioning vents, airborne contaminants—viruses or bacteria, and/or outgassing of furniture and carpeting (which usually contain formaldehyde and numerous other chemicals). Many of these chemicals easily pass into the bloodstream and the brain when inhaled. Symptoms include respiratory complaints (sore or burning throat, nasal irritation, cough), headache, nausea, cognitive problems, dizziness, heart palpitations, sleep difficulty, and rashes. The range of symptom severity is wide, and a working diagnosis has not yet been established. The agents that cause SBS may also be a causal or precipitating factor in CFIDS; similar pathologic processes may be shared by both illnesses.

• **Silicone gel breast implants** may cause symptoms and abnormalities found in CFIDS, FM, and EI, particularly body pain, lymphadenopathy, granulomas in the breast and liver, and abnormal sedimentation rates and liver function tests. Symptoms may develop five to twenty years after the implantation of silicone. Immune abnormalities are often found, suggesting immune dysregulation, possibly an autoimmune response to the silicone. Researchers are investigating possible links between silicone and autoimmune disease as well as long-term effects of silicone compounds on immune system functioning. This disorder may be related to such illnesses as scleroderma, lupus, rheumatoid arthritis, CFIDS, and MCS. These may be overlapping syndromes or they may exist on a single continuum, representing a range of related disorders.

• **Sjögren's syndrome** is characterized by dryness of the mucous membranes (especially evident in eyes, mouth, nose, throat, and vagina) and a variety of autoimmune phenomena. Symptoms include fever, pharyngitis (sore throat), lymphadenopathy, xerostomia (dry mouth), tooth decay, myalgia, arthralgia, neurocognitive and other central nervous dysfunctions, headache, sleep disturbance, fibromyalgia, burning throat, difficulty chewing or swallowing, gritty- or filmy-feeling eyes, and depression or other psychiatric symptoms. It is possible that a subset of PWCs develop this syndrome over time and that the two may share a causal relationship, or they may be distinct disorders. This syndrome is considered an autoimmune disease and is diagnosed by a biopsy of the lips or salivary glands. A retroviral cause has been speculated.

• **Systemic candidiasis** is a condition characterized by overgrowth of or infection by candida albicans, a yeast normally found in the body. Symptoms include fatigue, thrush, vaginal yeast infection, digestive problems (intestinal gas, abdominal pain, diarrhea, constipation), weakness, dizziness, headaches, sweats, sore throat, muscle and joint pain, numbness, asthma, chronic sinusitis, allergies, irritability, rashes, carbohydrate cravings, and chemical sensitivities. It is possible that immune abnormalities cause both candidiasis and CFIDS. Although there is little question that this syndrome exists, its presence in PWCs is a controversial issue. Some CFIDS physicians routinely prescribe an "anti-candida" diet and medications, and many patients are helped by these because candidiasis is present and responsive to treatment and/or because the medications have immune modulating effects.

RULING OUT DEPRESSION

Although depression almost invariably accompanies CFIDS, it is not the cause of the illness. Common to both CFIDS and major depressive disorder (MDD) are fatigue, lethargy, anhedonia (inability to experience pleasure), sleep disruption, lowered activity level, impaired concentration and memory, decreased libido, and weight changes, but MDD shares only some of the features of CFIDS. Researchers at the National Institute of Health, however, are reluctant to dismiss the psychological angle, ignoring most clinical research and insisting that CFIDS is an illness of psychoneurotic origin. Unfortunately, many physicians cling to the "psychologized" notion of CFIDS, continuing to misdiagnose and mistreat their patients.

In order to distinguish between depression and CFIDS as the primary cause of an individual's symptoms, the following differences should be noted.

1. Onset. CFIDS begins in a majority of patients with a flu-like illness, but acute onset is not characteristic of MDD. The vast majority of PWCs do not have a history of major depression. Although many PWCs experience depression (as do those with other chronic illnesses), some PWCs are not depressed. In many cases depression decreases later in the course of the illness.

2. Incidence. CFIDS occurs in both epidemic and endemic forms, that is, outbreaks occur but individuals may develop it any time. Depression has never been known to exist in epidemic form, but pockets or local outbreaks of CFIDS are common.

3. Major symptoms. The primary symptoms of depression are feelings of hopelessness and helplessness. The exaggerated feelings of guilt and the tendency to be overly self-critical that are characteristic of primary depression are not usually characteristic of CFIDS-related depression. Although such feelings are experienced by many PWCs, they are not the primary symptoms of the illness. Those with MDD generally do not wish to be active; most PWCs would like to be active but are physically unable. A depressed individual would not generally experience most of the physical and neurological deficits found in CFIDS: sore throat; tender or swollen lymph nodes; unusual headaches; body pain; nausea; irritable bowel syndrome-type symptoms; unusual sensitivities to medications, odors, and other substances; decreased blood flow to the brain following exercise; memory disturbances; photosensitivity; word-finding difficulty; visual discrimination and sequencing problems; altered spatial perception; abstract reasoning difficulties; aphasia and dyscalculia (difficulty using words and numbers); disequilibrium; and so forth. On various memory tests, PWCs perform poorly as compared to depressed patients and to healthy controls. Depressed patients exhibit slower motor speed than PWCs, who evidence decreased mental speed.

4. Attribution. Individuals with MDD often describe feelings of guilt, inadequacy, and low self-worth, and they tend to view depression as a personal failing or defect (internal attribution). Those with CFIDS, however, are more likely to attribute the development of their symptoms to external forces (external attribution).

5. Laboratory test results. Immunological, neurological, and endocrine measures yield different results for the two disorders. Neuroendocrine studies have indicated hypothalamic pituitary axis (HPA) (the combined neuroendocrine system that regulates the body's hormonal activities) dysfunction in both MDD and CFIDS, although the types of dysfunction are believed to differ. Most notable are the differences in corticotropin releasing hormone (CRH), cortisol, and adrenocorticotropic hormone (ACTH) levels, all of which are elevated in MDD. CFIDS findings are opposite: decreased CRH, cortisol, and ACTH, and inadequate response of the hypothalamic pituitary axis (HPA) to stress. More metabolic defects have been found in CFIDS than in MDD.

Certain immune and neurological abnormalities found in CFIDS, such as increased antibody production to viruses such as Epstein-Barr virus (EBV), cytomegalovirus (CMV), and Human

Herpes Virus number 6 (HHV-6); decreased natural killer cell (NK) function; decreased IgG subsets; elevation of TGF-beta; and abnormal 2'–5' synthetase/RNAse (antiviral pathway) are not known to occur in MDD.

Changes in cerebral perfusion (blood flow to parts of the brain) as measured by the NeuroSPECT scan are common to both disorders, but the areas and degrees of hypoperfusion differ significantly. Other brain scans have shown abnormalities in CFIDS that are believed to be absent or different in MDD.

6. Response to treatment. Although the medications used to treat MDD are helpful to PWCs, they do not cause the type of overall improvement found in those who are depressed. In addition, the amount of antidepressant medication commonly administered to PWCs for symptom relief is extremely low as compared to dosages for those with MDD. It is believed that certain antidepressants administered in doses much lower than those used for treating MDD create improvement in CFIDS by exerting immunomodulating properties, affecting certain neurotransmitters, exerting an antihistaminic effect, and creating improvement of various symptoms. Other medications that are beneficial in the treatment of CFIDS do not cause improvement in depressive disorder. The symptoms of depression in PWCs disappear or decrease significantly when overall symptom improvement is accomplished. Dependence on alcohol and psychiatric medications is commonly characteristic of depressives; it is unusual for PWCs to be able to tolerate alcohol or such medications.

7. Sleep disorders. Sleep disorder is a prominent symptom of both depression and CFIDS but the disorders are different in the two illnesses. Characteristic in CFIDS is the delayed onset of dreaming sleep, the opposite of findings in depression, which show abbreviated onset of dreaming, and alpha-EEG sleep anomaly, which is also not known to be present in depression. Additional findings in CFIDS but not in depression include breathing difficulties, involuntary leg movements, increase in certain interleukin levels, and a drop in natural killer cell activity during sleep (Demitrack 1991; Moldofsky 1991).

8. Psychological and neuropsychological testing. The Minnesota Multiphasic Personality Inventory-2 (MMPI, Version 2), a test that is widely used to diagnose psychological/psychiatric disorders, shows different scale elevations (or "profiles") for MDD and CFIDS. A unique MMPI-2 profile consisting of elevation of scales 1, 2, 3, occasionally 4, 7, and 8 has been identified for CFIDS. The profile for chronic illness (elevations in scales 1, 2, and 3) overlaps with the profile for the CFIDS group (Iger, 1992). This finding is highly significant in that this profile is unique to CFIDS and has not been seen in any other disorder, including depression, malingering, hypochondriasis, or other chronic illnesses. By contrast, the profiles found most often in depression are 2; 2, 7; or 2, 4, 7. Thus, the MMPI-2 is a useful tool for differentiating between CFIDS and depression.

When "neurological" items were removed from the test and the tests were rescored, all scores dropped to within the normal range; that is, no elevations were found. This finding provides evidence of neurological dysfunction rather than psychopathology as the cause of many CFIDS symptoms.

Other test results that differentiate between CFIDS and MDD include the WAIS-R IQ test, memory tests, and certain neurological test battery subscales as previously described.

Depressives tend to underestimate their performance on tests, probably due to decreased self-confidence, whereas PWCs overestimate their abilities, most likely because they are accustomed to their pre-illness performance levels.

9. Suspected cause. It is likely that depression and CFIDS are both multifactorially caused; that is, each is the result of an interaction of various factors in an individual's life. In the case of CFIDS, an infectious agent of some type is suspected and will most likely be found to be a virus or viruses, in conjunction with individual susceptibility, genetic factors, stressful events, toxic exposure, etc. No such agent is suspected as a cause of MDD, although genetic factors and stressful events may be causal or triggering factors.

10. Contagion. Although it is unknown how CFIDS is spread, there have been cluster outbreaks of the syndrome for many years and the disease may be contagious, especially in its early stages. Depression is not known to be contagious or to occur in clusters.

11. Exercise intolerance. Exercise intolerance is characteristic of CFIDS but not of MDD. PWCs who exercise will generally experience a return or intensification of symptoms. Although those with MDD may be reluctant to exercise, their symptoms are generally improved by an exercise program.

12. Course of the illness. CFIDS tends to persist for many years even when treated, which is not generally characteristic of MDD. CFIDS tends to follow a waxing and waning pattern not usually seen with depression.

13. History. Most PWCs do not report a history of mood disorder in themselves or their families; the opposite is often true in MDD.

14. Other differences between MDD and CFIDS are related to age at onset and other demographic characteristics. Depression occurs increasingly with age; the age range for CFIDS is childhood to late adulthood with a predominance of cases in the middle years (thirties and forties). Those in certain professions are believed to be at greater risk of developing CFIDS, a phenomenon not found in MDD.

To summarize, chronic fatigue in and of itself is a common complaint and may be symptomatic of any number of problems; chronic fatigue *syndrome* is a distinct illness of which fatigue is one of myriad symptoms. Depression is a symptom of CFIDS but not its cause. Immune abnormalities and other findings and characteristics of CFIDS are not known to be found in mood disorders such as depression. Most PWCs were emotionally stable and not depressed prior to the onset of CFIDS.

Note: This summary of the differences between CFIDS and MDD is based upon my clinical observations and on the work of such researchers and clinicians as Drs. Bastien, Demitrack, Goldstein, Hickie, Iger, Jacobson, Lottenberg, Mena, Moldofsky, Sandman, and Wakefield.

FINALLY, A LABEL

It is well-established that the mere fact of knowing
what hurts you has an inherent curative value.

Hans Selye, M.D., *The Stress of Life*

Obtaining a diagnosis is a good news-bad news proposition. The good news: this is a physical, organic illness. "I'm not crazy. There's a name for this miserable condition. I'm not the only one with this disease. This compact label replaces the long, difficult description of what's wrong. I was right to listen to my body; it really is telling me something is wrong. I have some control now that I know what I'm dealing with." One patient said, "I was so relieved to know I *had* something." A diagnosis gives us permission to be sick and offers validation of our complaints. It helps to explain the peculiar symptoms and sensations and alters our perspective on our lives and life changes. I summarized the initial postdiagnostic double bind in my journal: "Oh good, I'm really sick. Oh shit, I'm really sick."

The "honeymoon period," the initial relief of having obtained a diagnosis, is short-lived, and we are left once again to deal with the symptoms, the losses, the lack of understanding of those around us. And we wonder, "Knowing is good—but now what do I do to become well again?" realizing that the answer to that question is not included in the diagnosis. We are labeled, put into a cubbyhole: I am a PWC, a person with chronic fatigue immune dysfunction syndrome. And the aftershock: the illness is real. It isn't going to go away overnight, if at all. I will have to make many changes in order to cope and maximize recovery potential; these changes will involve considerable sacrifice. Having obtained a diagnosis becomes a mixed blessing—first relief and then acknowledgment of the forthcoming journey into an unknown realm.

Acknowledging CFIDS means losing a large degree of perceived control over one's life. The illness continues to be unpredictable and unwelcome. The diagnosis brings with it a sense of betrayal, anger at one's body, feelings of fear and insecurity. And the inevitable question: *Why me?* The emotional aspects of diagnosis are varied and confusing as we ride the emotional roller coaster: denial, shock, truth, disbelief, numbness, anger, relief. We don't go through these emotions in any particular order and keep returning to the ones that are most difficult. Since the illness is chronic, its emotional effects are continuous and variable.

COMMUNICATING THE
DIAGNOSIS TO THE PATIENT

The way the diagnosis is communicated by the doctor can have a profound influence on the patient. Norman Cousins asked, "Is it possible to communicate negative information in such a way that it is received by the patient as a challenge rather than as a death sentence?" Many physicians tell CFIDS patients such things as, "Just accept this and go on with your life," or "You have a chronic illness. There's nothing I can do for you. It will probably never go away." This is incomplete information, delivered insensitively with a closed-minded attitude.

CFIDS is not a death sentence but it may be a life sentence. Once a diagnosis has been made, it is constructive to discuss options, various treatment modalities and coping mechanisms, and the hope for a cure in the future. Physicians should try to motivate their patients, working together toward symptom alleviation. A dose of hope delivered along with the diagnosis is vital. Newly diagnosed PWCs need to hear such statements as, "You have quite a struggle ahead of you, but there is hope. We can experiment with treatments to see what works for you. You will probably get better over time and you may or may not fully recover. Numerous resources are available to you."

Despite the lack of a cure or even a reliable or specific treatment program, patients should consult only competent, open-minded, CFIDS-educated physicians and stay well-informed about current CFIDS theories and treatments. Patients who remain actively involved in treatment are more likely to do well than those who crawl back under the covers.

Chapter 5

Symptoms

The symptoms of CFIDS vary among patients, and in individual patients over time. As new symptoms crop up, we may find it hard to determine whether they are part of the syndrome or something unrelated. The illness often begins with an odd assortment of symptoms, later joined or replaced by others. Early in the illness the PWC is likely to experience swollen lymph glands, frequent infections and illnesses, fever and chills, sore throat, depression, and persistent headaches and myalgias. As time goes on, additional symptoms, especially neurological symptoms, may develop or become worse. The pattern varies widely among individuals.

Betty, a PWC, reported:

> I had laryngitis all the month of December. I had to make long-distance calls at work, and I could hardly talk. Later in December I noticed difficulty in walking. My legs felt heavy and they ached. I thought, "This is weird. I feel like I've been running around a tennis court for two or three hours, when in reality I've been sitting at my desk." My legs ached; I took labored steps and thought, "I'm not old enough for this to be happening." I didn't know what it was but I ignored it because there were things I had to take care of. My throat hurt all the time, I ached; I was still pushing myself.

In my case, the illness began with a bout of what I thought was the flu: fatigue, malaise, and lethargy. Within a few months these symptoms were joined by others: tinnitus (ringing in the ears), sore throat, equilibrium problems, irritability, morning nausea, weight gain, and shortness of breath. Additional symptoms developed over time: lymph node tenderness, unusual headaches, a tendency to become "overloaded" easily by activity or sensory stimulation, brief periods of severe depression, a periodic inability to find the right words as I spoke, and slowed speech and thinking. I tried to ignore other odd symptoms: photosensitivity, transient facial numbness, night sweats, "broken thermostat" (random sensitivity to heat and/or cold), heart palpitations, and general weakness. I popped vitamins and continued the hectic pace of my life as mother, therapist, workshop presenter, college instructor, and jogger. I attempted to ignore or overcome my symptoms because they didn't make any sense and because they got in my way. I did what I had always done: I pushed hard and fought aggressively.

In retrospect my approach was misguided and inappropriate. Dogs have the good sense to rest an injured paw by using only the other three until it is healed. I used to think symptoms were a signal to do *more* of what I was already doing. As is common in early CFIDS, I didn't talk to many people about what was happening to me because I felt too wimpy, vulnerable, and crazy to risk other's judgment. I simply wasn't allowed to have such things happen to me. I am not a weakling, hypochondriac, somatizer, hysteric, or victim to whom such things happen. In fact, as a psychologist, I am a provider of help—not a recipient! So I tried to ignore my symptoms, hoping they'd disappear. Sometimes they did, only to return accompanied by other symptoms.

Other PWCs relate similar stories in which various unusual, bewildering symptoms occur, disappear, and reappear. In the past many had experienced allergies, colds, and viral illnesses from which they had typically recovered within a few weeks. They assumed that their new symptoms would follow a similar course. But all of us have been astounded at the variety, unpredictability, and duration of the symptoms we have experienced. Toni Jeffreys described the symptoms as a "cafeteria in a nightmare" with each patient experiencing a "horrendous array of horrors" (1982).

LISTS OF SYMPTOMS

The following list of symptoms is grouped into three general categories with approximate percentages of PWCs who experience them. These percentages are based upon information reported by Drs. Bell, Cheney, Fudenberg, Goldstein, Jessop, Komaroff, Peterson, and two surveys (Kansas City and Phoenix). Grouping symptoms into categories is done for convenience. It is likely that all symptoms are related to neuroimmune dysfunction.

In the lists below, symptoms marked with a * do not have statistics available at this time; symptoms marked with a ** are probably underreported and more prevalent than indicated.

General or Physical Symptoms

Fatigue, often accompanied by nonrestorative sleep, generally worsened by exertion: 95–100%

Nausea: 60–90%

Irritable bowel syndrome (diarrhea, nausea, gas, abdominal pain): 50–90%

Chronic sore throat: 50–90%

Fevers/chills/sweats/feeling hot often: 60–95%

Muscle and/or joint pain, neck pain: 65–95%

Bladder/prostate problems, frequent urination: 20–95%

Low blood pressure: 86%

Recurrent illness and infections: 70–85%

Malaise: 80%**

Heat/cold intolerance: 75–80%

Painful and/or swollen lymph nodes: 50–80%

Systemic yeast/fungal infection: 30–80%

Fungal infection of skin and nails: 71%

Weight gain: 50–70%

Increased/severe PMS (premenstrual syndrome): 70%

Swelling, fluid retention: 55–70%

Shortness of breath: 30–70%*

Subnormal body temperature: 65%**

Severe allergies: 40–65%**

Sensitivities to medicines, inhalants, odors, and foods: 25–65%*

Difficulty swallowing: 55–60%

Heart palpitations: 40–60%

Sinus pain: 56%

Rash or flushing of face: 35–45%

Chest pain: 40%

Hair loss: 20–35%

Eye pain: 30%**

Pressure at the base of the skull: 30%

Weight loss: 20–30%

Tendency to bruise easily: 25%
Vomiting: 20%
Endometriosis*
Dryness of mouth, eyes*
Pressure sensation behind eyes*
frequent canker sores*
Periodontal (gum) disease*
Pain in teeth, loose teeth, and endodontal problems*
Cough*
TMJ syndrome (jaw pain or locking)*
Mitral valve prolapse*
Carpal tunnel syndrome*
Serious cardiac rhythm disturbances*
Pyriform muscle syndrome, causing sciatica*
Impotence*
Thyroid inflammation*
Hypoglycemia or hypoglycemia-like symptoms*
Swelling of nasal passages*

Neurological/Central Nervous System-related Symptoms

Confusion; inability to think clearly: 75–100%
Concentration/attention deficit: 70–100%
Sleep disorder/disturbance (insomnia, unrestorative sleep,
    unusual nightmares): 65–100%
Muscle weakness: 85–95%
Headache: 75–95% (daily headache: 50%)
Memory problems (especially short-term memory): 80–90%
Photosensitivity: 65–90%
Disequilibrium, spatial disorientation, dizziness, vertigo:
    60–90%
Spaceyness, light-headedness: 75–85%
Muscle twitching, involuntary movements: 55–80%
Aphasia (inability to find the right word, saying the wrong
    word) and/or dyscalculia (difficulty with numbers): 75–80%**
Alcohol intolerance: 45–75%**
Seizure-like episodes: 70%** (seizures: 2%)
Coordination problems/clumsiness: 60%
Paresthesias (numbness, tingling or other odd sensations in
    face and/or extremities): 25–60%

Visual disturbance (scratchiness, blurring of vision, " float-
   ers"—harmless spots behind the lens of the eye): 45–55%**
Episodic hyperventilation: 40–45%**
Fainting or blackouts: 40%
Strange taste in mouth (bitter, metallic): 25%
Temporary paralysis after sleeping: 20%
Earache: 20%
Decreased libido*
Hallucinations*
Alteration of taste, smell, hearing*
Tinnitus*

Emotional/Psychological Symptoms

Anxiety 70–90%
Mood swings, excessive irritability, overreaction: 70–90%
Depression: 65–90%
Personality change: 55–75%
Panic attacks: 30–40%
Isolative tendencies*

These figures represent a range of percentages of reported
symptoms in different studies. Patients do not necessarily experience these symptoms all the time. In most cases only one-third to
one-half of those reporting individual symptoms indicated that
they experienced the symptom at all times. In my survey of the
Phoenix area group, figures were compiled to indicate the average
total number of symptoms each patient experienced all of the time
(11 symptoms) and the average total number of symptoms experienced by each patient some of the time (18.6 symptoms).

PWCs may experience symptoms other than those listed
above. Some of the symptoms reported may have been experienced
prior to the onset of CFIDS in a milder or different form. Additionally, other illnesses or conditions may exist simultaneously
with CFIDS, complicating the diagnostic problems and often causing lack of clarity as to which symptoms are attributable to which
conditions. The major symptoms in each group are discussed below
in some detail.

GENERAL OR PHYSICAL SYMPTOMS

Fatigue

A hallmark of CFIDS, and often the first symptom to appear, is chronic fatigue. To the healthy, fatigue means tiredness, feeling worn out, or needing a nap. CFIDS-related fatigue is of a different magnitude: it spans feeling debilitated, disabled, exhausted, drained, washed out, weak, wasted, zapped, and unable to function mentally or physically. The degree of fatigue varies over time. CFIDS fatigue defies description and cannot be measured.

CFIDS fatigue is often accompanied by a sense of feeling totally overwhelmed, along with general malaise, or feeling "sick all over." In some cases the fatigue comes and goes, often unpredictably; in others, severe fatigue is constant. Some patients are literally unable to get out of bed. Some describe the experience of waking up, showering and dressing, and then getting back into bed, having drained the day's energy supply in these simple activities. What used to be preparation for the day can become the day's major activities; even the simple act of brushing one's teeth can become a monumental chore. Although this may sound dramatic and exaggerated to a healthy individual, it is all too real and very discouraging to the PWC.

Fatigue is worsened by physical, cognitive, or emotional exertion. Although some PWCs find that stretching exercises or yoga are helpful in alleviating fatigue, others are unable to exert themselves even minimally without danger of collapse. Exercise tolerance varies considerably among PWCs.

Just as the Eskimos have many different words for "snow," we need more precise words for the phenomenon we call "fatigue" to indicate the type of fatigue and its severity. One may be extremely fatigued but not sleepy. One PWC in her seventies said that at certain times of the day she would "just need to go flat." She didn't need to sleep but only to rest in a horizontal position for about thirty minutes before resuming even mild activity.

Many PWCs describe a type of fatigue referred to as "sensory overload," which is detailed in the "Neurological Symptoms" discussion. Sensory input of a specific type or of a combination of types (noise, light, motion, etc.) becomes overwhelming and debilitating.

Sleep does not necessarily relieve CFIDS-related fatigue. Although the perceived need for sleep may be great, even many hours of sleep may not be refreshing, and the PWC may awaken still tired. In his book *Waiting to Live*, Gregg Fisher described his need for sleep:

> I have often slept for twelve hours or more, only to wake up feeling much sicker than I did the night before. I believe part of the reason for this is that I did not get a good night's sleep. Sometimes I wake up two or three times during the middle of the night, totally disoriented. Other nights I toss and turn so much, I use more energy than I gain. (1987)

Extreme fatigue may be accompanied by an inability to sleep. Sleep problems include difficulty falling asleep, early awakening, or frequent awakenings during the night. One patient complained that she felt tired all the time but was unable to sleep more than a few hours per night. Inactivity compounds the problem, but increased activity may lead to relapse.

Aches and Pains

> I'm old too soon, yet young too long;
> Could Swift himself have planned it droller?
> Timor vitae conturbat me;
> Another day, another dolor.
>
> Ogden Nash, "A Man Can Complain, Can't He?"

Lots of things hurt. Ellen described waking up each morning wondering, "What's going to hurt today?" Sometimes it was her arms, other times her legs, and sometimes she hurt all over. On rare days, nothing hurt. Her problem had been diagnosed as arthritis, but her other puzzling symptoms did not fit with that label, and ultimately CFIDS was diagnosed.

Betty says:

> I'd pushed [the pain] aside because it was something I didn't want to come to grips with, something I told myself wasn't happening. All of a sudden I had acquired arthritic symptoms. I started swelling. My hands, my legs, my joints, between the rib cage and the sternum. They took thermograms.

It's been one test after another. I don't know if it's arthritis or symptoms of arthritis attributable to [CFIDS]. My doctor doesn't know. If I don't take my arthritis drug, I feel worse; I ache all over. Every now and then I test myself by going a couple of days without it, and I start hurting. I know enough now to know it's not psychosomatic. It hurts; I ache all over.

PWCs describe various types of pain: in their joints, muscles, and lymph nodes (notably those in the neck and armpits). In some cases pain is the predominant symptom, and the illness may be diagnosed as fibromyalgia or fibrositis. (Fibromyalgia is diagnosed when 11 of 18 specific trigger points are present.) Some PWCs report increased pain when they are most fatigued. The onset of even mild pain can serve as a warning sign: time to stop and rest.

Many PWCs complain of localized sore spots, often called tender points or trigger points. Even gentle pressure on one of these spots can cause anything from a wince to a trip right through the ceiling.

Patients may complain of swollen or tender lymph nodes. There may be extreme soreness without any swelling, or slight swelling noticeable to the patient but unremarkable to the physician. Soreness in the nodes in the back of the neck is commonly reported; some patients describe difficulty turning their necks. Such neck pain may be accompanied by headache, backache, sinus pain, or eye pain.

The headaches described by CFIDS patients are of varying types. Some are migraine-like, in that the headache is unilateral (on only one side of the head), and sometimes accompanied by nausea and sensitivity to light and noise. Others describe headaches accompanied by severe pain behind the eyes and/or sinus pain. Patients may refer to their headaches as "CFIDS headaches" to distinguish them from "normal" (previously experienced) headaches. CFIDS headaches may last for several hours or several days. They may develop in one side of the head, moving to the other side on the following day. Here, too, the patterns vary considerably as does the pain level. Excruciating ones have been described as Lizzie Borden headaches, chisels-behind-the-eyes headaches, and "ten pounds of shit in a five pound bag" headaches, the latter referring to the sensation of increased pressure.

Sore throat is another common complaint: the pain ranges from mild to severe. Like other aches, a mild sore throat may serve as a warning signal, heralding a "crash." Severe exacerbations of CFIDS may be accompanied by a strep-like sore throat, especially early in the disease.

Some patients without sore throat complain of difficulty swallowing. Those with this complaint may have to cut their food into small bites and crush large pills and vitamins. Some patients complain of choking or a fear of choking.

Allergies and Sensitivities

About two-thirds of the PWCs I surveyed indicated a history of allergies. Most of them, as well as many previously nonallergic patients, report more severe allergic symptoms and an increased sensitivity to various environmental substances, foods, and plants. It has been speculated that all CFIDS patients have allergies and sensitivities of which some PWCs are not aware. Many PWCs are sensitive to the odors of perfumes, exhaust fumes, cleaning products, and other chemicals. Exposure to these substances may produce overall discomfort, nasal congestion, headache, equilibrium problems, and a return or increase of other symptoms.

Some PWCs report new sensitivities to food additives, such as preservatives, colorings, and flavorings. Some report particular sensitivity to sulfites (commonly found in diet soda, wine, prepared foods, produce, and fresh or frozen fish). A few patients report a negative response to sodium benzoate or to aspartame (Nutrasweet).

Sensitivity to Temperature Extremes

Many PWCs become extremely sensitive to heat and/or cold. Kyle says, "I get cold. Other people say they're hot, and I say I'm freezing. I feel like an idiot carrying a sweater around all the time. My bones are cold."

It is like having a broken thermostat. Some patients can tolerate only a very limited temperature range, becoming unusually uncomfortable with small variations in either direction. Like Kyle, they may feel cold most of the time, even when others feel warm or it may be just the reverse. Feeling unusually hot or cold often may be attributable to brain dysfunction, causing dysregulation or metabolism and other aspects of basic body functioning.

Low Body Temperature, Fever, and Sweats

Subnormal body temperature is reported by many patients. In some cases the problem is thyroid-related, although routine thyroid tests may yield normal results. Some doctors routinely prescribe thyroid medication for patients with low body temperatures and other symptoms of hypothyroidism, even when test results are within the normal range, while others disapprove of this practice.

A possible explanation for low body temperature was offered by John Reed, M.D., who stated at a Phoenix support group meeting in March 1988: "Microorganisms do things to slow the body down to make a happy home for themselves." Viruses are quite fond of and replicate best at temperatures slightly below normal body temperature.

Body temperature may jump around madly at times. One day I remarked to a friend that my temperature had jumped from 96.6° to 99.4° in just a few hours. (His advice: "When it gets to 100, *sell!*") Someone whose body temperature is "subnormal" (below 98°) will feel feverish at a "normal" temperature of 98.6°.

Some PWCs report low-grade fevers either intermittently or constantly over long periods of time. They may experience night sweats resembling hot flashes: an abrupt rush of heat and sweating, especially in the upper portion of the body.

Weight Gain and Loss

When CFIDS was thought to be chronic Epstein-Barr virus syndrome, the assumption was that most patients would lose weight, as is the tendency with EBV-caused mononucleosis. Weight *gain*, however, has turned out to be a more common problem in CFIDS.

In our society, being overweight is equated with a weak-willed, out-of-control person who has "let herself go" (go where? to the refrigerator?). Stigma city: the assumption is that being overweight connotes emotional weakness rather than a physiological problem. It is common for PWCs to experience weight gains of 30–60 pounds during CFIDS, and some patients have gained 100 pounds or more. Although the weight gain is attributable in part to inactivity or to increased carbohydrate cravings, most PWCs experience weight gain without increased food consumption or significant change in eating habits. Weight change is another baffling CFIDS symptom, one most likely attributable to alterations in brain chemistry and/or dysregulation at the cellular level relating to the body's ability to convert calories into energy.

Many PWCs experience decreased self-esteem, helplessness, and anger regarding weight gain. "I have no control over my weight," remarked one. "It's on its own little program." Another lamented, "I'm heavier than I've ever been in my life. I've gained a great deal of weight and am so dissatisfied with my size, but my doctor told me not to worry about it. The weight will come off later, he says." This gaining trend is a leading cause of High School Reunion Syndrome (HSRS), which is summarized as "I don't want them to see me like this."

In an article called, "Weight-ing to Lose," (her title a likely takeoff on Gregg Fisher's *Waiting to Live*), Connie Steitz Fox laments her increasing girth with mirth. She claimed that "even a dead person's metabolism is higher than mine" (*The CFIDS Chronicle*, August 1988). I have speculated bitterly that any illness that causes years of daily morning nausea coupled with weight gain is likely to result in the birth of a large mammal.

Some PWCs have lost weight, particularly those with severe food intolerance and digestive problems. In extreme cases, individuals have become almost skeletal in appearance. This excessive weight loss, although problematic for them, is unlikely to elicit understanding and sympathy in our society, which values thinness.

Bladder and Urinary Problems

Interstitial cystitis is an inflammation of the space between the bladder lining and muscle. Men as well as women may develop this condition, which causes pain on urination and sometimes during sexual intercourse. Unlike a bladder or urinary tract infection, interstitial cystitis is not caused by bacteria, so antibiotics are not helpful in treatment. Larrian Gillespie, M.D., believes that such cofactors as hormones, certain drugs, and viruses may play causal roles; additional cofactors, if any, remain unknown. It may be an autoimmune disease. Gillespie regards interstitial cystitis as an environmental disease that is progressive, in which the bladder has become ulcerated and scarred (1986). It is treatable but not curable. Chemical sensitivity may contribute to this problem. Male PWCs may develop prostatitis (inflammation of the prostate gland), a condition that is treatable.

Abdominal Pain and Digestive Problems

Jenny reports having been diagnosed by various specialists as having not only irritable bowel syndrome but also arthritis, Ménière's disease, anxiety disorder, and depression before anyone put the symptoms together and saw CFIDS (like the story of the blind men and the elephant). This situation is not unique.

Irritable bowel syndrome has been diagnosed in many PWCs with such symptoms as nausea, gassiness and bloating, diarrhea, abdominal cramps, and constipation. Like other symptoms, these may be constant or intermittent, mild, or severe.

Yeast Overgrowth

Candida albicans, or yeast, is normally present in the body, particularly in the intestinal tract. Under certain conditions, yeast cells proliferate out of control in the intestines and elsewhere in the body, causing a host of uncomfortable symptoms including rectal or vaginal itching, gas and bloating, feelings of spaceyness or disorientation, and other symptoms often associated with CFIDS. Although the relationship between CFIDS and yeast overgrowth is not clear, some practitioners believe that the two often occur simultaneously. Others view candidiasis as a "fad" diagnosis of no significance.

This diagnosis remains controversial and unproved. However, many PWCs report feeling better on an antiyeast diet, one that eliminates sugars, alcohol, other refined carbohydrates, and sometimes yeast and dairy products.

Other Illnesses

Some CFIDS patients report that they have developed a series of infections and illnesses and are prone to catch "whatever is going around." One woman complained, "I came down with two different kinds of flu in one month. I threw up; I had diarrhea. I passed out." Another said, "I get everything that comes down the pike." Others state that they have been less prone to catching other illnesses. It is common for other illnesses and infections to appear in early CFIDS but to become less frequent over time.

CFIDS and Pregnancy

In many cases pregnancy brings about a temporary remission of CFIDS symptoms, beginning several weeks after conception and lasting until several weeks after delivery. PWCs considering pregnancy should keep in mind that they will have to curtail the use of medications during pregnancy and may have difficulty caring for an infant in terms of the energy required. They should also be concerned about whether CFIDS, or a predisposition toward developing it later in life, can be passed on to an infant. For this reason, Charles Lapp, M.D., recommends bottle- rather than breast-feeding. The rate of first-trimester miscarriage is higher than normal for PWCs. However, babies born to PWCs usually thrive and do well. All of this information is anecdotal and is based upon the observations of Drs. Behan, Cheney, Hyde, Jones, and Lapp.

NEUROLOGICAL SYMPTOMS

Initially viewed as a viral disorder and later as immune system dysfunction, CFIDS is now being considered a neurological illness, or a psychoneuroimmunological one. Psychoneuroimmunology describes the interactions of the three systems of the body—psychological, neurological, and immunological—that are often involved in illness and healing. Neurological testing and patient reports reveal numerous cognitive deficits, reflected in lower-than-expected scores on tests of intelligence, performance, achievement, and other aspects of neurological functioning.

PWCs describe perceptions of neurologic changes in interesting terms:

I've got cotton in my synapses.

I'm reacting backwards to everything.

I've got brain fog.

This feels like Alzheimer's, or maybe just "Halfheimer's."

My brain is on strike.

I become so disoriented. Sometimes I don't know where I am, even when I'm in my own neighborhood.

I feel like a camera lens that can't focus.

I feel like a VCR on "pause."

I've been short-circuited.

I feel like there's an infection in my brain. It just isn't working right.

Neurological problems include visual disturbances, vestibular (balance) problems, numbness and tingling, light-headedness, abnormal movements, seizures or seizure-like episodes, visual sensitivity and distortions, speech disturbance, confusion, difficulty concentrating, impaired short-term memory, and other cognitive impairments to be discussed in the next section. Such symptoms may appear with the onset of CFIDS but usually emerge months later. Neurological deficits range from mild to acute, varying in severity over time. Sheila Bastien, M.D., refers to CFIDS as an "atypical organic brain syndrome" (April 1990).

Many doctors dismiss such complaints as manifestations of emotional problems or hypochondriasis. However, the consistency among patient reports of such symptoms, uniform test results showing a predictable pattern of abnormalities, and the lack of evidence of previous psychiatric problems among CFIDS patients suggest that these neurological symptoms are CFIDS-related.

Cognitive Problems

> Unusual cognitive complaints are, increasingly to me,
> the single most important symptom.
>
> Paul Cheney, M.D., *The CFIDS Chronicle*

Each of us has developed a concept of how we normally function based on past abilities and characteristics. When our brains aren't working right or functioning as they used to, we become frustrated and frightened.

Cognitive problems include difficulty with speech (e.g., word-finding and word transposition, using the wrong word—often an incorrect term from the right category, such as saying "hot" when we meant to say "cold"), difficulty with numbers and mathematical computations, problem-solving difficulty, attention deficit, problems absorbing and remembering information, directional problems, gross and fine motor problems, abstract reasoning deficits, sequencing problems, and difficulty gauging time and distances (visual/spatial problems).

Betty describes her neurological deficits and related fears:

> I would have to read and reread because I had forgotten what I had read. For a person doing research and writing for professional journals and the media, this became disconcerting, and I was scared. I was so frightened that I did not want to tell my family, my coworkers, anybody. I thought this must be presenile dementia; I had the telltale signs. At meetings, I was quiet, because it was so difficult for me to concentrate; I didn't know how to say what I wanted to say. I couldn't always figure out which words to use. I became reclusive because I was afraid others would find out.
>
> When I was driving, I'd have to force myself to focus so I wouldn't wreck my new car and myself. I'd forget where I was, where I was supposed to be going, and why. I was afraid to pull over because someone might find me and discover what had happened. It was hard for me to remember where my office was. When I remembered and got there, I wondered what I was supposed to be doing and I was afraid to ask my secretary. My aide asked, "Are you all right?" I thought, "Dear God, this is it. I can't continue." I didn't know if I was going to break down or what.

Many patients report similar experiences of being unable to ascertain their whereabouts in familiar territory, rereading because of an inability to absorb information, losing track of their train of thought, or forgetting how to perform simple tasks.

Susan reported a typical experience of becoming lost while driving in her own neighborhood. She asked her five-year-old son to direct her home, pretending it was a game. Other patients whose impairments are more consistent have given up driving and now rely on others for transportation. Many no longer trust themselves behind the wheel of a car because of poor judgment and a tendency to become lost in familiar areas. Those who experience this strange phenomenon feel embarrassed and stupid and are often reluctant to tell others, even their doctors. One patient explained, "I feel drunk when I drive," and another stated, "I feel like I'm in another dimension. It takes all my concentration to drive."

We live in a society where faster is better, and slowness at anything is not accepted. PWCs react more slowly and speak more slowly, like 45-rpm records being played at $33\frac{1}{3}$. We fear that others will notice, that we will be ridiculed and lose our jobs and our identities as intelligent, functional human beings. One woman said sadly, "My life is not the same. I have an above-average thinking process and now I feel so dull and slow. My mind is no longer sharp."

"My brain is broken," laments Kyle. "I can't even say things that are important to me any more. That's when I get angry. I answer the phone at work and then can't remember who is calling; I have to ask someone two or three times and still forget."

"I depended on this wonderful tool that I have, my brain, and it just doesn't work very well any more," reports a now-unemployed patient who has neither the energy nor the cognitive ability to work any longer.

"My memory doesn't work well, my brain doesn't work well, and I get spacey and lose pieces of information," says one PWC, and Betty adds:

> The forgetting is hard. I lose track of myself. I test myself periodically to see if my mind is still working. When I can't recall something, I feel devastated. I used to have an excellent memory; it was frightening when it failed me. I was losing myself. All of a sudden, I didn't know who I was, or what I was becoming. I tried to train my mind to remember; I made lists every day. I was hopelessly lost; I couldn't think. I couldn't read or write or knit because I kept losing track. All of a sudden my mind was gone. It was awful.

Reading had been an important leisure pastime for Betty, who experienced a double loss: inability to work and inability to pursue an enjoyable pastime. (Update: several years later, Betty reports considerable improvement, although she has not yet returned to work.)

Normally an avid reader, I use my comprehension level as a cognitive-function barometer. When I was sickest I had no desire to read. As my health and cognitive functioning have improved over time, I have regained my former comprehension level and reading habits. My cognitive improvement has been consistent over time but is still mildly affected by exacerbations. Intermittent memory problems persist.

Forgetting is a common problem: Where did I put my keys? How did I "lose" the paper that was right in front of me? What did I come into the bedroom for? What is the name of the person to whom I was just introduced? Have I already told you what I am about to say? What is that word on the tip of my tongue? What are my shoes doing in the freezer? Several PWCs echo the lament: "Of all the things I've lost, I miss my mind the most." Knowing that adequate cognitive functioning will most likely return over time is helpful during relapses, when it seems our minds are gone forever.

In her well-known article in *Rolling Stone*, Hilary Johnson wrote about her inability to concentrate, hold a conversation in a group, use appropriate and often simple words, sustain a train of thought, and recall such familiar things as names of her friends and schools she had attended. She described such behavioral errors as picking up the wrong object (a comb instead of a pen), trying to replace a drawer in a space that was actually a shelf, and being unable to fasten her seatbelt on an airplane (July 1987). Another PWC described forgetting how to turn on the headlights of his car, and many report similar inabilities to do common, daily "simple stuff."

Many describe this confused state as brain-spin or trance-like states of altered perception. "I feel dizzy, light-headed; my brain spins. My vision changes a lot; sometimes things look closer than they really are or everything will look unusually crisp and clear," says one. "I get an intense buzzing feeling throughout my system. It varies in intensity. It's not a noise, it's a drugged-like feeling, it's systemic. It's in my head mostly, but I can feel it throughout. It affects my thought processes," says another.

Many report distorted thinking and unusual thought patterns and images they never experienced prior to the onset of CFIDS. They describe vivid, often disturbing dreams that may be accompanied by strong sensations lasting into their waking hours.

Photosensitivity

Most PWCs are sensitive to light. Many avoid bright sunlight, wear dark sunglasses outdoors, and keep indoor lighting dim. Many are especially sensitive to fluorescent lighting, describing it as harsh, eerie, and disturbing. Fluorescent light sensitivity may be associated with balance disorders.

Symptoms associated with exposure to bright light include dizziness and other equilibrium problems, nausea, sensory "overload," and headache. One patient reports feeling "blinded" by bright sunlight, needing to cling to a friend's arm for support. Although some patients are acutely aware of this problem, others recognize it or associate it with CFIDS only when asked if light sensitivity is experienced.

Vision Problems

David J. Browning, M.D., a North Carolina ophthalmologist, states that numerous vision problems have been reported, ranging from mild to severe: floaters, impaired depth perception, dryness, bouncing images, transient blurred vision, transient double vision, extreme light sensitivity, burning, and pain. A very small minority of patients may develop serious conditions such as multifocal choroiditis and panuveitis, which are inflammations thought to result from viral infections.

Although the patient may report experiencing the more common problems to an ophthalmologist, most of them are not readily apparent upon examination. Dr. Browning recommends seeking a doctor who takes such complaints seriously and is willing to initiate a trial-and-error approach to symptom treatment. He stresses that in most cases the eyes will appear normal upon examination, and that the problems may be due to "the immunoneurological problem causing the fatigue, inability to concentrate ('focus'), and increased sensitivity to noxious stimuli" (*The CFIDS Chronicle*, October 1988).

Vestibular (Balance) Problems

Included in this symptom category are: dizziness; vertigo; spatial disorientation; difficulty navigating (e.g., loss of balance, frequently bumping into things, or listing to one side); nausea, with or without vomiting; and tinnitus (ringing in the ears). These problems may be associated with feelings of anxiety, often accompanying phobias and panic disorders. Usually transient, these problems may fluctuate with other symptoms, but in a minority of patients, vestibular symptoms are constant. Sara Reynolds, M.D., a Phoenix physician and PWC, wrote:

> Occasionally, *tinnitus* (ringing or buzzing in the ears) is associated with vertigo, and again the level of sound is usually not constant and varies from person to person, and from time to time. It may interfere with normal hearing and is usually unilateral (in one ear only). (*The CFS Bulletin*, May 1988)

Patients report a variety of sensations typical of vestibular disorders: a sense of unreality or disorientation, or of feeling "foggy" or "spacey"; light-headedness; episodic momentary loss of equilibrium; increased disorientation in the dark; inability to concentrate; increased distractibility; and a need to restrict motion. Some must remain perfectly still in bed; others are ambulatory but must restrict head movement, or may not do well on escalators, elevators, and some forms of transportation. These sensations are often described as trancelike and may be produced or worsened by certain types of motion, noise, odors, or bright light.

Harold Levinson, M.D., associates such sensations with malfunction of the cerebellar-vestibular system (CVS), which is responsible for processing and making sense of external sensory input to maintain orientation and balance. If this "filter" malfunctions, incoming messages become scrambled, resulting in the sensations described above. He discusses this concept at length in *Phobia Free* (1986) and spoke at the 1987 CFS Convention in Portland: "It's not just a balance problem. The inner ear system doesn't control just a balance and coordination output, but acts as a sort of a fine-tuner to the whole brain. It fine-tunes the whole sensory input, sort of like what a fine-tuner does to a TV set."

Levinson has tied certain learning disorders, many symptoms of anxiety, and many phobias to CVS dysfunction, reporting a corresponding decrease in self-esteem as these problems occur. Levinson believes that a viral illness such as mononucleosis can trigger vestibular problems, resulting in the symptoms reported by so many CFS patients: tripping, stumbling, dizziness, slurred speech, impaired coordination, and so on. He discussed blurry or scrambled input, which is not appropriately filtered or sorted out by the brain and results in distorted signals and thus confusion. Overload is the phenomenon of too much input, causing even small amounts of additional input to create exaggerated responses, resulting in an increase in vestibular symptoms.

Situations with high levels of sensory input that are difficult for many CFIDS patients include shopping in crowded stores or malls where they are bombarded with motion, lights (which may be bright, fluorescent, and/or flickering), colors, shapes, odors (foods, perfumes, or cleaning solvents), people talking, music playing, and so on. Large amounts of visual, auditory, and motion-related input result in overload and such symptoms as spaceyness, imbalance, disorientation, anxiety (sometimes with panic attacks), inability to navigate properly in space, stumbling or falling, hyperventilation, concentration impairment, nausea and vomiting, motion sickness, and mental fogginess. These symptoms, like most others, tend to wax and wane.

EMOTIONAL SYMPTOMS

The notion of mind-body duality has fallen into disfavor. Although we can distinguish some primarily physiologically-caused problems, such as a bone fracture, from emotional problems, such as depression following the loss of a loved one, emotional and physical problems are interrelated. So-called physical problems have psychological manifestations and vice versa. Illness is a function of the "mindbody," an integrated system.

When we seek medical help for symptoms whose "physical" cause cannot be found, we may be told that it is an "emotional" problem, that it is "all in our heads." What exactly does that mean? That we have fabricated symptoms? That we want them? That we are crazy? That we seek attention for imaginary ills? To regard an illness with both emotional and physical symptoms as such is inappropriate and insulting. Phrases such as "all in your head" and "mind over matter" add insult to illness. Emotional symptoms are no less real than physical ones, and there is no real distinction between the two.

Typical CFIDS-related emotions include depression, anxiety, anger, frustration, and disappointment. A majority of patients report mood swings that may be abrupt and are triggered by minor events or occur without apparent cause. These mood swings lead to out-of-control feelings; the way we react makes no sense to us. The reaction is out of proportion to the stimulus and is not typical of past responses.

We may call such mood swings "emotional overreaction," or being "too sensitive," or "going crazy over nothing." The overload phenomenon described earlier may help to explain such reactions. When an individual's tolerance threshold is low, any stimulus may become too much to process logically. Even healthy people experience busy, frustrating days during which minor incidents become major problems. This phenomenon in CFIDS, though, is radically different in kind and in degree. Our short fuses may result in sudden, intense angry outbursts, surprising to others and to ourselves. Angry outbursts may be triggered by dysregulation of the limbic system, an area of the brain associated with anger and aggressive behavior. Outbursts may be inappropriately directed at someone in the immediate environment, such as a spouse, family member, or coworker. Exhaustion makes anger more difficult to direct constructively.

When PWCs are sickest, even the mildest frustration or sensory input is intolerable. Music or conversation (especially in combination) becomes grating. At such times we are more prone to react very strongly to any sort of demand, frustration, or problem. Our tolerance threshold is lowered considerably, and our responses to such events are often quite extreme. The reactions we experience are out of proportion to the events.

The emotional aspects of CFIDS can be devastating and crazy-making because our reactions are not typical of us and don't make sense. Others in our environment may be more puzzled and disturbed by our emotional changes than by our other symptoms.

Anxiety

"I always feel nervous now, all the time," says Bill. "I'm nervous when I get up in the morning. I'm nervous right now. My nerves are so whacked out; maybe there's something actively attacking them."

"In response to almost nothing . . . my heart was pounding, my skin was burning, my anxiety level was skyrocketing," remarks Yolanda. "What the hell is the matter? I just can't handle stress. This is really guilt-provoking." Other patients comment:

> My heart starts to pound, and I feel as if I'm going to pass out—for no reason! I can't figure out what causes this; I really don't feel anxious about anything in particular.

> I've never had this problem before. Sure, I've gotten uptight about tests or interviews, but never for no reason.

> I get all worked up about nothing, or about something really minor.

> Things I could handle easily in the past seem to really get to me now; I get anxious and upset so easily.

Joe describes his panic reaction as a series of symptoms beginning with a feeling of danger, followed by panic when he cannot determine the cause of the anxiety. He feels a surge of adrenalin and strange sensations, including a fear of dying or going insane. At such times he feels safe only at home because of the unpredictability of the sudden onset of symptoms, particularly those that provoke anxiety. Harold Levinson, M.D., links the anxiety, panic, and phobia symptoms to the "internal state of alarm" that "results when the brain receives scrambled information," attributing the emotions to malfunctions in the cerebellar-vestibular system (1986).

The fight-or-flight response is a normal response to stressful stimuli, and its symptoms include shortness of breath, internal chemical changes, increased muscle tension, and circulatory changes. These changes are accompanied by feelings of light-headedness and fuzzy thinking. When this response occurs in the absence of dangerous stimuli, the unexplained sensations can cause us to feel even more anxious and uncomfortable.

Depression

The medical profession often views depression—and/or an inability to cope productively with stress—as likely causes of any symptoms for which a physiological cause cannot be determined. Thus, psychiatry becomes the dumping ground for those with unexplained illness. Although the fields of psychiatry and psychology are valuable in the treatment of many disorders, indiscriminate referral of those with illnesses of unknown cause is inappropriate. It is wrong to assume that symptoms for which no cause is found on standard medical tests are due to psychological problems.

Depression almost invariably accompanies CFIDS. Because many of the symptoms of depression and CFIDS overlap, it is important to differentiate between depression alone and depression that is a manifestation of CFIDS. The appropriate diagnostic guidelines should be used to make this determination.

Depression may be of the endogenous or exogenous types. In most CFIDS cases it is a combination of the two. Endogenous depression, or depression from within, is thought to have a physical origin, an imbalance in brain chemistry, and may have a genetic basis. The onset of endogenous depression may be abrupt or gradual and is generally unexplained. Exogenous depression (also called reactive depression) is depression "from without" and is attributable to an external event, such as a loss or chronic illness. This type of depression is more common in the general population. In CFIDS, disturbed body chemistry combined with deprivations, losses, changes in lifestyle, and the lack of understanding and empathy of others can produce profound depression. The incidence and severity of the depression may vary, sometimes in rhythm with other CFIDS symptoms.

Symptoms of depression include the following:

Fatigue and loss of energy
Feelings of hopelessness, helplessness, emptiness, and loss of
     control over one's own life
Loss of pleasure in life, especially in activities once enjoyed
Feelings of worthlessness, self-deprecation, and guilt
Inability to concentrate; memory problems
Changes in appetite and weight
changes in sleeping patterns (sleeping too much or too little; frequent awakenings; early-morning awakening)
Loss of interest in the outside world
Loss of interest in sex
Thoughts of suicide, or planning one's suicide.

Some CFIDS patients described their feelings of depression:

It comes on me out of nowhere, like I'm suddenly enveloped in a black cloud. It may last a day or two. I hole up in my room; I don't want to talk to anyone. I hate myself, and I'm not fit company. I have no interest in other people or in my normal life activities. I just don't care about anything, least of all myself. It lifts as suddenly as it hit.

When the depression hits, I try to get out of it. Sometimes I can't, but I try. It takes so much effort to be depressed and so much effort to try to get out of it. In the past, when I'd become depressed, it was situationally caused. This is different.

Depression is different from anxiety. . . . Depression is more debilitating.

Even when I have good days and feel on top of the world, later it's back down again, sometimes worse than before. Other times it's not as bad and I can come out of it again.

I have reached the point of planning my suicide. I realize that something must be done but I don't have the energy to do anything. I can't work, can't pay my bills, or keep my personal life going. This is very difficult for someone who has always done everything, who carried twenty-one or twenty-two semester hours per semester and graduated summa cum laude.

I feel crazy and out of control, and I really don't give a shit about anything. Life just seems so hopeless.

Others may react strangely to our depression, often not understanding that it is beyond voluntary control, that we cannot simply think positively and snap ourselves out of it. Their attempts to cheer us up may backfire by causing us to feel terribly misunderstood.

Depression is not a sign of unworthiness, incompetence, or weakness. It is more profound than the sense of discouragement that is likely to accompany any exacerbation of symptoms. Depression is a serious matter; its severity and debilitating effects must not be minimized. If depression is prolonged, severe, or accompanied by suicidal thoughts, treatment should be sought immediately.

Chapter 6

Exacerbations
and Remissions

W hen asked what he thought about the exacerbation-
remission cycle, one patient said, "I'd rather have a
Harley."

It's like riding the waves: slowly we climb and climb . . . and
then, crash! But ocean waves are somewhat predictable; they follow a pattern. CFIDS symptoms come and go unpredictably, without regard for any other plans we may have made. Sometimes we can
identify the events or exertions that trigger an exacerbation, and at
other times they occur for no apparent reason. We seek to identify
a catalyst, both to have something to blame (in the absence of
this, we often blame ourselves) and to determine what activities or
substances to avoid or minimize in the future. On the other hand,
some patients experience a steadier illness course with fewer dramatic fluctuations. There may be periods of relative calm interspersed with crashes, or an overall level course of feeling unwell.

EXACERBATION TRIGGERS

Exacerbations may be triggered by changes of almost any kind—
physical, emotional, or environmental. Some of the factors that
can precede relapses are:

> Changes in weather, temperature, barometric pressure, alti-
> tude, humidity, or general climate (especially abrupt or
> severe changes)
> Overexertion: periods of intense or increased physical activity
> Emotionally stressful events, such as family problems or in-
> creased demands at work or elsewhere
> Allergy season, or exposure to allergens or substances to
> which one is sensitive

Changes in diet or water source
Pregnancy (which also causes remission in some cases)
Immunosuppression
Other illnesses or infections
Surgery
Antibiotics
Air travel

Many PWCs experience relapses, often severe ones, following air travel. Although the reason for these relapses is unknown, many hypotheses exist. Air quality on airplanes is often poor; fresh air circulation is reduced to decrease costs. Recirculating stale air means exposure to every germ on the plane and breathing air with lower oxygen content and higher levels of carbon dioxide than the air we normally breathe. The air is dry, making passengers more susceptible to disease, and air pressure is low. Newer planes are often the worst culprits. Many filters used by airlines can remove dust, bacteria, and viruses but not gases or odors. Tests of airplane air indicated the presence of high levels of particulates, implying that filters are not being used properly if at all. The Federal Aviation Administration (FAA) has no ventilation standards according to an article in *Consumer Reports* (August 1994, pp. 501–506), and there is a separate ventilation system for the cockpit. Infections have been known to spread widely on flights, and on some occasions a number of people on the same flight have developed the same illness; in one case the illness was tuberculosis. Flight attendants frequently become ill, some with minor respiratory problems and some with more serious illnesses, such as CFIDS.

Airplanes are sprayed with pesticides (especially on international flights, but many of the same planes are used for domestic flights as well), sometimes with passengers on board. Pesticide residues remain in the air and on surfaces inside the cabin. The *Consumer Reports* article mentioned air contamination with "aromas of perfumes, aftershaves, cooking, fuel, de-icing chemicals, cleaning fluids, pesticides, carpeting adhesives, or upholstery finishes," all toxic to those with allergies, asthma, or chemical sensitivities. One study of interior airplane fumes found low concentrations of a number of contaminants that resembled the air found in sick buildings.

Various PWCs describe exacerbations of symptoms preceded by triggering events:

I've always been the family caretaker, the peacekeeper, every-one's confidante. When there's family stress, like relationship problems between my parents, I get sicker.

I have to be careful to guard against exhaustion. Reading about this illness makes me feel morbid and anxious; this focus worsens the illness. I'm unable to determine an appro-priate activity level. When should I crusade? When should I rest? What can I handle?

I did real well when I was working full time and wasn't smok-ing. I started smoking again about eight months ago, and my health has deteriorated gradually. There have also been stressful events since then in my personal life: a divorce, a new relationship, and changes in my work schedule. I think all of these things that have happened to me have made this decline happen.

I went for a job interview. I was thinking about how I'd have to organize my life in order to work. Then, at the interview, the room was spinning; they wanted focused answers, con-centration. It was a draining experience. When it was over I wanted to go home and collapse, and they wanted me to do an extra test. By then I was totally out of it: the room was spinning, I was exhausted and fatigued. [Before this inter-view] I had been feeling better and then I realized that a focused, short period of stress . . . could quickly catapult me into that deadened zone. Just because I had something stress-ful for a day or two, I was wiped out. It took several days at least before I was back to where I was before I started the whole thing.

Having been advised to resume normal activity levels by a doctor who was unable to diagnose his problem, Bill says:

I took his advice, got out of bed, and went back to the office. It was very poor advice; I got worse again. I was not ready to go back to the office. I'm self-employed, which makes me tend to work harder. I probably would have been better off in bed.

UNPREDICTABLE EXACERBATIONS

Acceptance is undone by nasty surprises.

Cheri Register, *Living with Chronic Illness*

In the preceding cases, the triggers were known or suspected. At other times, an exacerbation may occur for no apparent reason. Toni Jeffreys wrote in *The Mile-High Staircase*:

I sank down rather less gracefully than a dying duck . . . . Once again I was hauled up those stairs to bed. I was quite hysterical. Hysterical with the horror of finding myself back in the nightmare. Every cell was crying out. My body was leaden. My head was in agony. I cried and screamed with what little strength there was left. And then I lay staring at the familiar hateful bedroom wall . . . .

The unthinkable had happened. Again. Every cell in the body, in the brain, was once again crying. Crying out for want of some absolutely necessary chemical, or else suffused with the wrong ones. I was by then battling with the deepest depression. Was I to spend yet another year feeling not dead/ not alive? Was there no end to it? . . . I was vulnerable, vulnerable.

PWCs describe unpredicted and unwelcome exacerbations:

Some days I feel really good and calm and relaxed; things are going well and the world is nice and rosy. There are other days, the downers, when I don't want to put forth any energy or mess with anything; I just want to feel good.

Every morning I wake up and think, "I wonder how I'm going to feel today."

It's a crapshoot. When will I feel worse and when better? I can't figure it out. As the little girl next door used to say, in response to a question for which she didn't have an answer, "I can't know."

This is such an up-and-down thing; you feel like you're getting better and you feel like you can handle it, and then— Boom! Problems again, you start from scratch again, you lose hope again. How many times can you go on the roller coaster?

Warning Signs

Although relapses are usually unpredictable, some PWCs have discovered a particular exacerbation-remission cycle. For example, Bill reports attacks every two to three weeks that last four or five days. Others report a six-week cycle: six "up" weeks followed by six "down" weeks. For most the cycle is not consistent, but preceding the exacerbations they notice warning signs such as fatigue, headache, paleness, muscle aches, visual disturbance, food cravings, or slowed speech, movement, and reactions. Other people may notice these changes before the PWC is aware of them. One of Sara's friends can tell in the first few seconds of a telephone conversation that Sara is having a "tired" or "down" day, and other CFIDS patients report the awareness of people close to them of signs of symptom fluctuations.

I am often surprised when my husband says, "Your speech and movements are slowing down. Do you need to rest?" Most of the time he's correct; I do need to stop and rest and may be starting an exacerbation—but he saw the signs before I did. At other times I am aware of vague warnings: mild muscle aches, fatigue, or equilibrium difficulties. The sooner I pay attention to my body's request for a time-out, the less severe the relapse is likely to be, although sometimes it doesn't seem to matter what I do or how soon I do it. The sick and tired feelings come back full force, and I again feel victimized by a mysterious force outside my control.

Emotional Fallout

It's tempting to assign blame when exacerbations occur. We search for a cause or a scapegoat, but sometimes there is none to be found, and we end up blaming ourselves. "It is quite common to feel ashamed or guilty when the illness worsens," writes Cheri Register about illness cycles. "Most of us would rather believe that mind has authority over matter, if we can only learn how to enforce it." So we heap the self-blame on top of the devastating disappointment of the crash, creating a bitter stew of fear, guilt, betrayal, and helplessness. Our feelings run the gamut from hope to desperation, from guilt to anger, as our lives bounce between harmony and discord.

AH! REMISSIONS

To feel good again is exciting—to feel that the virus, or whatever it is, has gone away forever or disappeared into hiding. It feels so good to feel good! Still, the doubt lingers: how long will this last? We learn to savor the moment, pushing back our fears of plummeting again as we enter a period of tentative optimism. We're ever-cautious, alert for signs that the grace period is over and it's time to be miserably sick again.

We hope the remission is permanent; the disease is over. We don't ever want to return to that other state. During a remission I wrote in my journal:

> The exacerbation is a black hole. I'm acutely aware of every second—difficult, dark, empty, painful. Then when the sun breaks through, the pain becomes a blur. I wonder where I've been all that time, where my self has been. I am so grateful to have the kind of day that was once only average. An almost-normal day reminds me that I am still myself.

Another excerpt, different remission, several years ago:

> Oh shit, I'm feeling better and getting hopeful again. Maybe I'm really getting over this—but I've thought that before and then crashed. Each time, like now, I get scared. Each crash is more difficult than the one before it. Now it's scary to feel this good. However, I sure know how to appreciate the value of feeling normal, feeling good, which I used to take for granted. Do I dare believe I'm getting well, or am I just buoyed up by this temporary semi-security, waiting for a fall?

Like most PWCs, I have experienced improvement in my health over time. Symptom severity continues to fluctuate, but my baseline (the way I've learned to expect to feel each day) has improved. Exacerbations still occur, but they are not as severe or long-lived. Looking back on some of the difficult ones, I'm amazed I got through them.

But just as the exacerbations are horrible, the remissions are wonderful. The freshness and energy of remission are invigorating. Hope is rekindled; life matters again. We get back in touch with the pleasant sensations of living and are able to appreciate beauty and joy. No longer wrapped in a cocoon, we are able to see beyond our own boundaries. In remission, I laugh more. I listen to music. I play music and sing. I am able to feel good about others because I am able to feel good about myself.

We notice other people and become more aware of their needs. We receive joy from giving to others—willingly and lovingly. We know remission is probably a temporary reprieve for an unspecified period of time. The trick is to enjoy it without tainting the good feelings with a sense of impending doom, and pacing ourselves to ward off the lurking, unpredictable menace.

When feeling better we tend to overdo, thinking that feeling okay grants us permission to make up for lost time. Such behavior leads to an excessive amount of activity that may put us back in bed. Of course, being careful doesn't guarantee indefinite postponement of an exacerbation, but at least it doesn't invite one. A moderate activity level is difficult to achieve, and the temptation to overdo is enormous.

Exacerbations inevitably occur, despite self-care and preventive measures. The crash produces the familiar sense of defeat and discouragement, and grueling self-questioning about what we've done wrong, what we've done to deserve *this*. Still, as pleasure-seeking human beings, we want to go for it; we try to enjoy the good times while remaining ever-cautious, almost superstitious.

Andy Rooney wrote in a piece entitled "The Flu": "It's difficult to remember how you felt when you were well while you're sick; and difficult to recall how you felt when you were sick when you're well." When I'm feeling better, I can remember feeling horrible, but I can't recapture the true misery and pain of the awful times. Perhaps that's best. We have built-in mechanisms for forgetting pain. (Otherwise everyone would be an only child.) But when the misery returns, the memory is quickly rekindled: back in the black hole, hoping for another reprieve.

Chapter 7

In Search of a Cause

THE IMMUNE SYSTEM: A CRASH COURSE

In an important sense, the immune system
is far greater than the sum of its parts.

Mizel and Jaret, *The Human Immune Systems:
The New Frontier in Medicine*

Immunology is a relatively new field of medicine; many doctors practicing today didn't even study it in medical school. In the past twenty years progress in technology has allowed us to study the immune system, which is far more complex and important than previously imagined. It had been believed that the immune system was complete in and of itself, with little connection to other body systems. This notion has proven false. The immune system is integrated with all other bodily systems and our understanding of it is still rudimentary.

The immune system has no central regulating organ, as do other body systems (e.g., the circulatory system has the heart as its central organ; the respiratory system, the lungs). Its components are located throughout the body. Communication takes place among immune cells and between the immune system and other organs.

The primary function of the immune system is to be sensitive to invaders, to distinguish between "self" and "nonself." Anything foreign to the body is "nonself": a potential enemy, called an *antigen*. The immune system is capable of identifying a tremendous number of different antigens. Once an enemy is recognized, a complex process is set in motion.

Functioning of the Immune System

What follows is a simplified explanation of a very powerful and complex process by which our bodies defend themselves against invasion.

There are three basic types of immune cells: *Phagocytes* are white blood cells, the body's scavengers or garbage collectors that gobble up invaders; *T-* and *B-cells* are types of lymphocytes. B-cells mature in the bone marrow, T-cells in the thymus gland. Lymphocytes flow through lymph nodes, small lumps of glandular tissue along lymph channels, which are the "organs" of the immune system. Lymph nodes are found throughout the body: in the throat area below the tonsils, in the armpits and groin, behind the knees, in many joints, at the base of the lungs, and in the abdomen.

Phagocytes find and attempt to destroy foreign substances ingested from the environment, such as chemical toxins and pollutants. If enemy cells are multiplying so fast that the phagocytes can't keep up with them, they can sound an alarm to alert the rest of the troops. When viruses, bacteria, protozoa, fungi, and other organic invaders attack the body, a complex battle ensues.

The Players

• **Antigens:** Substances recognized by the immune system as "non-self," triggering a complex immune response. In the example following these definitions, the antigen is a virus.

• **Viruses:** The invaders—bundles of genetic material in search of a home where they can find host cells in which to reproduce. A virus that is too successful will sabotage its own life by killing its host. If it is just successful enough, it will coexist with us so that we will survive and serve its needs.

• **Macrophages:** One type of circulating phagocyte that roves the body on the lookout for invaders, which it attempts to gobble up, while summoning additional help from helper T-cells.

• **Helper T-cells:** The stars of the team that orchestrate the battle. Helper T-cells circulate throughout body tissues, like sentries. When T-cells become aware of an enemy invasion, they begin to multiply and alert the spleen and lymph nodes to encourage the production of other immune cells by means of *lymphokines* (immune system "communicator chemicals"). Each of the many varieties of helper T-cells is programmed to recognize a specific enemy.

• **Killer T-cells:** Cells summoned by the helper T-cells that act as their name implies: they rush to the site of the invasion and at-tempt to kill the invaders.

• **B-cells:** Munitions factories in the spleen or lymph nodes. Ar-riving helper T-cells stimulate production of B-cells, which pro-duce antibodies designed specifically for the type of invader.

• **Antibodies:** Protein molecules produced by B-cells that are de-signed specifically to combat particular invaders. Antibodies rush to the war zone to neutralize or destroy enemy cells.

• **Suppressor T-cells:** After the invaders have been conquered, the suppressor T-cells call off the attack by stopping the B- and T-cell activity.

• **Memory cells:** These circulate in the body with a memory of a previous attacker so that a subsequent attack by the same type of enemy can be more easily conquered, even many years later. Vac-cines stimulate production of memory cells. When antibodies to such substances as pollens or cat dander are produced, we are said to be allergic to these things.

The Process

The process of a viral attack begins when the virus enters the body. Macrophages notice its presence and attempt to destroy it. They call for helper T-cells, which become active and multiply. Specific killer T- and B-cells are produced to launch an attack on the invader. The B-cells produce antibodies against the invader. Since some of the invading viral cells have infiltrated host cells, killer Ts attempt to kill the invaded cells. Antibodies then neu-tralize the viruses by attaching to them (to prevent them from invading other cells) and producing substances intended to poison the infected cells.

After the infection has been halted, other T-cells call off the battle, shutting off the immune response. Memory cells memorize the chemical identities of the conquered attackers so they can recognize them should they reattack in the future. Although this is the basic program by which the immune system is believed to fight off infection, the process is actually much more complex, and much of it is not currently understood.

Note: This summary is based in part on a section of Peter Jaret's excellent article "The Wars Within," *National Geographic,* June 1986.

Immunological research has led to a knowledge of protein substances called lymphokines, the immune messengers that cause the production of such symptoms as fever and inflammation, indicating that the immune system is at war with an invader. Some lymphokines are thought to be able to kill enemy cells, such as some cancer cells, directly. Examples of lymphokines are interleukins (ILs), B-cell growth factor, B-cell differentiation factor, and the interferons. Lymphokines are now recognized as extremely important parts of the immune response, and they are being used in the treatment of cancer and other diseases. Some researchers feel that a better understanding of lymphokine functioning and identification of currently unknown lymphokines will provide the keys for understanding and treating immune problems as well as some psychiatric disorders that may be immune-related.

Because CFIDS involves dysregulation of the immune system, many of its symptoms may be caused by an immune imbalance, specifically in levels of various lymphokines. When the immune system is constantly turned on, it reacts to all types of substances perceived as "nonself," producing the various discomforts of CFIDS. (Keep in mind that our symptoms may be caused by our bodies' *reactions* to particular agents, such as viruses, rather than by the direct action of those agents.)

IMMUNE DYSFUNCTION

When the immune system is not functioning perfectly a number of problems may develop, some apparent and others subtle. Immune dysfunction is probably a contributory factor in many currently unexplained illnesses. Improper immune functioning occurs when the immune system underreacts, overreacts, or reacts inappropriately to an invader. When it reacts appropriately, we are able to fight off, or resist, infection. When the immune system's attempts are inadequate, illness results. We are constantly exposed to many antigens; only when the antigens "win" do we get sick.

The interaction of helper and suppressor T-cells is the on-off switch of the immune system. The ratio of helper to suppressor T-cells is normally 2:1 or 3:1. The balance between them is critical to proper immune response and functioning. During and following illness, this ratio varies.

In *autoimmune disorders*, the immune system has lost its ability to distinguish between "self" and "nonself," and the body attacks its own tissue as if it were an antigen (enemy). In the process healthy cells are attacked and destroyed. Multiple sclerosis, rheumatoid arthritis, some forms of thyroid disease, and systemic lupus erythematosus are considered autoimmune disorders. The incidence of autoimmune diseases is thought to be higher in women, possibly due to hormonal factors or immune systems that respond more aggressively to invaders.

A state of *immunosuppression* allows enemy cells, such as viruses, to reproduce actively. The situation may be a "stand-off" in which the immune system is unable to rid the body of invaders but keeps them somewhat in check. When the immune system is rallying, symptoms subside. When the disruptive agent becomes stronger, symptoms increase. Neither side is able to sustain a victory and end the war. As the war continues, the infectious agent retains a degree of control; if the agent "lost," it would be killed. If the agent "won" it would kill the patient, thus destroying itself. So it is to the invader's advantage to stay in control by using the host but not killing it. In the process, it attempts to disrupt the host's functioning in ways that will make the invader's life happier—and the host's life more miserable.

Immune dysfunction can be caused by a variety of factors. Primary immune deficiencies (those that are congenital, or present from birth) may not become apparent until later in life when exposure to certain antigens creates symptoms. Secondary immune deficiencies are acquired; they develop as a result of nongenetic factors such as nutrition, age, amount of sleep, surgery and general anesthesia, infections, injury, certain drugs, emotional state, hormonal imbalance, stress level, and exposure to various environmental toxins and allergens. Such deficiencies may be transient; for example, when an infection has been successfully resolved or when exposure to a toxin is discontinued, the deficiency may also resolve.

Negative emotional states, such as loneliness and depression, can impair immunity to a significant degree because of alterations of neuroendocrine function (the connections between the brain and the glandular system). Intense and/or prolonged stress adversely affects immune functioning. Constant stress response (the fight-or-flight reaction) and negative emotions affect hormonal, neural, and endocrine function, which in turn cause the immune system to function less efficiently. Conversely, positive emotions and a hopeful outlook are believed to enhance immune functioning.

When the immune system is out of balance, some parts become overactive and others underactive. The problem is not that the immune system isn't reacting *strongly* enough but that it's reacting inappropriately. The signals being sent between the parts of the immune system, and between the immune system and the rest of the body, may be distorted, creating malfunctions in the entire body system. Excessive, futile attention focused on a benign invader (such as pollen) while a more significant threat is ignored is analogous to an individual shooting bullets at a harmless fly while ignoring a burglar who is looting the house.

So far there has been a lack of consistency in findings regarding immune dysfunction in CFIDS as well as great difficulty in correlating measurable abnormalities with the patient's symptoms. Immune abnormalities are a piece of the CFIDS puzzle, but it is still not known whether the abnormalities are a cause or effect (or both) of the illness. Techniques for measuring immune function are fairly rudimentary and we are unable to measure the strength of an individual's immune system. We are able to measure certain types of immune functioning but these measurements are not comprehensive (or able to be generalized) and are often inaccurate.

A landmark medical journal article entitled "Phenotypic and Functional Deficiency of Natural Killer Cells in Patients with Chronic Fatigue Syndrome" reported abnormal activity and ratios of natural killer cells, a "first line of defense in animals against viral infections." The researchers were not able to determine whether this aberration was a cause or effect of CFIDS but it was significant in that it was the first documented immune abnormality (Caliguiri et al. 1987). Since that time other immune abnormalities have been noted in PWCs (as described in Chapter 4) but, unfortunately, such abnormalities are difficult to test for, test results are inconsistent, and findings vary among patients. But the types of abnormalities found in PWCs yield insight into the mechanisms involved in CFIDS and offer additional treatment options.

The essential question, then, is not simply, "What goes wrong with the immune system that makes us sick?" or "What is the virus or causative agent that makes us sick?" but the more complex question, "How do these various factors interact to make us sick?" The cause(s) and contributing factors are likely to include the following.

Viruses

'Virus' is a word used by doctors a great deal.
It means, 'Your guess is as good as mine.'

Bob Hope

Viruses are submicroscopic, protein-covered bundles of genetic material containing blueprints for self-reproduction. Viruses are covered with a capsid, or coat, and/or a special envelope, which they use to attach to the cells they subsequently enter. In fact, many antiviral drugs work by damaging or destroying these coats so that attachment cannot take place. Unlike bacteria, which are living organisms, viruses are neither alive nor dead. Incapable of reproduction on their own, they search for hosts whose cells they can invade to accomplish this purpose. Although we view viruses as our enemies, they are not, in reality, malicious. Their only goal is to replicate—not to cause trouble. In the process, they invade our cells (like checking into a motel) and give genetic orders, turning our cells into virus factories. Their offspring burst forth, destroying the previously invaded cell and seeking out new healthy cells for their continued reproduction. These tiny, elusive viruses are capable of hiding, mutating, and combining.

There are many types of viruses, probably hundreds of thousands, only some of which have been identified. Because viruses are adept at escaping detection, viral illnesses are often diagnosed on the basis of symptoms and by exclusion of other possible illnesses. We can guess about them based on the damage they do, and we identify them based on the antibodies produced in reaction to their presence.

Polymerase chain reaction (PCR) is a relatively new and sophisticated technique that allows us to amplify DNA or RNA sequences in viruses to aid in viral identification. It has the potential to make this determination for virtually any viral sequence for which a specimen can be obtained. Various techniques are employed in performing PCR, and there is often disagreement among results, especially in attempting to identify new viruses. PCR is a sensitive method of detecting viruses but it is not sufficiently specific to identify them well. As PCR technology improves, we will be able to identify greater numbers of viruses directly, rather than having to rely on indirect measures, such as antibody titers. This task of identifying individual viruses is made more difficult by the ability of viruses to alter their identities by mutating.

Many viruses can remain in latent (nonreproducing) form in our bodies for long periods of time without producing symptoms. Viral agents that may produce latent (inactive) infections include herpes simplex, herpes zoster, cytomegalovirus (CMV), human herpesvirus type 6 (HHV-6), and retroviruses. Many viruses are capable of producing chronic illnesses by alternating dormant and active (replication) phases. Their versatility allows viruses to exist in an active, dormant, or low-level state, producing varied immune reactions in our bodies. Factors that facilitate reactivation of latent viruses include infections (for example, infection with one virus may trigger activation of another dormant virus), exposure to certain chemicals (allergens, toxins, immunosuppressive drugs), fever, corticosteroids, physical or emotional stress, ultraviolet light, and local trauma.

Certain viral disorders are believed to be linked with disorders elsewhere in the body, for example in the nervous system, the endocrine system, and the immune system. Future research will likely reveal the nature of these links.

Several viruses are being studied to determine their possible roles in CFIDS. They fall into various classes. Adenoviruses can infect cells and can persist for long periods of time. They can reproduce slowly but consistently, producing low-grade infections. Slow viruses have long incubation periods and can cause persistent disease (often neurological) after being in the body for a long period of time. Viruses in the herpes class demonstrate a particular ability to remain latent for long periods of time. Herpesvirus infections include cold sores, herpes encephalitis, influenza-type illness, chicken pox and shingles (both caused by the varicella virus), cytomegalovirus-related illness (which occurs mainly in fetuses and babies, but which can also produce a mono-like illness), and mononucleosis. Certain herpes viruses are believed to play a role in some forms of cancer.

The Epstein-Barr virus (EBV) is a herpes virus that infects virtually everyone; 90–95% of the adult population have antibodies to it, meaning that they have been infected at some time during their lives (in many cases, without obvious symptoms). Once the virus has infected an individual, it persists for life, generally remaining inactive following the initial exposure, probably because we have developed enough antibodies to suppress the virus but not kill it. EBV infections in children are generally asymptomatic. Young adults initially exposed to it may develop mononucleosis, which typically lasts about six weeks, although symptoms may persist for months. Reports of chronic mononucleosis (mono that doesn't clear up after six weeks to six months) have been documented. EBV may play a role in CFIDS, although not a causative one. Chronic mononucleosis has never been known to appear in epidemic form. In CFIDS and other illnesses, a weakened immune system may allow replication of EBV and other previously dormant viruses. It is also possible that we are faced with a new strain of EBV in CFIDS.

Human herpesvirus type 6 (HHV-6) was initially isolated in 1986. It is a common virus, although infection is often asymptomatic. Like other herpesviruses, it may remain dormant for many years until reactivated by some type of trauma, such as stress, infection with another agent, or changes in the immune system. A high frequency of HHV-6 reactivation is found in PWCs. It may play a causal role or may be an epiphenomenon of immune dysfunction, perhaps causing increased production of cytokines, activating other viruses, and destroying natural killer (NK) cells.

Other viruses that may play a role in causation and/or symptom production are cytomegalovirus (which causes symptoms similar to those caused by EBV, notably neurological ones); coxsackie virus; herpes zoster (which causes chicken pox and shingles and remains dormant in the nerve cells thereafter); and other herpesviruses, such as herpes simplex I and II and gamma herpesviruses. All of these viruses tend to become more active when the human host is under increased stress.

Byron Hyde, M.D., of Canada speculates that CFIDS, or ME as it is called there, is caused by an enterovirus, a category of viruses that includes coxsackie and polio. There is some speculation that CFIDS is another form of poliomyelitis or is caused by a nonpolio enterovirus—or that enteroviruses do not play a causal role but are reactivated by immune dysregulation, as are the herpesviruses, for example.

Another suspect is a retrovirus—possibly human T-lymphotrophic virus type 2 (HTLV-2). Retroviruses contain an enzyme called reverse transcriptase that allows them to reverse the order of genetic information processing—hence their name. Retroviruses have been implicated in such illnesses as AIDS, a rare type of leukemia, and certain forms of cancer. Research findings by Dr. Elaine DeFreitas at the Wistar Institute, in conjunction with Drs. Bell and Cheney and other researchers, were presented at the Eleventh International Congress of Neuropathology in Kyoto, Japan, in September 1990. In a large percentage of the small number of cases studied they reported the presence of certain viral sequences that resemble HTLV-2 but which also might be a new, previously undiscovered retrovirus that shares a common gene sequence with HTLV-2. Attempts to replicate these results, however, have been unsuccessful. It is also possible that a retrovirus interacts with other viruses to cause CFIDS.

John Martin, M.D., made the news when he prematurely announced his discovery of a retrovirus (an RNA virus) called a Spumavirus, or "foamy" virus, which he believed to be related to CFIDS. Martin is currently working on isolating a "stealth" virus (a DNA virus), which may infect the brain and play a part in CFIDS and other diseases with a neurological component. The exact identity of this virus is not clear; it may be a herpesvirus—perhaps a mutated cytomegalovirus, which infects the brain without causing inflammation and hence escapes detection.

The significance of the early retrovirus studies is the finding of rare viruses in PWCs, according to Dr. DeFreitas, who believes that retroviruses are suggested as causal agents because they are neurotropic (they live in the brain and other parts of the central nervous system) and because retroviruses are associated with immune dysfunction (November 1991). However, to make any causal assumptions about these preliminary findings would be premature. The possibility of retroviral involvement in CFIDS is a first significant step in what will doubtless be a lengthy research process that may yield a breakthrough—or another blind alley. Such findings have served the important function of alerting the medical profession and the media to the existent seriousness of CFIDS.

We don't know whether CFIDS is virally caused. CFIDS acts like a viral illness: it comes and goes and produces a dazzling array of symptoms that vary over time. CFIDS patients often have high levels of antiviral antibodies that are assumed to indicate viral activation. In our attempts to determine viral involvement in CFIDS, we operate under many handicaps. It is difficult to measure viral activity directly; we are unable to measure antibodies to many viruses, and we don't even know how many varieties of viruses actually exist. In future study, molecular biology will allow us to gain a better understanding of viruses and their involvement in CFIDS.

A virus may be only one of the causal or triggering agents. Nonviral triggering factors that interfere with immune functioning may allow viruses to move from dormant to active states so that viral activation is an effect, rather than a cause, of CFIDS. The cause may turn out to be a newly discovered virus, a more virulent strain of a known virus, a recombinant virus, a faulty immune system reacting inappropriately to a "normal" virus, all of the above—or none of the above. And, of course, CFIDS may be an umbrella term for a number of different but similar illnesses with various causative factors. Even if the cause of CFIDS is viral, there may be no one particular virus that is causal in all cases.

And if a virus or viruses are implicated, what to do? Detection, the first step, is very difficult. Treatment, the next step, is also difficult. Only one virus, smallpox, is believed to be completely eradicated. There are vaccines for a few viral illnesses: polio, rubella, hepatitis B, and some strains of influenza virus. Another approach to treatment is aimed at increasing our immune effectiveness: immune-enhancing drugs are currently used for treating CFIDS and new ones are being developed and tested.

Genetic Predisposition

Many PWCs report medical histories indicative of long-term, low-level immune dysfunction. The following comments are fairly typical:

> I've always thought of myself as a healthy person, but over the years I've had numerous infections and problems with fatigue. But until now I've always recovered uneventfully.

I've had something in my system all my life; periodically, it flares up. I've had diphtheria three times, Legionnaire's disease, viral pneumonia twice, and cancer. I get sick after stressful events.

I've had low body temperature all my life, and I've always needed lots of rest.

I had asthma as a child, measles three times, pneumonia during my third pregnancy, sinus trouble, hepatitis, Legionnaire's disease . . . . But I've always been active and considered myself healthy. Then, in 1985, I slowed down more and more, stopped ice skating and running, dropped the aerobics classes I was teaching, one at a time. I felt like a balloon that lost its air.

I had mono when I was 36 [present age 53]. I've had a history of colds, throat problems, allergies. I had rheumatic fever as a child. I've had low stamina all my life. I've always gotten motion sickness and have a tendency to faint.

My immune system has never worked right.

I've had frequent infections all my life, but I've always recovered from them—until this one.

One patient, a retired university professor, speculated that those most prone to get CFIDS have a history of such illnesses as cradle cap, eczema, asthma and other bronchial problems, whooping cough, chicken pox, rubella, measles, allergies, depression, and viral illness, with periodic illnesses and periods of "not feeling well" throughout their lives interspersed with times of relatively normal functioning. He believes that such a history, combined with the stress of Type A behavior and a busy lifestyle, contributes strongly to the development of CFIDS. Many patient interviews support this impression, but it is dangerous to draw conclusions from such sketchy data.

Such histories suggest that an incompetent immune system, either genetic or acquired, may contribute to the development of CFIDS in susceptible individuals. However, many other PWCs report a history of good health, rarely missing school or work, with little tendency to get colds or flu.

Environment

> ... [T]oo many major American industries dig up the good things out of
> the earth, spit out what they can't use and produce poisonous waste
> by-products that are eventually going to kill the land and then us . . . .
> While the leaders of government everywhere are worrying about the
> Big Bomb, mankind everywhere is poisoning the ground and
> the waters we depend on for life.
>
> Andy Rooney, *The Dead Land*

Hippocrates stressed the importance of viewing the human body within its context—its geography, climate, diet, and so on. Our environment is a dangerous place to live. We are subjected to pollutants in the air we breathe, additives in our food, and contaminants in our drinking water. We ingest harmful chemicals in startling amounts daily. We are poisoning ourselves slowly with substances whose potential damage we can only estimate. The so-called safe amounts of these chemicals are mere guesses; their synergistic effects are totally unknown. Government regulations are inadequate and poorly enforced.

In recent years the number of new chemicals introduced into our bodies has increased dramatically; our bodies have become chemical processing plants that are heavily and unreasonably taxed, affecting all levels of functioning. In the name of progress we have created compounds that are both helpful and harmful, and the immune system bears the brunt of their assault. Just a few of the culprits found in air, soil, and water are pesticides (insecticides and herbicides such as chlordane), food additives (such as preservatives; flavoring and coloring agents; steroids, veterinary medicines, and antibiotics in meat and poultry; waxes; thickening agents; emulsifiers), and air pollutants (such as sulfur dioxide).

Anyone would refuse a cocktail made of arsenic, aldicarb (a pesticide), vinyl chloride (used in making plastic), polychlorinated biphenyls (PCBs), hazardous industrial solvents, radioactive wastes, and heavy metals (such as chromium, lead, and cadmium)—yet we ingest these substances frequently. They may affect our immune systems adversely, but we fool ourselves with a game called, "What I can't see can't hurt me."

In "The Poisons Within," a six-part series which appeared in *The Arizona Republic*, Mike Masterson, investigative team leader, wrote:

Americans are consuming an unprecedented number of hazardous chemicals in their food, water, and air. Some are becoming ill and dying from this relatively new threat, but no one knows the extent of the long-term effects. (January 29, 1989)

Scientists are concerned that sustained low-level exposure to many different types of manufactured chemicals will damage *immune or neurological functions* and elevate cancer rates over the coming decades. (January 29, 1989) [italics added]

Ground water in at least portions of every state is contaminated with cancer-causing pesticides, solvents or other hazardous chemicals. New contamination sites are being discovered every year. (January 31, 1989)

The federal agencies that once told Americans they could ingest small amounts of the pesticide DDT [now banned for its toxicity] without fear today assure them it is all right to ingest minuscule levels of many pesticides that have yet to be thoroughly tested. (February 1, 1989)

Some pesticide residues, or metabolites, are present in almost all American adults. One 1987 study showed evidence of three potent pesticides in 72 percent of the urine samples taken from 28,000 people in 64 communities. (February 1, 1989)

Federally permissible traces of various pesticides and drugs exist in much of the meat and poultry that Americans consume, resulting in a cumulative effect on the body when they combine with other chemicals in fruits, vegetables and water. (February 3, 1989)

Each month many new chemicals are registered, adding to the existing risks. "Americans routinely ingest thousands of these man-made chemicals created, ironically, to enhance the quality of life. Many compounds remain in the body for years" (January 29, 1989). Many banned substances continue to be used either in the United States or in countries from which we import food.

The toll on human life is gradual and subtle, but alarming. Even if we were to begin an aggressive cleanup program on a national level, much of the damage cannot be undone because many of these dangerous substances are stored indefinitely in adipose tissue (fat), the cumulative and synergistic effects are unknown, and irreversible genetic changes may have already taken place. In addition, a comprehensive program to make dramatic changes in our use of these chemicals would be politically unpopular because of its astronomical cost. Our government is more responsive to market pressures than to social welfare; because the use of harmful chemicals is economically profitable, its impact on health is almost ignored. The long-term damage to our bodies cannot be assessed but these dangerous substances are believed to cause immune and nervous system disorders. Unless we make massive cleanup efforts a priority, the damage will continue to compound.

Disease symptoms related to the ingestion of toxic substances in the workplace show up in many occupations. For example, daily exposure to solvents has produced cognitive dysfunction, aggressiveness, mental fatigue, and disturbances in social relationships (Orbaek and Lindgren, 1988). Office personnel in large, sealed buildings are subject to increased exposure to viruses and bacteria as the air endlessly recirculates. Daniel Peterson, M.D., commented on the closed-building phenomenon in relation to the CFIDS outbreak in Lake Tahoe, stating that the incidence of CFIDS in local schools with poor air exchange had been significantly greater than its incidence in schools with better air circulation (May 1991). However, the possible connection between closed buildings and CFIDS has not been studied systematically. Another unknown is the effect of electromagnetic pollution. We are subjected to electromagnetic fields created by power stations, power lines, and home appliances daily, but little research regarding their effects has been done.

Radiation is another suspected risk factor in the development of CFIDS and other diseases. The increased susceptibility of the younger population to various immune disorders such as CFIDS, cancer, and HIV may be related to the release of low-level ionizing radiation into the environment. These releases began in the 1940s with nuclear weapons plants, bombings, above-ground bomb tests (underground tests started in the 1960s), and later nuclear power plants. Radioactive fallout, especially resulting from above-ground tests and leakage from radiation energy plants, is released locally and may be carried to other parts of the country by winds and precipitation. Is it a coincidence that many PWCs are in their middle years, having been born in an era of extensive above-ground nuclear testing which affects infants and children strongly? Radiation may work synergistically with other environmental and personal factors to increase susceptibility to disease, but no formal testing has been done.

Environmental pollution and illness, immune dysfunction, and CFIDS may be inextricably related.

Stress

Stress is natural and necessary. In and of itself stress is not bad, it is simply continual adaptation to demands from without and within. In a positive sense, stress is the force that urges us forward, allowing growth and progress. Even positive events—a promotion at work or a new addition to the family—are stressful in that adaptation is required. When stressors are numerous, severe, and constant, or when we fail to adapt successfully, the result of stress can be bodily damage. Sources of stress are everywhere in our lives: too much or too little activity, the demands of families and employers, responsibilities, excessive noise and environmental pollution, and so on.

The amount and nature of the stressors and our individual ability to adapt successfully determine the toll stress will take. If we neglect self-care (sufficient sleep, moderate exercise, relaxation, and adequate diet) and constantly push to get ahead, our health will be affected. Our society doesn't regard self-care as a priority. To push harder as stressors accumulate is the norm; to pull back and rest as needed is frowned upon. Often we neglect ourselves and our needs because we're on autopilot, putting out lots of time and energy as we're programmed to do, and not caring for ourselves because self-care may not occur to us, or because we may be unaware of its importance.

Many of us live in a state of constant tension and anxiety. Stress activates the fight-or-flight response, a protective process in which bodily changes take place and numerous chemicals are released. Some of these chemicals are hormones that inhibit immune system function. As the body continually taps its resources for coping with stress, certain chemicals become depleted and exhaustion may set in, rendering us susceptible to illness. In the face of continuing challenges we push (rather than rest, as our bodies urge us to do) and our self-neglect compounds the problem. Essentially, we are drawing from an account that has dipped deeply into credit reserve.

The total stress load on an individual consists of stress from within and without, including major life changes and personal crises (identity crises, relationship problems, low self-esteem, disappointments). Unmet needs, challenging events, and the ongoing daily grind contribute to the total load. Unrelenting stress or a series of sudden highly stressful events is taxing even to the strong and hardy.

Many PWCs have described stressful events that preceded the onset of illness: death of loved ones; divorce or breakup of significant relationships; other illnesses (their own, or those of family members or close friends); childbirth; career or job changes; health problems including illness and surgery; financial problems; moves to different geographical areas; and other individual or family crises. Many stressful events involve some type of loss, and the average number of major stressors reported in a survey of Phoenix PWCs was 3.2 per person in the eighteen months preceding the onset of CFIDS. In addition to these events the majority reported highly active, busy lifestyles, which presented chronic stressors: rapid life changes at the individual and societal levels, economic instability, changing roles, anxieties about spiritual and existential concerns, various life dissatisfactions, time pressures, lack of social structure, and difficulty relaxing.

Many of us have taken on a number of professional and personal roles: we may work several jobs and balance hectic schedules. Recent years have brought a dazzlingly accelerated rate of technological change. Keeping up with the fast pace of life and barrages of sensory input can be overwhelming. We live a crazy lifestyle in which denial of personal needs is considered heroic. We travel widely, diet frequently, intersperse dieting with junk food pig-outs, try to force rapid recovery after surgery or illness, ignore the problems and symptoms that are trying to give us messages about our needs, and spend so much time "taking care of business" that we neglect to take care of ourselves.

One PWC, a former actress, says:

> You put a car in a garage and it will last a lot longer than if you put it in a grand prix all the time. It's going to get worn out; my immune system is worn out. My body is a very important vehicle and I've abused it by overachieving, always being on the go without sufficient food or sleep. I had two surgeries, marital problems and a divorce, and then I got this illness.

Yolanda relates her high stress level to graduate school pressures, family responsibilities, divorce, remarriage, and her self-concept as a superwoman who could and should handle these pressures and transitions easily. She admits that she put others' needs before her own and had always had unrealistically high self-expectations. She developed CFIDS in her last year of graduate school and barely made it through finals. Now unable to work, she wonders if she wasted her time and money to prepare for a career she may never attain.

Another PWC states, "I was going to school, caring for my four kids, and building a house. I lost several friends. My parents became ill and died. I'm in the process of adopting two more kids. I don't have time to be ill." And when she developed CFIDS, her illness became another stressor.

Once the diagnosis is made, the CFIDS label is an additional stressor, as is the search for treatment. What would have been minor events in the past become more stressful because of the illness: physical or mental activity, travel, chemical exposure, hormonal fluctuations, and any type of family problems. The body becomes exquisitely sensitive even to minor assaults.

Psychoneuroimmunology

Psychoneuroimmunology (PNI) is an age-old, newly embraced interdisciplinary approach to understanding the interconnectedness of all body systems—the central nervous system (brain and spinal cord), the immune system, and behavior. All illness is psychosomatic, involving both mind and body (the "mindbody") for they are inseparable. The mindbody exists in a delicate balance called homeostasis; its disruption results in symptoms or disease. The term psychosomatic, however, is commonly used incorrectly to denote an illness that is self-created or "all in one's head," often implying an illness more imagined than real. Illnesses such as CFIDS must teach us to recognize and respect the importance of the integration of mind, spirit, and soma (body), to see them as inextricably interconnected.

Recurrent symptoms indicate that something has interfered with homeostasis, the ability of the mindbody to maintain its delicate balance. The communication among body systems is amazingly complex; the mind, brain, immune system, and other systems send constant back-and-forth chemical and electrical messages. A malfunction in one area creates imbalance, causing malfunctions in other areas.

Psychosocial and environmental events take their toll on the immune system, but the way in which this occurs is not fully understood. In *The Healer Within*, Locke and Colligan discuss the tendrils of nerve tissue from the brain that run through the most important parts of the immune system: the thymus gland, bone marrow, lymph nodes, and spleen. Hormones and neurotransmitters secreted by the brain have an affinity for immune cells. There are active lines of communication between the brain and the immune system, and brain chemicals have both positive and negative influences on immune functioning. The brain–immune system link works both ways; changes in either entity affect the other because they are inextricably bound. Neither controls the other but each influences the other. The links among all body systems present the opportunity for our emotions to influence how well the body is able to defend itself.

The limbic system, for example, helps to maintain internal homeostasis by acting as a buffer between the internal and external worlds and by integrating bodily processes. Jay Goldstein, M.D., believes that it plays a central role in CFIDS. The limbic system is a complex neural network, a rim of cortical structures above and highly interconnected with the hypothalamus, the area of the brain that controls the endocrine system and the autonomic nervous system, which generates the drives and instincts that promote survival of the self and the species. The limbic system affects most aspects of bodily functioning, including emotion and mood (and their connection with behavior), respiration, memory, appetite and weight, fatigue, sleep, libido, immune and endocrine systems. The limbic system serves the necessary function of integrating internal and external events (that is, coordinating input from the inside and outside worlds and determining our behavioral responses).

Goldstein conceptualizes CFIDS as "a limbic encephalopathy in a dysregulated neuroimmune network," stating in his book *Chronic Fatigue Syndrome: The Limbic Hypothesis*, "No matter what the cause of the syndrome, the symptoms are transduced through the limbic system." That is, in the complex intercommunications between the central nervous system and the immune system, many of the symptoms associated with CFIDS may be of central (brain) origin, rather than peripheral (local) origin. This does not explain the cause of the disease (although certain viruses have an affinity for the brain), but it does explain many CFIDS symptoms, including: fatigue; sleep disorder (initiating and maintaining sleep, sleep-phase disorder, hypersomnia, nightmares, thermoregulation disorders such as nightsweats, frequent awakenings, apnea, nonrestorative sleep, irregular sleep-wake patterns, alpha-EEG sleep); cognitive dysfunction (e.g., memory); vision problems; anxiety and panic attacks; rage; affective (mood) disorders (e.g., depression); headache; fibromyalgia; lymphadenalgia (painful lymph nodes); tinnitus; vertigo; muscle weakness and difficulty walking; nasal allergies; chemical sensitivities; metabolic rate changes; rapid weight gain (limbic modulation of brown fat thermogenesis); irritable bowel symptoms; increased PMS or PMS with onset after developing CFIDS due to hormonal factors; respiratory complaints such as dyspnea on exertion, air hunger, and hyperventilation; thirst; urinary problems; libido; impotence; endometriosis; disorders of temperature regulation; alcohol intolerance; cardiac rate and blood pressure changes; lower basal temperature; and lack of immunoregulation, including recurrent illness.

Unfortunately, the medical profession as a whole has not embraced PNI and holds fast to the outdated notion of mind-body duality. Increasing numbers of medical specialties and subspecialties offer more effective treatment of certain disorders, but also indicate considerable fragmentation, causing the importance of the interconnections between body systems to be minimized. This simple cause-and-effect view hampers our understanding of such complex illnesses as CFIDS.

Other Suspected Causes and Contributing Factors

• **Systemic yeast/fungal infection.** Whether systemic candidiasis is related to CFIDS or not is a controversial issue. Yeast overgrowth may be a causal contributor to CFIDS, or vice versa—or both may be attributable to immune dysfunction. Contributing factors to both conditions may include nutritional deficiencies, overuse of antibiotics, extended use of birth control pills, environmental toxins, and emotional stress—all of which are believed to have detrimental effects on immunity.

The fact that anti-yeast medications and diet are helpful to many PWCs does not prove a causal relationship but does indicate that further research is warranted. Perhaps both yeast overgrowth and CFIDS symptoms are the result of dysregulation of the immune system.

• **Vaccines.** Routine immunization has obliterated several life-threatening illnesses but may also have negative effects on the immune systems of susceptible individuals. Vaccines contain attenuated (weakened) viruses to stimulate the production of antibodies so that the individual will not get an active infection if exposed to the virus at a later time. However, the injected viruses, although attenuated, may be transmitted from those vaccinated (usually children) to others who are sufficiently sensitive to react to the virus and become ill.

SELF-RESPONSIBILITY FOR ILLNESS?

We were all being assaulted now with the verbiage of self-help guerrillas who said gay men had brought AIDS on themselves. "I'm taking a course in miracles, " as one Hollywood airhead shared with me on the phone one night. "People pick their own diseases," he said, bragging that his lesions had faded to inconsequence . . . . But nobody picks his own disease —except, perhaps, the more rabid religions.

Paul Monette, *Borrowed Time*

Humans are unwilling to believe that great suffering and disaster can be inflicted without moral justification.

Rita Mae Brown, *High Hearts*

Some of us have been led to believe that we have "made ourselves sick." Are we responsible for our illness? Is it something we have chosen? A punishment for not living right? A sign of weakness or personal failure? The result of an inadequate spiritual belief system?

And what does it mean that we have remained sick? That we haven't triumphed, conquered? That we're weak rather than strong? That we have failed to learn the right lessons?

In a *New Age Journal* article, Ken and Treya Wilber discussed the downside of New Age spiritual belief systems that blame patients for their illnesses and insist that new, correct attitudes and beliefs are a primary curative force. According to this new way of thinking, we are supposed to "think" or "will" the disease away. Our inability to rid ourselves of illness can become a source of shame and inadequacy. The Wilbers do not view illness as a punishment or life lesson but as an opportunity to make life changes and achieve greater harmony.

"I blame myself for having gotten sick," says Bill, who thinks a medicine he took might have caused CFIDS. "I'm angry at the doctor who prescribed it and at myself for taking it. I haven't gotten over the guilt and I don't know if I ever will." Kyle comments, "I think we create our own realities and our own diseases. I think there are accidents, but I'm wondering if we didn't create those, too." Yolanda says, "I still feel the guilt of wondering if [CFIDS] is my own fault."

Is illness something we bring upon ourselves as a special challenge, a signal of a particular deficiency needing to be grappled with, a sign that we have not handled our emotions properly? Susan Sontag (1977) believes that the punitive notion of disease causation has been long-standing and counterproductive, encouraging the patient to engage in self-blame for having become ill and then for not getting well. These feelings may retard rather than speed healing. In writing about AIDS, Paul Monette lamented the "growing 'empowerment movement,' which tended to start with the assumption that people brought on their own illness," and suggested that developing the proper attitude would allow the virus to "evaporate like a fog" (1988).

We have all questioned ourselves similarly. The verdict is: *Not guilty*. To blame ourselves—or anyone—for our illness is not only erroneous, it's destructive. I don't believe that illness is part of a divine plan, that it is our karma, that we somehow chose it and should be able to will it away. I've been through all that, questioning my attitudes, beliefs, and lifestyle. I've wanted to have someone or something to blame (we're conditioned that way), but I've drawn a blank. I am able to identify some factors that contributed to my susceptibility to this illness, but I no longer look for the cause within myself.

Judging ourselves for being ill is self-defeating. It is essential to develop a sensible belief system about illness, preferably one that includes the following concepts:

Illness is not a test of character strength or a sign of personal deficiency.

Life is not fair.

Bad things do happen to good people. (Conversely, good things happen to bad people!)

Just because I don't know exactly what caused my illness, that doesn't mean I should blame myself—or anyone.

Question: *Why me?* Answer: *Why not me?*

There are some questions to which we don't have, and may never have, answers.

Having participated to some degree in the origins of an illness is not the same as having caused it or being to blame for it.

Illness did not occur in our lives to present a growth opportunity we needed or invited. But since it has happened to us, we can learn from the experience. We can grow in ways we could not have anticipated and find new meaning and goals in life. Taking the illness as a given, something that happened for a number of reasons that have nothing to do with personal volition or worth, we can decide what to make of it—whether to give in to it or to learn from it, whether to neglect or take care of ourselves to maximize our chances of regaining health. We don't have a choice about whether or not to be sick. It's an opportunity to grow, one we can accept or refuse. But we can't go back to the way we were.

PERSONALITY TYPE AS
A CAUSE OF ILLNESS?

Many of those diagnosed with CFIDS were once energetic, driven, aggressive, intelligent, perfectionistic, goal-oriented people with busy lifestyles. Phillip Rubin, M.D., said at a Phoenix support group meeting, "Most of you do in your impaired state more than most people do in their normal state."

Many PWCs fit the "magic caretaker role." In their personal and professional lives they have always taken care of others, often at their own expense. They have felt most comfortable when providing, even sacrificing, for others and they feel a very strong need to "be good." Others depend on them. They are often overextended. These are the people-pleasers who make such statements as:

I have taken care of other people all my life.

Everyone has always relied on me.

I feel like I was addicted to stress, to the adrenaline rush. Relax? No—I just wore myself out because I never let up.

I didn't take vacations . . . and I loved what I was doing, even though the hours were long.

I've never been accountable just for me. I've been working for a long time now, going to school, raising kids. You make up your mind to do something; you do it. And all of a sudden I couldn't. Nothing had ever stopped me.

I was very self-sufficient, very independent. I didn't need anybody's help.

To assess changes in personality characteristics pre- and post-CFIDS, I administered a checklist of personality traits to 59 PWCs at a meeting of the CFS Association in Phoenix. The changes indicated were dramatic and are consistent with the suspected typical CFIDS profile:

	Pre-Illness	Currently
Outgoing personality	82%	26%
Introverted personality	11	50
Easygoing	47	21

	Pre-Illness	Currently
High achiever	87	18
Energetic, always "on the go"	87	18
Competitive	87	8
Perfectionistic	76	21
Assertive	68	26
High self-confidence	63	26
Caretaker of others	84	34
Independent	92	18
Dependent	11	47
Physically fit	63	3
Financially secure	79	32
Have difficulty asking others to meet your needs	53	53
"Yuppie" lifestyle	39	5
Frequent exercise: vigorous	37	5
Frequent exercise: mild	45	21

Note: It is not known whether PWCs in this group are a representative sample of all PWCs, or if they are those most likely to have pursued a diagnosis, seen multiple doctors, joined support groups, and volunteered for studies, thus skewing the results. More passive PWCs may remain undiagnosed, see fewer doctors, and be less likely to become active in organizations and studies.

Kenneth Pelletier views the "Type A" person as competitive, driven, hostile, impatient, accomplishment-oriented, aggressive, extroverted, and internally insecure. The Type A person feels a constant sense of time urgency, often places great emphasis on monetary success, is easily aroused, has a difficult time relaxing, and focuses single-mindedly on present achievements rather than on the overall view of life. The Type B person feels less time urgency, values leisure time and uses it without guilt, is more likely to be committed to meaningful life goals, reacts more slowly, is more self-accepting and less self-critical, and is more thoughtful, relaxed, and contemplative than the Type A counterpart. The Type B lifestyle is thought to be more conducive to health. Recent theories regarding A-B duality have been carefully scrutinized, especially in reference to increased health risk. Many of the original assumptions have not held true, but the high achiever with a stressful lifestyle often ignores bodily needs and is still thought to be at a higher risk for illness.

Some popular yet controversial current theories associate specific personality traits with certain illnesses. Recent literature has examined the question of a "cancer personality," the individual described as nice, accepting, polite, passive, sensitive, and subservient. Those with colon diseases are thought to be rigid, compulsive, and anxious. Those with rheumatoid arthritis are unable to express anger and are self-sacrificing, compliant, depressed, introverted, and tense. Migraine sufferers are viewed as compulsive, perfectionistic, hostile, self-righteous, and rigid. Those prone to coronary disease are egotistical, unable to express resentment, and performance-oriented (Pelletier 1977).

Such theories remain unproved. Whether certain personality traits precede an illness or develop as a result of the illness is also unknown. To associate an illness with a certain personality type is to run the risk of oversimplifying. However, it is highly possible that a busy, active type of person is predisposed to illness because of the high stress level in this type of lifestyle, and that in some people the immune system is inclined to be vulnerable for genetic or other reasons. On the other hand, Sara Reynolds, M.D., comments, "I know of no study of active overachievers with stress to see what proportion *don't* develop CFIDS."

PUTTING IT ALL TOGETHER

The microbe is nothing; the terrain everything.

J. Achterberg, *Imagery in Healing:*
Shamanism and Modern Medicine

We tend to oversimplify the problem, believing that a germ causes an illness, so conquering the germ will allow us to become well again. The illness process is actually a complex interaction between a susceptible host and a triggering agent. The agent alone doesn't cause the illness; it acts as a catalyst in provoking the vulnerabilities of an organism.

The single-cause approach is tantalizingly simple. All we have to do is identify the culprit, kill that rotten germ, and be well again. But as in any war, the problem is not as simple as merely obliterating the immediate enemy. There will always be other enemies. Interaction between such factors as environment, heredity, behavior, infectious agents, immune functioning, central nervous system functioning, coping strategies, self-expectations, and stress are likely determinants of who will get ill and who will not. Other determinants of disease resistance include psychosocial factors such as lifestyle, job, place of residence, cultural background, personality factors, race, sex, and social status.

Causal Hypotheses

Numerous hypotheses have been suggested about the cause of CFIDS. These are not mutually exclusive; many of them fit together nicely. Among them are the following:

- There is a single causal agent of CFIDS, probably a novel virus, that affects only those who are predisposed due to constitutional and environmental factors.

- There is one causal agent of CFIDS, but it is a ubiquitous (common) virus to which only some people are susceptible.

- There are several causal agents of CFIDS, which is actually a spectrum of diseases. The different agents account for the variability among cases.

- Infection with one or more agents triggers disease by affecting various body systems, but the agent itself does not cause any symptoms.

- CFIDS is a "two-hit event"; that is, one must be infected with two viruses, for example HHV-6 plus a retrovirus, to become ill with CFIDS.

- The infectious agent presents a "hit-and-run" situation in which it infects the individual, causing immune dysregulation and symptoms, and then disappears, while its effects continue.

- An agent causes an initial infection, dysregulating the immune system and thus allowing previously dormant viruses (e.g., the herpesviruses) to come out of their latent state and actively reproduce. The reaction of the immune system (e.g., increased cytokines) causes CFIDS symptoms.

• A massive environmental assault (toxins, stressors, etc.) or a defect in the cells' energy production (e.g., mitochondrial defect) allows an already damaged immune system to succumb to an agent it cannot fight off.

• CFIDS may be part of a spectrum of neurological illnesses caused by one or more pathological agents. Manifestation of the disease is related to the location and severity of the brain infection.

A combination of these theories may explain the illness better than any one theory. The infectious agent may disappear, leave the body, hide within the body, or remain active in the body but escape detection. The central nervous system may be the site of infection, with symptoms caused by its dysregulation.

The lack of a unified hypothesis means that research will be divergent, that many possible etiologies must be studied. We need to learn more about identification of viruses and interconnections among body systems and between organism and environment. A multifaceted, multidisciplinary research approach to CFIDS will contribute to our understanding of the pathophysiology of this baffling disorder.

Part II

CFIDS:
What It Does

Chapter 8

Effects of CFIDS on Patients' Lives

Let me tell you that from a purely experiential, sensory
perspective, CFIDS lives in the brain, and in the soul. It cripples
the mind and the spirit as much as it does the body.

Marc Iverson, *The CFIDS Chronicle*

According to a recent poll of [CFIDS] sufferers, 40 percent have been
forced to leave their jobs or schooling. Marriages fall apart. Depression is
a common complication. To these stresses add the unsympathetic skepticism of
much of the medical community. "Massively overdiagnosed," "a vogue disease,
like hypoglycemia," and "wastebasket diagnosis" are just some of the
professional judgments that have found their way into print.

William Boly, "Raggedy Ann Town"

CFIDS seems like the type of incomprehensible thing that
happens to other people. We become ill with a sense of
disbelief and betrayal. And as the illness lingers it becomes more difficult to deny its foothold on our lives.

Just as a senseless death is a tragedy, so is a senseless life. As
many PWCs have noted, AIDS kills you whereas CFIDS kills your
lifestyle, your hopes and ambitions. Periodically you get some of it
back, only to lose it again. The unpredictability of CFIDS presents
a horrible challenge. The most severely affected people lead a day-
to-day existence in which they are capable of taking care of only
their most basic needs. Bedridden, they must depend on others
financially and emotionally. In others the illness is cyclical:
"down" periods are interspersed with more productive days.

Some PWCs describe the devastating effects of CFIDS:

With this illness, you don't have the concrete thing to look
at, like a big lump on your arm. It's invisible. Not only is it

invisible to everybody else, but you begin to think that maybe it really doesn't exist. I've tried to pretend that sometimes. My body had just crumbled. It was out of my control; that's the scary part. The ear thing, then the motion thing, then I couldn't drive anywhere, couldn't study, then I just couldn't function. Am I going to be incapacitated? Do I need a mental hospital? Am I dying? What is going on?

CFS has totally disrupted every aspect of my life!

It's been a two-and-a-half year nightmare experience.

This is a boring illness.

I feel like I've got permanent jet lag.

I used to watch kids in my home, but I kept falling asleep, and that's dangerous. I drank a lot of [caffeine] just to keep myself going through my routine without falling asleep. Sometimes my heart raced, or I got the shakes. I gained weight. I'd lose it, then get tired and gain it again. It seems to be a roller coaster; it never levels out. I can't control it. I'm used to controlling my life. Even when I do the things that I know are good for me, I expect that it will help, but sometimes nothing helps.

Life is passing me by.

I used to look forward to every day. Now I wake up and think "Oh shit, I'm awake." I wake up totally exhausted. I guess I only feel good when I'm sleeping.

My body is a traitor.

"[CFIDS] is capable of destroying the *experience* of life," wrote Hilary Johnson. "For me, [CFIDS] has been the most wrenching, discouraging episode of my life, changing my relationship with the world. ... [It is] a kind of endless mononucleosis with a touch of Alzheimer's disease." In Part II of her *Rolling Stone* article, she described fruitless attempts to maintain a positive attitude, but most often her mood was black and gloomy.

And everybody says, "I'm sick and tired of feeling sick and tired."

Many PWCs awaken feeling as tired as they felt the night before, wondering, "How bad am I going to feel today?" We pay

close attention to the nuances of our physical and emotional functioning, alert for the development of new symptoms, or old symptoms subsiding, or to a particularly "good" or "bad" day, seeking
some sense of how well or poorly we will be able to function.

A good day (or week or hour) is to be treasured, its energy
spent wisely, its pleasures fully savored. We are on leave from being
sick but can be called back at any moment. We must be careful
not to overdo, which will cut our good time short. We are always
alert for overt or subtle signs of a relapse.

On a bad day (or week or hour), time is interminable, life is
bleak, and our goal is just to survive. Basic, routine activities, such
as getting the mail and making minor decisions, turn into major
tasks of enormous complexity. Kyle says, "I feel overloaded, overwhelmed. There are many days when I feel like I can't handle one
more thing. I've made so many major decisions in my life. Now
'What am I going to wear today?' is a major decision."

An excerpt from my journal reads:

> On a good day I feel like I've got this thing licked for good.
> I know it can come back, but I figure I can roll with the
> cycle. On a bad day I think I'll never in my whole life feel
> good again. I feel useless, worthless, drained, fat, and stupid.
> I hate being sick, and I hate myself, and I figure anyone who
> loves me is even crazier than I am.

Fortunately, my relapses are now less frequent and less severe.
In retrospect, I am amazed to have survived these ordeals intact.

It is impossible to prepare for continual readjustment. It is
impossible to plan in advance or to make major commitments.
Every tentative plan is carefully qualified with "maybe." My husband asks me if I would like to go for a walk later, and I have no
way of knowing if I'll be up to it.

Trying to make plans with someone who also has CFIDS is
weird. "Would you like to come over on Saturday night about 8:00
if we're both feeling okay?" And the response: "Sure. I mean,
maybe. I'll let you know on Saturday at 7:55."

When we feel sickest, we don't even care about getting together with friends or doing other things we used to enjoy. Lacking
motivation and goals, we feel lazy and awful. We're too tired to
want to want to do anything. "Deprivation of motivation is the

greatest mental tragedy because it destroys all guidelines," wrote Hans Selye (1974).

What's left? Who cares? How long will I continue to feel this way? Forever? Pain, fear, and uncertainty. And then another breakthrough. Maybe this time it's really over. Maybe I'll just continue to improve from now on. It wasn't *that* bad feeling sick. And so it goes.

Uncertainty and unpredictability become the hallmarks of the new lifestyle, the one we grudgingly adopt. These themes permeate every aspect of our lives: self-image, self-esteem, career, finances, education, relationships, and recreation. Our roles in our families change, our feelings change, our bodies function strangely, doing unpredictable and uncomfortable things. Others don't understand. Friends, family, and doctors are puzzled by our altered behaviors and feelings. Our social roles change. We no longer contribute as we had and instead feel dependent and demanding. We lose a large degree of control over our lives. We have been sabotaged from within. Or from somewhere.

When questioned about the effects of CFIDS on their lives, PWCs in Phoenix, Arizona, responded:

	Positive Effect	Negative Effect
Employment	4%	91%
Relationship with significant other	18	70
Relationships with family	18	55
Relationships with friends	18	66
Financial status	2	74
Lifestyle in general	7	89
Personality in general	2	92

(The remainder reported no change.)

Andy Rooney described having the flu as wanting only one thing: to recover. He noted how difficult it was to do such simple things as turn over and get up to go to the bathroom. "I'd lie in bed wondering how I'd feel if this were a disease I'd never get over." (1985)

That's where we're stuck. This is like a flu that might get better, or better and then worse, or just stay the same. Everything we've ever planned is up for grabs.

ECONOMIC EFFECTS

Chronic illness creates financial dependency on others: spouse, parents, friends and families, and in some cases on private insurance and/or Social Security disability benefits. Because our abilities vary with the severity of the illness, dependency is a matter of degree. PWCs who filled out questionnaires and who discussed their situations with me expressed embarrassment, frustration, and helplessness because of their need to depend on others.

The results of a second questionnaire administered to Phoenix-area PWCs indicated a dramatic change in work status since the onset of CFIDS.

	Pre-Illness	Since Illness
Work full time	76%	11%
Work part time	16	32
Not working	8	58

Another survey of 100 CFIDS patients indicated similar findings:

> ... [A]lthough 92% of the patients had been employed before they were diagnosed, only 65% were employed following onset of the illness. And, while 76% of the patients worked 40 or more hours per week before they became ill, 73% report working fewer than 40 hours after they became ill. (Staver 1989)

A survey published in the Summer 1990 *Mass. CFIDS Update* indicated that 12% of PWCs worked full time, 52% worked part time, and 36% cannot work.

These figures show an especially marked shift in the numbers of people who worked full time prior to the onset of CFIDS and who now work either part time or not at all. The effects of CFIDS on patients' ability to participate productively in the work force have been drastic.

Men who are unable to work suffer the stigma of no longer being the breadwinner, wage earner, achiever—in short, an inability to fulfill the traditional male role. Women who fought the stereotype of the passive nonachieving female by becoming high achievers now find themselves disappointingly dependent on their spouses or families for support. PWCs in their late teens and early twenties, normally a time for establishing independence, find themselves thrust back into the role of dependent children. Giving up the roles and goals that helped to define us and give our lives meaning is difficult. And on a more practical level, the financial crunch ranges from difficult to devastating.

With her career plans interrupted indefinitely, Yolanda decided to apply for a low-stress job she felt she might be able to handle. Frustrated by her inability to continue with her original plans, she reluctantly lowered her sights.

> I'm not doing what I want to do, and I don't know how to accept that. I haven't given up on my career goals; I'm trying to be positive. I don't know whether to push myself or berate myself, to feel guilty because I couldn't cut it . . . . You need to feel successful at something. I always wanted to do something other people saw as worthwhile to validate my self-worth. Out of guilt and self-incrimination, I've applied [for a menial job] for which I was overqualified. They asked why I wanted the job, and I couldn't just say, "I have this virus." It was like, "I'm not the only one who wonders why I'm here." Other people wonder, too. I did a good rendition of "I've got to get on with my life."

Six months later Yolanda was relieved that she hadn't gotten the job because she wasn't sure she could handle its demands. Still, she felt that "If you're not earning a paycheck, you're not worth shit. My husband and even my children feel that way about it. I just feel useless." Her self-esteem had crumbled. Six years later Yolanda is divorced and remains unable to work.

Since so many of us had been strong, responsible people and since we still usually appear healthy, others' expectations of us remain constant. Our ability to achieve is severely impaired, however, and others are continually disappointed in our failure to function as we had previously.

Betty describes her difficult situation:

> The head of the agency for which I worked really disappointed me. He kept saying, "You need to rest and take care of yourself because we need you. You've always produced for us." I thought, "You son of a gun," but I just said, "I can't

right now. I can't concentrate. I can't absorb what I read."
[He demanded] a lot of me, researching and drafting important information. He said, "It's just a virus, so just work for a
couple of hours and go home and rest and you'll do all right.
You come back in the morning, and the work will just come
pouring out. Don't do anything at home. Rest at home; don't
cook, don't do the laundry." He was making more and more
demands. One of my close friends said, "Tell him to go fuck
himself. Why are you letting him do this?" I said, "I can't let
him down. I can't let my family down. I can't let anybody
down."

But she was letting all of them down, and by disappointing
others she was also letting herself down. Quitting her job and
learning to relax was a difficult but eye-opening experience for
Betty, who found that her department did continue to function in
her absence. She learned to take it easy and to enjoy her life more
fully. Six months later, Betty reported a considerable degree of
recovery, but she wasn't nearly ready to return to work. The good
news: she no longer felt responsible or guilty for her inability to
work.

Kyle describes a different predicament: previously an energetic worker, and now with limited energy and poor health, she
was about to separate from her husband.

Now I'm getting ready to live on my own, and I don't think
I can do that because of the disease. I'm just not strong
enough to make it on my own because I just can't think the
way I used to or do the things I used to do. What if I have a
relapse and can't work? What am I going to do?

Other PWCs commented:

I was at the height of my career when this thing struck. [This
statement has been made by countless PWCs.]

I'm the kind of guy who never falls apart. I'm always fair and
honest and was always a good problem solver and a hard
worker. I can't do that now; I can't do the kind of job I can
feel good about, so I don't work at all. It's a big hurdle for a
Type A, workaholic, hard-driving, very successful, polyphasic
thinker who loves what he does to change the rules. These

are abrupt changes, and you can't make them . . . very easily. Nothing like this has ever happened to me before.

My worst fear is being dependent.

My security got taken away.

I'm terrified that it will never go away and I will lie in bed the rest of my life with only the TV, magazines, and pets. There is no joy or fun in my life; I'm a burden. I can't participate in work or community activities. I can't get out of bed.

I no longer feel productive. What's left?

My life has become centered only in work because that's all I have energy to do.

I will have to retire earlier than I had planned.

These people have expressed some of the common reactions among those of us who can no longer function as we used to and whose careers, educational plans, and incomes have been drastically affected by CFIDS.

Whether to continue with work and/or school, and to what degree, becomes a matter of individual judgment. It makes sense to continue meaningful activities to the extent possible but not to the point at which chances of recovery are jeopardized. To continue what you are doing to whatever degree is comfortable for you at a given time requires difficult evaluations, flexibility, common sense, and guesswork. It means being honest with yourself about what is feasible, shedding unrealistically heroic self-expectations. Inability to work usually causes loss of benefits coupled with soaring medical expenses. Even when a PWC has health insurance, many treatments are not covered. Some policies contain a catch-22 clause stating that only standard, Food and Drug Administration (FDA)-approved treatment for an illness is covered, and there is no standard FDA-approved treatment for CFIDS at this time. Many PWCs have exhausted their incomes and savings accounts seeking effective treatment.

Self-esteem plummets along with income, and the loss of one's identity as a productive worker is significant. One option for those who can no longer work is to apply for disability benefits.

However, the application process is long and frustrating, and reliance upon insurance companies and the government for support is difficult to accept for those who are career-oriented.

Social Security Disability Income (SSDI) benefits have been difficult to obtain for many PWCs who are often denied benefits in the first two stages, which are handled at the state level. If benefits are denied in stage two, the next step in requesting reconsideration is a hearing before a Social Security Administration administrative law judge. It is imperative at this stage that the PWC is represented by an attorney who specializes in SSDI work and is CFIDS-educated. The process is long, arduous, and frustrating. Ultimately, many PWCs are able to obtain benefits but there is a long time lapse between the initial application and the final decision.

Similar problems may be encountered with private disability insurance claims. Become familiar with your policy; in many cases benefits for a "psychological" disability are of shorter duration (often only two years) than benefits for a "physiological" illness. Therefore, be certain that the disabling condition is considered CFIDS or CFS rather than depression.

CFIDS can devastate one's lifestyle, bank balance, career, and educational plans. Illness can force us to incur large debts (because of decreased income and increased medical expenses) or to move to less expensive housing or "back home." Most PWCs have experienced a decrease in their standard of living, and many find their financial futures disturbingly uncertain.

EFFECTS OF CFIDS ON SELF-IMAGE

Self-image is the way we view ourselves. Self-esteem is how we feel about ourselves, our sense of personal value and worth. CFIDS affects both dramatically. "Before I got sick," says Lorna . . .

I was vivacious, outgoing, always "up." I was the achiever, the giver, the caretaker. I was a successful salesperson. I felt I could do anything I wanted to do. Now I have mood fluctuations, I become depressed, and even have thoughts of committing suicide. I'm vulnerable; I've lost my identity and my self-esteem. I can't work, and I can't even be a good mother to my two-year-old son. I feel guilty because I have nothing to give to others. We're having financial problems because I can no longer work. I can't concentrate, I have blackouts, I lose my train of thought. I'm weak and numb much of the time.

Suddenly everything is different; we are unaccustomed to the new, unwelcome feelings and perceptions. We must redefine ourselves and our lives. I wrote in my journal about my lost sense of self. I felt like a victim of bizarre internal circumstances beyond my control, having become in essence a stranger to myself.

Paula says:

My self-esteem went right down because I couldn't do things. It wasn't that I didn't want to. I did want to, but I couldn't. I'd never been helpless in my life; I've always been fiercely independent, radically so. I never needed any help. So when I started having to ask, I didn't ask. I kept struggling to try to do it all and got angry at the people around me. And their expectations of me, because this is what I'd trained them to expect: that I could do it . . . better than anyone. All of a sudden, I couldn't. This was my whole lifestyle, my mindset, my whole core of who I am . . . and now I'm not who I was. I can't do it.

Are we victims? We feel a loss of control regarding our plans for the present and the future. Helplessness feels alien, uncomfortable, and dangerous. Martin Seligman (1975) has written about the loss of control that accompanies certain life events, pointing out the correlations between helplessness and depression. When we lack control and predictability in our lives, we begin to feel hopeless, helpless, and weak.

The onset and continuation of CFIDS provokes such feelings, which exert a negative influence on the illness process, compounding the problems and crushing our self-perceptions, self-expectations, and hopes. In the words of PWCs:

I am so much less myself.

I want to be productive. I used to think I could be perfect if I tried hard enough.

I was this superperson. Under stress, I just pushed harder. It worked for all those years.

I feel so stupid now. My brain doesn't work. I can't even do simple things, like type.

I was taught to be strong. Now I don't have the strength to get up off the floor. I feel I have failed my family, my co-workers, myself.

The uncertainty is awful. Will I be an invalid for the rest of my life? [Feeling like an invalid means feeling "invalid."]

My sense of humor . . . I don't think I've lost it, but I have to fake it; life has become a lot more serious. I'm overly sensitive now. I can't joke because my brain can't come up with anything smart.

The worst thing that could happen has happened. My mind's functioning has been impaired. I can handle pain or other kinds of physical discomfort. This affects me, myself; it's the hardest thing to handle. The uncertainty of not knowing if I'm going to be me again.

I used to be successful, aggressive, fast-moving, and I thrived on it. My profession was lucrative. But I can't function like that any more. I can hardly function at all, period. I do the best I can, but I'm not the same guy I used to be.

I don't know what I'm capable of doing. I wish someone could tell me what to do and what not to do. Then I wouldn't feel guilty about all the things I'm not doing.

My psychiatrist told me I may never be well enough to [resume former activities]. I have trouble with "never" and "may never," with not knowing.

I was trained to be "fine." You're supposed to always be fine.

We define ourselves largely in terms of what we do. Indeed, this is usually the first question new acquaintances will ask each other. In college it was "What's your major?" Later in life it is "What do you do?" How do we answer that question when we can no longer function in accustomed roles? Options: *I sleep. I stay in bed a lot. I do what I can. I work part time. I collect disability payments. I complain a lot.* These are all true, but embarrassing. Who am I without my former roles? We have become human doings rather than human beings, as John Bradshaw explained in his PBS lecture series, and without something specific to *do*, we are unsure who to *be*.

Everything we knew about ourselves before is now uncertain. We apply new labels to ourselves, many of them hurtful and self-deprecating. *Am I a hypochondriac?* (I'm certainly obsessed with my body and its functioning.) *Am I a dependent person?* (I am needier than I've ever been.) *Am I a sickie?* (This illness dominates my life to an uncomfortably great degree.) *Am I a patient?* (I hate that passive-sounding word, and I'm not at all patient about this illness.) *Am I a pessimist? Or a realist?* (It's hard to be hopeful sometimes, especially when symptoms hit unpredictably.) *Am I a survivor?* (Or does that mean I'm pushing too hard and risking self-harm?) *Am I a martyr?* (That's how I feel when I perform resentfully, out of a sense of duty, even though I'm too drained to function well.) *Am I a grouch?* (I get angry over nothing, and I'm very angry about being ill.)

Like the labels, our self-messages are often negative and irrational, reflecting changes in self-image and self-esteem. Examples of damaging, irrational self-messages are:

I can't do anything any more.

I'll always be this way; I'll never get better.

I brought this on myself. It's my fault that I'm sick.

If I could think positively, I could banish this illness.

I should fake it, play the "I'm fine" game. I'm acceptable to myself and others only when I'm well.

I need to be taken care of, and that's a sign of weakness.

I shouldn't complain.

I used to be superwoman, superemployee, superfriend, superparent. Now I'm superwimp.

I shouldn't be so down, so depressed.

I should be able to change this, make it go away.

I'm supposed to be strong, capable of anything, able to handle the responsibilities of the world.

I'm too sensitive. I shouldn't feel or react as I do.

I used to think I was smart, but now I know I'm stupid.

My life is over.

Such distorted, unrealistic, perfectionistic self-statements compound the already numerous problems of chronic illness. Kyle summarizes her situation well:

I'm not the same person. I can't think and speak like I could before. I can't make the decisions I used to make. I'm different than other people, and people don't understand what's going on with me. I want to say, "Hey, I'm not really stupid. I have this virus." I want to wear it on a badge: *Please don't think I'm an idiot.*

I had a real full life, and I don't any more. My brain isn't the same anymore. Things are fragmented, and sometimes I even have trouble talking, putting sentences together. I'll be in the middle of the most profound thing in the world, and I'll forget what I was saying.

I feel really ripped off. I can't lead a normal life. I don't have a whole lot of energy. I don't have a normal social life. I have to go to bed at nine o'clock. I live a pretty one-dimensional life where I go to work and come home and spend the evening in my recliner . . . .

I feel like my brain will never be the same and I'll never be the same person I was before, even if I recover.

Each of us has already coped with tremendous stress, misfortune, and pain. We've been to hell and back, and back and forth again, and we've made it through. We are survivors, and we deserve full credit for our endurance.

FEELINGS

Feelings are pure emotion, irrational by definition. We can't talk ourselves out of them, but we need to define and understand them and their effects. It's also helpful to know how others in similar circumstances feel, so we don't feel so alone and crazy.

The gamut of CFIDS-triggered emotions include feeling:

• **Guilty.** Did I cause my illness? Did I choose to become ill? Is this "mind over matter"? Am I being punished for a wrongdoing? Am I somehow keeping myself from getting well? Is there something else I should be doing, or something I'm not doing right? I can't work any longer, or I don't work as productively as I should. I'm spending too much money on treatments that might not even work. I shouldn't have so many special needs. I'm letting everyone down, disappointing them—family, friends, employer, and myself. Maybe those who think I'm not really sick are right after all, and I'm just copping out. I don't have fewer responsibilities when I'm sick, just extra guilt for not carrying them out.

• **Misunderstood.** No one else really understands what I'm going through, except (maybe) the others who have it, too. Those close to me may try to understand, and think they understand, but they really can't. If I didn't have CFIDS, I wouldn't be able to understand what it's like, either, I suppose. I feel isolated and rejected.

• **Overloaded.** Even simple tasks overwhelm me. I can't make decisions. I can't sort things out. I can't trust myself to judge the degree of a problem or to know how to react in proportion to its significance. Molehills become mountains, and I don't always know when I'm distorting.

• **Depressed.** Sometimes things are so bleak, disappointing, and pointless. I feel incapable and unlovable. Sometimes I cry over nothing; other times I need to cry but can't. There's nothing I value or enjoy. Life is just one empty moment after another, interminably. Everything takes too much effort; nothing is worth doing. I'm not spontaneous or creative or fun-loving or silly any more. I'm a blob.

• **Desperate.** There's no hope. I've tried various remedies and interventions, even weird stuff, and nothing has worked well enough. Maybe nothing ever will. If only I knew what to do, I'd do it—whatever it was.

• **Suicidal.** Why don't I just die now? There's nothing left; my life is the pits. If I can't lead a useful life, I might as well not exist. I'd rather die than continue to exist like this. I need to get well or die.

Marc Iverson, president of The CFIDS Association of Charlotte, North Carolina, says:

I have never known a person with full-blown CFIDS who has not considered suicide at some point in his or her illness. I have known a number of individuals with this disease who have chosen death . . . . CFIDS steals so much of their lives that life is simply not worth living. (November 1990)

• **Isolated.** Sometimes I don't want to be alone, but I don't want to be with anyone either. Others can't possibly understand my feelings; I have no way of explaining them. Come closer; go away. Accompanied or alone, I live in a private hell. There's an invisible wall between me and the rest of the world.

• **Crazy.** Is this real? Have I lost my mind? CFIDS is a hall of mirrors from hell, distorted and freaky. I was level-headed and able to cope, but I've gone off the deep end. I don't even know who I am. Awake and asleep, my thoughts are distorted. I don't understand my thoughts, my feelings, or myself. I'm not normal now, not myself anymore.

• **Sad.** I've lost so much. This is so difficult. I've been taught to look on the bright side, but right now there isn't one. Everything hurts—my body, but also my heart, my spirit.

• **Stunned.** I can't believe this is happening to me. I cannot accept this illness.

• **Deprived.** There are so many things I can't do and things I shouldn't do or eat or drink. What's left? I want a normal life back. My life has been pulled out from under me; so much has been torn away.

• **Uncertain.** Will this ever be over? Will I ever feel good again? When? How will I feel tomorrow? How will I feel in an hour? Why did this happen? Do I dare make any plans? Do I dare to have hopes and dreams?

• **Confused.** I don't understand what's happening to me. I can't make sense out of this predicament. I can't trust myself to think or react rationally and logically.

• **Helpless.** I feel like an out-of-control victim, an unacceptable role for me. I'm so vulnerable physically and emotionally. My whole life is now unpredictable. I'm being held hostage by something mysterious and elusive. You can't *see* an immune system or a brain to know what's going wrong. There's not a damned thing I can do about it, either. I'm trapped inside a body that doesn't work right and won't cooperate. I don't have any faith in my abilities, my competence. I don't have the resources to fix this or even to adapt. The rules keep changing and all I can do is react.

• **Dependent.** I'm useless, worthless. I am forced to rely upon others to do the things I should be able to do and used to do. It's hard to feel good about me or to view myself as capable when I'm so dependent on others. I used to be in the driver's seat; now I'm just a passenger. I used to be a giver; now I'm a taker. It's not okay to be so needy.

• **Self-absorbed.** I get so wrapped up in how I'm feeling that I lose awareness of how others feel or what they need. Or if I am aware, sometimes I don't even have the energy to care. That's not like me. All I think about is this illness and what it's doing to me. My entire focus is inward; I'm preoccupied with my symptoms, worrying and wondering what they mean and what lies ahead for me.

• **Debilitated.** I have no energy. I feel used up. The vital part of me is gone.

• **Angry.** Why do bad things happen to good people? Why me? I hate this; it's unfair. I've tried so hard, and I've done so well; why am I being punished? This illness doesn't follow the rules. I *hate* CFIDS.

• **Weak.** I can't take care of myself or my own life. I'm a wimp now. My body is weak; my mind doesn't work right. I'm inadequate, wimpy.

• **Afraid.** What will happen to me? Will I become sicker? Will I develop new, worse symptoms? Lose even more control? Will I get cancer? Die? My head is filled with frightening possibilities, and no one has answers; nobody can assure me the worst won't happen. I'm afraid I'll never get well. I'm afraid of what I can't identify and don't understand.

• **Numb.** I feel dull, flat. This may be a temporary escape from emotional pain, but I can't feel pleasure either. I feel nothing.

• **Resigned.** It will always be like this. It's endless. They'll never find a cure, or even a remedy. It's hopeless; I might as well get used to it. My life as I knew it is over.

• **Hopeful.** Maybe there will be a breakthrough. Some people recover; maybe I'll be one of them. I just have to get better; I have to believe I will. Someday I'll look back on all of this . . .

• **Relieved.** It is possible to feel good, even if only for brief periods of time. I haven't forgotten how. There's hope.

The feelings vacillate unpredictably and uncomfortably, often triggered by a symptom exacerbation and remission. All these feelings are natural reactions to an unpredictable, chronic illness. We must learn to recognize and express these feelings despite their seeming irrationality. There are no shortcuts, and feelings don't go away if they're ignored; they go underground. Unexpressed emotions fester and will ultimately spill out inappropriately, maybe damaging relationships. Repressed feelings may also worsen our condition by further compromising the immune system.

EFFECTS OF CFIDS ON RELATIONSHIPS

Today, who needs a physician
When every friend is a diagnostician?

Ogden Nash, "We're Fine, Just Fine"

With the onset of CFIDS, others in our lives are puzzled but often sympathetic. As time goes on, they may begin to doubt the existence of an invisible malady, wondering if the illness is real. The PWC may feel betrayed while experiencing self-doubt as well, compounding an already painful situation.

Once we obtain a diagnosis of "chronic fatigue syndrome" it's hard to get others to take it seriously. It sounds too much like "chronic complainer's syndrome." We finally get a name for it, but by then everyone's run out of patience, and the name itself doesn't add much credibility. Calling it CFIDS may help the credibility factor somewhat.

There are two aspects of chronic illness: the obvious, physiological, tangible signs, and the hidden difficulties. The obvious signs identify one as sick and are usually taken seriously. The hidden ones are made evident to others only by verbal reports. If there is a discrepancy between the two (no obvious symptoms but reports of feeling awful), others become confused and have a hard time grasping the true nature and severity of the illness. Our society looks for evidence; seeing is believing. If you can't see it, it's not there. The assumption is that the severity of one's illness is directly proportional to its degree of visibility.

During the years that I have had CFIDS I've looked okay most of the time. Those closest to me have learned to read my signals of impending fatigue, often before I'm aware of them. They notice paleness, a general slowing down, and/or increased sensitivity to sensory input. However, to the casual observer I appear fine. I even feel strange telling others how lousy I feel, so I don't unless there's a good reason. I know it's hard for them to understand what they cannot see and have not experienced. The most distressing aspects of CFIDS are invisible. With no bandages, casts, spots, bruises, or other obvious signs of illness, I am presumed well.

Since we may look fine while feeling horrible, others' expectations of us remain about the same. And often others may harbor erroneous assumptions about CFIDS:

• **If it's not terminal, it's no big deal.** Others sometimes think we should just get on with our lives as before and stop paying attention to symptoms, stop worrying, and stop pampering ourselves (i.e., resting so much). Yolanda says, "When I first got sick, everyone was concerned, but now it's last year's news. People feel like if it's not fatal, it should be gone by now." They run out of patience, just as we do.

• **It's a woman's disease.** Although a greater proportion of PWCs are female, women have not cornered the market on this disease. To call it "a woman's disease" is not only to misrepresent the patient population but also to infer that the illness is a gender-linked affliction of an hysterical, hormone-driven population.

• **It's an emotional disorder.** The theory that this illness is merely depression with a dash of anxiety is unfair and pejorative. It ignores a whole host of CFIDS symptoms that have never been linked to depression. Such comments as "You're probably over-stressed," "You're just depressed and/or anxious," "You're just not handling stress very well," or "It's an attitude problem" add insult to illness.

- **It's related to AIDS.** There is no known connection between CFIDS and HIV. Some patients report that others are afraid to be near them for fear of catching the illness. The stigma can result in needless fear and isolation. The unfortunate phobic response of many people to AIDS is thus transferred to CFIDS.

- **It must be curable.** There must be something you can do to function normally. You get sick, you take medicine, you get better, right? Doing the right thing should restore health. You obviously lack the proper resources—willpower, determination, the right diet, medicine, or exercise program.

- **If you complain, you're being negative.** But if you don't complain, you must be feeling okay. This is a double bind for the PWC, who must decide whether to fake it, ignore it, or describe the feelings and symptoms honestly. We're almost always aware of our symptoms and the reactions of others. We want our "invisible" illness to be acknowledged but sometimes it's simpler to play the game of ignoring it, which seems the acceptable thing to do. But when we put on an "I'm fine" act, others are fooled into believing that we are.

Our attempts to disguise or minimize our illness may backfire. Well-intentioned others often make insensitive comments such as:

You're sick? You look fine to me!

Maybe this illness is all in your imagination.

Do you *still* have that illness?

I've heard that CFIDS doesn't really exist.

There must be *something* you haven't tried that would cure you.

You're lucky to rest and sleep all the time and stay home from work.

Cheer up. Things could be worse.

Your symptoms are the same ones everyone has.

Maybe you just need more exercise or vitamins.

You just don't *want* to do stuff any more.

I think you just enjoy being sick—especially all the attention you get.

I know just how you feel.

Here's the one no one says, but it comes through loud and clear: *You're not allowed to be sick.*

People react in a variety of ways to chronic illness, depending upon their own psychological makeup and issues, their perceptions of illness, and their belief systems. Our society encourages denial of all things unpleasant, especially those we fear or cannot readily understand. A lingering and debilitating yet invisible illness can be a trigger for the need to avoid and establish distance. Our pain and helplessness—and the fact that it could happen to them—makes others back away, and we attribute such behavior to lack of caring. Others' reactions have more to do with them than with us, but it's difficult to see this when we're vulnerable.

Effects of CFIDS on Relationships with Spouses/Partners

"In sickness and in health" takes on a whole new meaning. We repeat that phrase automatically when we marry but have little insight into its implications. Initially, a shared tragedy may bring partners closer together, but as time goes on and the problem endures, the marriage may not. The divorce rate for couples in which one partner has a chronic illness is estimated at 75% (Pitzele 1986).

The PWC is needy, requiring attention, costly medical services, and financial and emotional support. The PWC is demanding, but not purposely so, usually feeling guilty for being burdensome, for not contributing as in the past, and for having so many needs. If the PWC had once been the primary care giver in a relationship and can no longer fulfill this role, a significant adjustment must take place for the relationship to survive.

Caregivers have special needs, too, which may remain dangerously unexpressed because, after all, they are well and may feel guilty about having needs. Thus, the needs of the healthy partner may be overlooked. Maggie Strong writes in *Mainstay* about the greater burden on the well partner, who must assume an increased workload while the ill partner occupies center stage with his or her additional needs (1988).

The major financial burden often falls upon the well partner. Sacrifices become necessary. Life with a sick person becomes monotonous and boring. Plans must be canceled, dreams and ambitions put on hold. Many major decisions are dictated by CFIDS, but the caregiver is expected to remain understanding and patient. One partner said, "It's awful being around a person who's always depressed and lethargic. She doesn't accomplish anything; she feels lousy all the time," adding that he really wanted to be understanding but just couldn't understand what she was experiencing or why she was so needy and so unlike her "past self."

Several spouses of PWCs complain about the dual financial burdens of decreased income compounded by high medical bills. While indicating a desire to help, they also distrust many health practitioners and costly treatment programs. The burden of providing financially means spending money on what some refer to as "quack remedies" that are expensive and of questionable value. The unspoken attitude seems to be, "With me spending all this money, the least she or he could do is get well," an understandable but unreasonable position. While some feel ripped off, others are determined to pursue treatment regardless of cost. All seem to be fed up with the illness that has destroyed their family's financial stability and, in some cases, their self-image as good providers.

Problems that existed in relationships prior to the onset of CFIDS will be compounded by it. Changes occur in role expectations—the part each spouse is expected to play—and couples do not make this transition easily. Too often the issues aren't even discussed. To push on grimly and silently is considered the heroic course, yet the unexpressed but mounting feelings of pressure and resentment damage the relationship.

Although stereotypical male and female roles are currently undergoing change, men have typically been regarded as the primary wage earners and women as the emotional caretakers in the family. When the husband is ill, the wife continues her caretaker role and may need to become the sole breadwinner as well. When the wife becomes ill, the husband is forced into a new role of emotional caretaker as well as financial provider. The financially and emotionally dependent spouse is prone to substantial guilt feelings.

If the ill spouse is a hard-driving female "achiever," illness may thrust her back into a dependent relationship with which she is uncomfortable. Having developed educational and career goals, and having obtained satisfaction, competence, self-esteem, and independence, she is once again thrust into a role from which she has been trying to escape: the dependent wife.

Many PWCs have been problem solvers, fixers, doers, and caretakers, often taking responsibility for finding solutions to others' problems. This codependency creates a bind when their own CFIDS-generated problems are not readily "fixable."

A partner who is a "fixer" may offer suggestions and advice. If the ill spouse does not follow the advice, the "fixer" may become angry at this lack of cooperation. If the ill spouse complies but the remedy is unsuccessful, the "fixer" may feel the need to blame either the ill spouse or himself or herself for this failure. Rather than letting this dysfunctional blaming situation develop, it is far wiser to examine one's self-expectations about problem solving. Some problems are just not easily fixed, even when motivation to pursue solutions is strong. Often, the fixer is unaware that what the partner needs is support and understanding rather than well-intended but often ineffectual advice.

Illness (or any other continuing problem) can become the primary focus of a relationship. Like work, the role of illness expands to fit the time (and attention) available. A great deal of a couple's attention can be focused on CFIDS but a functional relationship requires that priorities be balanced.

When asked about the frequency of sexual activity prior to and after the onset of CFIDS, 79% of the respondents in a Phoenix survey indicated that sexual activity was less frequent, and only 18% said sexual frequency was about the same. (One person indicated that sex was more frequent, and she wrote an explanation in the margin: "Just married!") Many PWCs report that their sex drive has diminished substantially; others indicate that they just don't have the energy to have sex. A few reported that they enjoyed sex because it provided a brief "escape" from illness, a time when they could forget, but others said that sexual exertion caused a mild relapse over the next few days, so they were forced to weigh desire against consequences. What a shame to waste all that time spent in bed!

There's also the "come close, go away" syndrome, in which the PWC needs to be touched and comforted and simultaneously wants to crawl into a black hole of isolation. This sends out a confusing double message that may cause the partner to feel rejected.

Many PWCs are afraid. What if my illness and I are successful at pushing my partner away? What if my mate becomes fed up with the "sickie" I've become and leaves me? Yolanda feared her husband would leave her, and that she would be both emotionally bereft and financially destitute, since she could no longer work.

> A few weeks ago, it blew up, and he said he just couldn't handle being around a sick person. I've tried very hard not to act like a sick person; I don't stay in bed; I try to do the household work. But I have so much guilt and feelings of worthlessness because I've been so goal-oriented all my life, and now I'm so insecure. He usually blows up periodically and then it will pass over, but I'm afraid one of these times, he'll just leave.

They have since divorced.

In some cases spouses ultimately learn how to understand and handle the stressors presented by illness and grow closer. But in the face of pre-existing relationship problems compounded by the effects of a chronic illness, many relationships do not survive when the need to distance increases and understanding runs thin.

At times the need to communicate is strong, but the words won't come. This is in part the result of an inability to express these new feelings, compounded by CFIDS-related cognitive difficulties: impaired concentration, memory, and word-finding abilities. "I know what I want to say to [my partner]," says Kyle, "but I get confused and screw it up, and it starts a fight." She has trouble getting to the point because she loses it. The words become jumbled. The message becomes distorted or is incomplete, and both parties end up frustrated.

The PWC who had been an active and contributing partner is now depleted, robbing the healthy spouse of a challenging companion. Communication becomes strained and difficult as cognitive dysfunction increases. The well partner may retreat from the PWC, whose conversation has begun to focus on symptoms, losses, and other trials of CFIDS. The result is loss and loneliness for both partners.

But many are weathering the storm well. Many PWCs have expressed appreciation for having understanding, supportive partners. Many partners express considerable caring, as well as the pain of being unable to make it okay for their loved ones. PWCs often refer to their partners as the strongest sources of support available, willing to listen, empathize, and problem-solve. Many caregivers read CFIDS literature and attend support group meetings with their ill partners. This willingness to learn, understand, and participate facilitates a couple's adjustment to CFIDS.

My husband has been my primary source of support. He tolerates my mood swings: often I snap at him about the dumbest things and later he will say, "I guess that was CFIDS talking." His understanding and tolerance make me feel valued and cherished, but also guilty. Would I be able to do the same for him? CFIDS has spoiled so many of our plans. In some ways he's been cheated as much as I have. But he sticks around, and we have endured it together. His caring overwhelms me at times. During exacerbations, accompanied by one of those life-shattering depressions, I don't understand how anyone could love me—but somehow he does. We have good moments to share, in fact more and more frequently, and I am so grateful for the good times, for being able to participate together and enjoy positive changes and events.

"My wife has been great," says Bill. "I'd like to think I'd be as good to her as she has been to me, but I don't know. What I've put her through is a very good test of [whether] she loves me."

But the illness remains a lurking enemy in our households, producing tension and disruption. Even with the knowledge that the problem is the illness rather than a lack of love between partners, old problems escalate and new ones develop. It's tough to hang together and work as a partnership with CFIDS in the way.

Effects of CFIDS on Families

Some of the changes produced by chronic illness are: PWC's inability to shoulder former responsibilities; changes in financial circumstances; a shift in family priorities; new needs; and the feelings of confusion, anger, and resentment that develop. The PWC may feel guilty for causing problems and being a burden. Healthy family members may feel guilty because they were spared and resentful that the patient was not. In addition, the family accompanies the patient on the exacerbation-remission roller coaster and family life becomes more unpredictable. The PWC's anger may become disruptive since we often vent anger inappropriately at those we love and spend the most time with. Even when we understand what's happening and why, we must deal with changes. Family members often feel guilty about expressing their own feelings and needs, trying to protect the sick person from feeling responsible for the changes and difficulties.

The family undergoes a difficult period of adjustment as it attempts to restore homeostasis, a sense of balance. This process is different for everyone, but it follows closely the pattern experienced in grieving. The family's ability to cope depends on its resources and pre-illness level of functioning. Adjustment requires flexibility, tolerance of change, and ability to acknowledge and communicate about what is happening. Family members are called upon to accommodate new needs and limitations of the PWC and to accept new responsibilities and roles. Together and individually they experience pain and disappointment. They must learn to do what is helpful for the ill family member without going to either extreme: denying the problem or becoming overprotective.

Family disruptions may impact the patient by causing an exacerbation of symptoms, which further stresses the family. "They were used to me always being in charge of everything," says Betty. "I went from supermom to superwimp." The transition is hard on everyone in the family.

My children experienced difficulty with several aspects of my illness: my tendency to overreact or to react unpredictably, limitations on activities and travel plans, and changes in financial circumstances. Not only was I financially unable to provide for myself and my children as before, but a messy battle with my ex-husband for increased child support ensued and the kids and my current spouse got caught up in the turmoil.

One patient's small son said, "When are we going to get Mommy back?" Their mother used to take the kids to the park daily despite a hectic work schedule; she laughed and played with them a lot. Now she cries often, and her husband has assumed many of her former responsibilities. She says her whole family feels robbed.

Bill found himself overreacting to the behavior of his three young children because of CFIDS-related mood swings:

> I haven't been a good dad; I haven't been able to discipline my kids appropriately. I haven't been able to spend the time I normally would have spent with the kids, and that's killing me. It's one of the saddest things I've ever experienced; it's the hardest thing I've ever handled . . . . Before I was sick I was able to get out with my oldest and do some things I haven't been able to do with the others. They're always energetic, jumping around; they always want to be doing stuff. I can't do it. I do push myself; I go out with them even if I feel crummy. I want them to have a good experience. I don't know how my wife can handle all this; she has a real even temper.

Feelings of denial, guilt, anger, jealousy, and depression are normal reactions of children to a parent's illness. Open discussion is helpful in allowing children to express these feelings and have them validated. Professional intervention may be required if their reactions are prolonged or particularly severe or if other danger signals are present, including rebelliousness, problems with school-work, substance abuse, and signs of depression.

We may resent the needs of our children at times, but it's a displaced resentment. What we really resent is our illness preventing us from parenting as we'd like to. We worry that our children will be deprived of what they deserve and would have had if we weren't ill. Will they look back on their childhoods and feel resentment? Probably—but all children feel resentful and must learn that many of their expectations will not be met. We can easily become overly concerned with pleasing our children. Unfortunately, they're subject to the same disappointments as the rest of us. We can't shield them, nor should we. They, too, must learn to cope.

Relationships with our extended families are likely to change. As we become adults, we perceive our parents as peers (with some parental undertones). When CFIDS intervenes, the roles change. Parents fall into their former parental roles again with the con-comitant worry, need to give advice, and feelings of responsibility. They still want to make it all better and may try to deny the illness because of their own feelings of helplessness.

A curious role reversal takes place. Parents, even retired ones, may be leading active lives despite the inevitable aches and pains that accompany advancing age, while their children with CFIDS experience memory loss, arthritic-type pain, a sedentary lifestyle, and other symptoms and deficits that, in the scheme of things, are supposed to happen to older people. The process reverses itself; I *feel* older than my parents *are*. I have many of the same problems with my illness that they have with advancing age. PWCs may feel ashamed to rely on our parents again: "Here I am again, needing more parenting—emotionally and financially." Illness interrupts the natural life cycle by making us feel like dependent middle-aged children.

As Paula's mother has gotten older, she has increasingly relied on Paula for emotional support. Paula's role has been that of the giver, the caretaker, the listener—and now she has CFIDS.

> It's been hard for me to say "I need." I've never said that. I'm still in a supportive role with my mother and grandmother. My mother is just beginning to understand that I can no longer do many things. I always tried to live up to her expectations, but now she has to understand that there's something going on that I have no control over. Prior to that, her attitude was, "I know you're sick, but you're still functioning," along with her usual expectations. Now it's "Are you up to it? Do you feel like you can make it?"—not a demand, but a request. In this way, my relationships with people have gotten better.

In all family relationships, illness presents a challenge. It shakes up the status quo and demands change. Families who are able to work together, drawing on collective resources to meet the new challenges, become stronger as a result.

Effects of CFIDS on Friendships

CFIDS makes us different from our friends and alters our former roles in friendships. We need to confide in our friends, but try to strike a delicate balance between our needs and theirs. We need their support and understanding, although at times we pull back from them because of relapses and isolative tendencies. We need friends to be flexible and not take some of the things we do personally. We become needier, less able to participate in social events, and more preoccupied with how we are feeling. Sometimes we are reluctant to reach out to others. Friendships become pressured and strained. Like other relationships, friendships may be strengthened in the process or may be lost, unable to withstand the changes.

Here is what some PWCs have said about friendships:

My friends have been real supportive of me. They take good care of me and yell at me to rest and take care of myself. Most of my friends are in the health care field; they are used to health issues being a part of their lives.

I have found out who my real friends are. There are those who understand and those who want me to push too hard.

My personal life has gone down the tubes, so to speak. I was dating and now feel unable to do that. I find that people are so afraid of catching something from me. I am upset most of the time.

I lost most of my friends and feel devastated.

Most of us experience a combination of reactions from others. Special efforts at communication are required, presenting a problem when our energy is limited. Friendship becomes a balancing act between their needs and ours, which have grown to astounding proportions. The test of a friendship is its degree of flexibility—how well it can withstand change and allow for communication about what both parties are experiencing. Can our friends accept our limitations without judgment? Do they accept that we are ill despite the absence of obvious signs? Will they accept us even when we are at our worst? Will our friends love us even though it is difficult for us to love ourselves?

Friends may disappear, stick with us unconditionally, or withstand only the early stages of the illness, distancing themselves as CFIDS lingers. Each friendship is different, but one constant remains: it is essential to talk with each of our friends not only about CFIDS but about the effects it is having on the friendship. Doing this will not assure longevity of the relationship but it's our best shot. Readjustment and rebalancing are necessary over time if the friendship is to survive.

Chapter 9

CFIDS in Children

The incidence of CFIDS in children has been greatly underestimated. CFIDS may be especially difficult for children because they have not yet fully developed their capabilities or identities and thus do not have a sense of what is "normal" for them. Children with a gradual onset of CFIDS often do not recognize the illness as an external event since they are still in their formative years. They may not even be aware that they are ill because they have never experienced a time when they were not having symptoms. They have incorporated illness into their concept of normalcy. Symptoms are also more difficult to assess in children.

David Bell, M.D., an expert on CFIDS in children, states that the illness is rare in children under the age of five. Onset of CFIDS in children ages five through twelve is usually gradual (representing about 25% of juvenile cases); onset during adolescence is usually acute (representing about 75% of juvenile cases). Because those with a gradual onset are less frequently diagnosed with CFIDS (and often assumed to have another illness or, more often, no illness at all), these figures may be somewhat inaccurate. Bell finds that the number of male and female children with CFIDS is about equal.

Bell bases his diagnosis of CFIDS in children on the following criteria:

1. Chronic fatigue: at least 50% reduction in overall activity for six months

2. Symptom pattern: at least 8 of the following 12 symptoms:
   Malaise
   Sleep disorder
   Headache
   Recurrent sore throat
   Lymph node pain

Muscle pain
Joint pain
Abdominal pain
Eye pain/light sensitivity
Neurocognitive problems (attention/short-term memory)
Balance disturbance/paresthesias/dizziness/light-headedness
Temperature regulatory symptoms (fever/chills/night sweats)

3. Absence of other disease processes to explain symptom complex

(Bell 1994)

The most prominent symptoms in children are fatigue, depression, headache, abdominal discomfort, sleep disorder, body pain, dizziness, lymphatic pain, and neurocognitive problems. Unlike adults, the symptoms may be almost equally severe with frequent symptom changes. Many children with CFIDS have histories of allergies and frequent infections. Immune dysregulation findings are similar to those in adults. Periodic follow-up examinations are important to monitor for other illnesses.

Children often have difficulty describing their symptoms, especially neurological problems, including attention deficit, dizziness and disequilibrium, memory impairment, word-finding problems, impaired visual/spatial perception and, less frequently, seizure-like episodes. Emotional symptoms such as depression and rapid mood changes are difficult for children to understand and manage. In addition, children with CFIDS may experience nightmares and sleep disorders, weight loss, weakness, lack of interest in work or play, behavioral disorders, and exhaustion following physical exercise, according to Byron Hyde, M.D. Hyde feels that many children remain undiagnosed because adults do not believe they are ill and that the resulting frustration is the cause of some child and adolescent suicides. These children are experiencing considerable trauma: CFIDS symptoms, coupled with the disbelief or misunderstanding of others and an inability to perform adequately to meet others' expectations (Hyde, February 1990).

Those with milder symptoms and/or an acute onset are more likely to recover spontaneously, according to Bell. Children with allergies or a more gradual onset of symptoms generally remain ill longer and are less likely to recover, although they may improve slowly over time. However, this information is speculative and has not been studied systematically.

Parents and school personnel may have difficulty understanding these symptoms and the resulting behavior, mood changes, and impaired school performance. Often the undiagnosed child is perceived as being resistant, seeking the secondary gains of illness, or being lazy, school-phobic, neurotic, psychotic, or having learning disabilities or attention deficit disorder (ADD). Or the child may be misdiagnosed with another illness based on individual symptom patterns.

Neurocognitive testing may reveal a characteristic pattern, according to Bell, and special learning plans should be developed by school personnel if necessary. Academic performance may be significantly affected; grades typically go down and school attendance is often spotty (October 1988).

Family disruption may be significant. Children with CFIDS are often unable to participate in family activities. If the child has not been properly diagnosed, the family is unable to understand changes in health and behavior. Even with a correct diagnosis, the child's inability to perform chores and to participate in family outings causes strain. Siblings resent the preferential treatment of the ill child, and the ill child may blame him or herself for the illness and feel like a burden to the family. The ill child may feel "abnormal" and "different" from peers and other family members, and this is a considerable blow to identity formation and self-esteem.

A woman whose young daughter has CFIDS called me to arrange a consultation, saying that her daughter Lisa, a fourth grader, was experiencing adjustment problems, as were other family members. Formerly an active, vivacious child, Lisa had begun to tire easily and to become reclusive. She retreated to her room for long naps directly after school each day, awakened to eat dinner, then returned to bed and slept until the next morning. Lisa had become "overly sensitive to everything and anything," according to her mother. She snapped at others with little or no provocation. She no longer participated in family activities and had no energy to do her chores, causing resentment among her siblings. The need for family counseling was clearly demonstrated so that all could learn to cope appropriately, problem solve, and adapt to Lisa's illness.

An intelligent, perceptive fourteen-year-old PWC has asked me to refer to him as "John Doe." He and his parents describe numerous symptoms; most prominent are fatigue, depression, and cognitive impairment. John is unable to attend school and is bored at home despite homebound instruction. He is isolated from his peers and uncomfortably dependent upon his parents, from whom he is trying to individuate—a normal developmental task. John is often unsure how much of his emotional turmoil is CFIDS-related and how much is attributable to typical adolescent development. Having experienced bouts of severe depression and suicidal ideations (with several suicide attempts), John wrote about his feelings:

Mirror Image

It was dark, not an ordinary dark but more of a heavy dark. He shivered, yet it wasn't cold at least not to him. It is here that the sensation came. The sensation of danger. It always startled him even though its presence was known. Panicking him into paranoia, the presence upset him. It upset him with its chaoticness and havoc. It was there, although he couldn't define it, but it was there. His thoughts always merged and the colors ran together. Leaving him threatened by defenselessness. He liked the aloneness of this play, blocked off from the world. He was scared, and needed help. But something blocked off the given, the presence blocked it off. Using the tasteful aloneness to make him not want the help. The presence was in control and he was torn between what he needed and what he wanted. He needed help, he wanted aloneness. So help never came, and he sank deeply into his mind, searching for what it didn't matter. What he found left him pale. For in the far reaches of his thoughts was a mirror. In the mirror was an illness, the illness was himself, his darker self. He screamed, maybe help would come now.

Once diagnosed with CFIDS, John began seeing a helpful and sensitive physician who referred him to a psychologist. John has made considerable progress physically and emotionally, but he remains ill and experiences frequent relapses.

Children who are told they are not really ill become confused; they experience daily symptoms that the adults in their lives do not acknowledge, expecting them to continue with school, chores, and recreation. However, their special needs must be addressed—by parents, siblings, friends, and by the school system, which is obligated to provide special services as needed. Home instruction or special adaptations may be necessary, and parents must serve as strong advocates for their children in obtaining appropriate resources.

Parents may feel helpless and guilty about their children's illness. Family education, understanding, and communication, as well as the services of a well-informed and compassionate physician are essential.

A minority of children with CFIDS experience a severe course of the illness, in some cases resulting in persistent disability. Generally, however, the prognosis is quite favorable; a large percentage of children recover or improve substantially. Although a child's social, emotional, and academic growth may be adversely affected by CFIDS, children are wonderfully adaptable and so they often learn to compensate and do well over time.

Part III

CFIDS: What to Do

Chapter 10

The Medical Profession

Men of the cure have been more cruel than the disease.

Miguel de Cervantes, *Don Quixote*

What's up, Doc?

Bugs Bunny

Those of us with chronic illnesses often get negative reactions from a medical community that deals primarily with acute problems. We fall through the cracks of medicine. When we are ill, we are expected to do one of two things: get well or die. Yet we do neither, nor do all of us respond in the same ways to treatment. We are a difficult lot to work with, and so are many of our doctors. The inability of medicine to deal productively with illness lacking a known cause and a specific remedy is apparent in the stories told by patients.

Some PWCs have been fortunate in finding good medical care, but many doctor-shop for years. Those who have been ill long-term, and even some whose onset has been more recent, may have seen 10 or 20 doctors before finding one who could diagnose the problem correctly. Some of our symptoms are those typically ascribed to neurotic, depressed people who are accused of enjoying medical and social attention for their ailments. That there are so many of us with similar symptoms (which developed over a period of time during which we didn't know anyone else in the world was similarly afflicted) suggests an organic illness.

Doctors usually form diagnoses based on laboratory tests and physical examinations. Since there is still no test for CFIDS and because many of the symptoms we describe are not apparent in a physical exam, the diagnosis of CFIDS requires special understanding and knowledge on the part of the physician. To diagnose CFIDS, the physician must be familiar with the diagnostic criteria, listen carefully to the patient's description, take a thorough history, and order tests to rule out other illnesses.

Unfortunately, this process takes time—a commodity that is in short supply in most doctors' offices. The time problem is a serious dilemma because insurance companies have largely taken over the political realm of medicine. As a result, many doctors are now seeing larger numbers of patients to make up for reduced fee allowances from insurance companies. At a time when patients are becoming more consumer-oriented and insisting that their needs be met, doctors are finding it increasingly difficult to spend adequate time with their patients. This serious problem is not easily solved.

Many of the patients who consult me report that they have been diagnosed on the basis of Epstein-Barr antibody panel results. Probably many more who reported similar symptoms but "failed" the blood test were told they were fine (or crazy) and sent home. Many doctors are still testing for EBV alone and diagnosing CFIDS inappropriately on that basis, rather than applying the appropriate diagnostic criteria. Although we cannot expect doctors to be aware of all the nuances of every current health problem, we can expect them to be attentive, thorough, and willing to explore.

Conventional medicine is challenged by today's medical consumers. Sources of patient dissatisfaction with allopathic (mainstream) medicine are many. First, allopathic medicine has become a high-tech maze, offering sophisticated equipment and procedures with both benefits and risks. Overreliance on technology and data alone results in decreased attention to the individual patient. Second, medicine has become big business, and insurance companies are now sufficiently powerful to exert financial control over the medical profession, keeping it on a tight leash. Third, patients are becoming increasingly disgruntled with the degree of medical specialization today and irritated about being shuffled among specialists while never being given an opportunity to present the whole picture or to be treated as a whole person. Fourth, the public has become more consumer-oriented, more aware of its needs and rights, and thus more demanding of time, attention, explanations, and alternatives in medical matters. Fifth, patients have become more openly resentful toward what they perceive as cursory and/or condescending treatment when their complaints are trivialized by their doctors. Sixth, medical consumers are now examining options, recognizing that allopathic physicians are not demi-gods practicing the only valid type of medicine, but simply one alternative among the types of health care available.

CONCEPTS OF ILLNESS AND WELLNESS

In our society, illness is viewed as something that happens to a person as a result of a germ or an accident. The body is broken and needs to be fixed. Something goes wrong at the biological level. But illness is not simply an interaction between a "bad" germ and a "good" body. When exposed to a germ, some people become ill and others do not. The larger picture must be considered: genetic makeup; environmental conditions; nutrition; our thoughts, beliefs, and feelings; social interactions; addictions; emotional stress and pain; abuse of our bodies; how we live our lives. Why do some people who are exposed to a germ become ill while others do not?

The very concepts of illness and wellness are poorly understood. "We know health well in its absence," wrote Andrew Weil. Apart from being merely the absence of illness, however, the term "wellness" connotes a harmony of mind, body, and spirit, and an appropriate style of living. It also connotes self-care—proper nutrition, rest, and exercise. Attention to these aspects of health have generated unfortunate health fads: we seek to purchase magic remedies in our instant-fix-oriented society. But the wellness we seek cannot be purchased or easily achieved.

One mistake I made in my quest for wellness is having the unrealistic expectation of too much too soon. I continued to pursue an instant solution, unwilling to accept the reasonable approach of achieving balance in my life by budgeting energy, learning to be less rushed and pressured, and making gradual changes in the way I lived as I explored and experimented with treatment options. We tend to think that there's *one* thing we should do, or a specific approach or philosophy to follow that will make us well, and we look for someone who can tell us what it is. If we can't find an allopath who can do it, we look for someone outside mainstream medicine who can. To seek professional care that will augment the healing process is sensible; to expect a magical instant cure is not.

THE SPECIAL PROBLEMS
OF CHRONIC ILLNESS

Wildly expensive medical care has made little advance
against chronic and catastrophic illness while becoming
steadily more impersonal, more intrusive.

M. Ferguson, *The Aquarian Conspiracy*

Doctors have a better success rate with acute illnesses than with chronic ones. Chronically ill patients have ongoing needs that present special challenges for health care providers. The chronically ill often do not look sick and tend to have unpredictable changes in health. We become experts on our illnesses and challenge our physicians. Doctors and other medical personnel often cannot comprehend what they can't see or measure. We claim to be ill, but our symptoms keep changing and most aren't obvious to other people. In requesting treatment for a problem that's invisible and difficult to define, we often feel rejected by the medical system on which we depend. In our frustrating quest to be treated as sane people with a continuing, crazy-making illness, we seek treatment from a system that doesn't welcome us, or we become hopeless.

Of course doctors prefer to work with easier-to-diagnose and easier-to-treat illnesses. Doctors are trained to cure people and that's what they like to do. When they can't fix what's wrong, they become frustrated; their professional identities are threatened. Once a series of expensive diagnostic tests has produced negative results, the patient may be referred elsewhere for what is then viewed as a "psychosomatic" (in an incorrect, pejorative sense) illness. The temptation to dump us on some other specialty such as psychiatry is great.

We are a huge inconvenience to practitioners who have the attitude that any illness involving unexplained symptoms and normal results on lab tests is not to be taken too seriously. Those of us with chronic illnesses *are* pains in the ass to our doctors. We don't get better, we don't go away, we just keep coming back with the same old complaints and additional new ones. We tell our doctors how awful we feel, and if they take us seriously, they have only two attitudinal choices: to feel badly about how little they have to offer us, or to harden themselves against their failure to make us well. The latter is a survival mechanism, born of the doctor's need to be a hero, a fixer, a curer of ills, and to see anything less as a failure. We present a challenge and a threat.

Most doctors don't state their frustration openly but demonstrate it in more subtle ways, which make their patients unhappy. Patients with CFIDS often feel rejected and neglected by their physicians; they either continue with their doctors while harboring resentment against them, or they seek medical attention elsewhere. Switching from one doctor to another or fragmenting care among several doctors is common among PWCs.

When the first case definition for CFIDS was published in March 1988, affording PWCs a legitimate status among the chronically ill, Marc Iverson, president of The CFIDS Association of Charlotte, North Carolina, wrote an article called "The Politics of CFIDS: A Salute for Some, An 'I Told You So' for Others."

> For good reason, many of us harbor feelings of anger and bitterness about the insensitive way these [non-believing] physicians treated us for so many years. Too many doctors . . . simply did not *listen* to us. With great arrogance, they concluded that just because they could not understand our illness (and their technology could not detect it) it did not exist and must therefore be 'in our heads' (i.e., 'psychosomatic'). How ironic it is that neuropsychological testing and MRI brain scans seem to indicate that for many CFIDS patients the illness literally *is* in their heads! For those of us who endured years of patronizing attitudes, demeaning remarks, and humiliating treatment at the hands of all-knowing, closed-minded physicians, I say to the guilty parties, damn it, you failed us and you failed yourselves. Most of us have emerged from this experience with our self-respect intact and our perspective on life enhanced. I wonder if this is true of those physicians who selfishly washed their hands of our difficult cases and dishonored their noble profession. (*The CFIDS Chronicle*, April 1988)

Doctors would like us to cooperate by getting well, and we'd love to comply—not for the sake of their egos but for the sake of our health. However, physicians must learn to treat chronic illnesses without blaming us for remaining ill or themselves for not curing us.

CFIDS PATIENTS TALK ABOUT MEDICAL TREATMENT

Most initial doctor visits involve recitations of symptoms and the inevitable question from not-yet-diagnosed CFIDS patients, "What's wrong with me?" Their inquiries may be met with a variety of discouraging responses, including accusations of hypochondria, inappropriate lifestyles, inability to handle stress, neurosis, menopause, laziness, a "bug," or generalized anxiety.

Some patients report helpful responses from their doctors:

I don't know. Let's run some tests and see if we can find the problem.

I've seen a lot of people with these symptoms lately. I'm not sure what's causing them.

It sounds to me like you have CFS/CFIDS. I don't really know much about it, but I'll see what I can find out. *Or:* I'll refer you to someone who has experience with treatment of this illness.

I can help you with CFIDS, but I can't cure you.

Other patients report upsetting experiences:

I've been sent to a separate specialist for each of my symptoms. None of them understands that all these things seem to be connected. They won't listen when I tell them this is all one illness.

I was tested by a psychologist [neuropsychological evaluation]. He was mad at me; he said a third grader could do things on the test that I couldn't do. He thought I was making it all up, that I just didn't want to work any more . . . . I had a cushy job that I loved, and I was making a lot of money. Why would I want to stop? And my doctor believed everything this guy reported to him; he didn't believe *me.*

The nurse in my doctor's office said, "You must know you're causing these problems yourself." I told her I was driving in a familiar street and just got lost. I didn't know where I was, and that was scary. She acted like I made it up. I told my doctor about it . . . but he didn't listen to me and didn't understand.

My doctor finally told me what's wrong. The advice I got was, "Just adapt to it. Rest a lot. Learn to manage stress. Persevere and be patient."

Such advice as, "Just accept the illness and go on with your life" is easier given than followed. It implies falsely that no treatment is available. Patients come away quite discouraged. Some give up passively and others decide to fight, to educate themselves about available alternatives.

PWCs have expressed anger, bitterness, and distrust toward the medical profession in general and certain doctors in particular. However, many have indicated that they found at least one physician with whose attitude and treatment approach they were pleased. Patients have indicated the qualities in a physician they deem most valuable: competence, honesty, warmth, concern, willingness to listen, being down-to-earth, spending adequate time with the patient, and a willingness to explore treatment alternatives. Patients greatly appreciate doctors who are willing to take the extra time to answer questions and offer explanations. Many patients have indicated being most satisfied with doctors who themselves had CFIDS or other chronic illnesses, or whose staff members, wives or family members had CFIDS. These doctors were more likely to understand what their patients were experiencing.

DIFFERENT SYSTEMS OF MEDICINE

Not all doctors practice the same type of medicine. This section discusses various approaches to medical practice. It does not advocate any particular form of treatment but simply describes options.

Physical Approaches to Healing

• **Allopathy.** Most mainstream doctors in the United States practice allopathic medicine. Allopathic treatment relies upon the use of pharmaceuticals and technology, which are often effective for acute medical problems such as trauma, acute illness, and repair or replacement of joints and organs. Sophisticated technology allows us access to the internal workings of our bodies, in many cases with noninvasive procedures. Many allopathic doctors are sensitive, caring, and open minded, but others have become rigid, closed to new ideas, or cynical because medical insurance companies are increasingly directing the practice of medicine. Sara Reynolds, M.D., adds, "Unfortunately, many physicians have learned from sad experience to beware of the apparent 'doctor-shopper' who goes from office to office until he or she gets the [desired] treatment or medicine."

Some doctors are more preoccupied with their machinery than with the health of their patients. Studies have shown that touch is very important in mobilizing healing, but technology pushes doctors farther away from their patients. The awe in which we hold hard science leads to a reliance on objective measures that is not necessarily in the best interests of the patient. Tests are most productive if used in conjunction with other findings.

The allopathic model draws artificial distinctions between illnesses of the mind and those of the body and tends to enforce the antiquated notion of mind-body duality. By ignoring the role of consciousness in the patient's states of wellness and illness, the allopathic doctor increases the distance between doctor and patient, and the two may fail to interact well.

Allopathic medicine is often accused of falling short in dealing with chronic illness. Drugs can offer symptomatic relief, but deeper causes of chronic problems are less easily detected or treated. Allopathy has also been criticized for a lack of attention to preventive medicine and health maintenance, although patients often do not follow advice regarding health maintenance. Fortunately many allopaths—usually the family practitioner or the internist—are attentive and responsive to their patients and treat them holistically.

Allopathic medicine has both strengths and shortcomings. "[A]lthough disenchanted with establishment medicine," wrote Locke and Colligan, "we must be aware of the danger of turning wholeheartedly to other forms of treatment. The risks of alternative practices are in some cases ignored or minimized" (1986). Sara

Reynolds, M.D., commented at a meeting of the CFS Association of Arizona: "Unfortunately, when anything is touted as miraculous or seems 'too good to be true' it probably is. Most allopathic [treatment] is based on scientific evidence. Most other therapy is anecdotal but may be valid."

• **Osteopathy.** Although this branch of healing is theoretically based on the structural aspects of the body (bones, muscles, and joints), osteopathy increasingly has come to resemble allopathy in the use of pharmacological drugs and other interventions. Osteopathic manipulation is used as a treatment approach (but not the sole approach to medical problems, a criticism leveled at chiropractic practice. Do not confuse the two!) Doctors trained in osteopathy (D.O.s) often pay more attention than allopaths to the whole patient and many stress the body's own healing powers.

Allopathic and osteopathic medical facilities are usually separate; however, the two types of medical degrees (M.D. and D.O.) are legally equivalent in all states. It becomes increasingly evident that sound medical practice and a positive relationship with patients rather than the type of diploma are the truly relevant aspects of quality medical care, and cooperation between the allopath and osteopath would be beneficial to practitioners and patients alike.

• **Homeopathy.** Homeopathic doctors seek to treat the whole body, to balance and to strengthen it, and to identify symptom patterns in each patient. Homeopaths emphasize the individual and the individual's manifestations of illness, seeking to stimulate healing by tapping the body's healing powers rather than by simply medicating symptoms. They do not rely heavily on lab tests to produce diagnoses; labels are not considered important. Rather than treating with pharmaceuticals, homeopathy works by isolating substances that tend to produce symptoms like those the patient is experiencing. These substances are then highly diluted and administered so that the body will react against them, thus fighting the symptoms. The theory is that a small amount of what caused the problem will fix it. A few scientific studies have been conducted, but it remains speculative why this approach is successful in some cases.

At present, some disenchanted mainstream physicians are considering alternatives and some are "converting" to homeopathy.

They feel that allopathic medicine has been ineffective in combating chronic and degenerative diseases, which abound today. They stress the need for prevention and education.

The practice of homeopathy is regarded with suspicion by most mainstream medical practitioners, and the American Medical Association (AMA) has taken an exclusionary view of homeopaths. Homeopathic treatment is quite expensive and is not generally covered by medical insurance.

• **Naturopathy.** Naturopaths believe in the ability of nature to heal. They focus on the body's innate healing ability and on curative properties of certain natural substances in the environment, such as plants and molds, which are the origins of many pharmaceutical products. Naturopathy seems to be gaining in popularity but remains unaccepted by most people as a viable approach to medical treatment. Although the healing power of nature is certainly real, naturopaths lack a consistent, shared methodical approach to treatment and some of their practices are unproven. Some PWCs have reported excellent results with naturopathic healers while others have not been helped.

• **Traditional Chinese medicine.** We usually associate Chinese medicine with herbal preparations, acupuncture, t'ai chi, and qi-gong, with mysticism and healing masters. Ironically, many regard traditional Chinese medicine as a fad, part of "New Age" medicine, but it is an ancient practice steeped in tradition. It takes an integrated approach, more subtle than that of Western medicine, combining physical and spiritual healing.

The unifying concept behind the tradition is the belief that the body has a number of meridians (circuits) that conduct energy throughout the body. Symptoms result from a blockage in these meridians, and healing is directed at removing the blockages so that energy can once again flow freely. The individual, rather than a particular illness, is the focus of treatment. Symptoms are viewed in terms of the functioning of the entire body, and the treatment goal is to locate and correct energy imbalances that manifest themselves as symptoms.

Acupuncture is a treatment process in which fine needles, sometimes along with heat, electricity, oils, or lasers, are inserted at various trigger points along the body's meridians. The energy points chosen depend on the nature of the patient's complaint or the treatment goal. Some PWCs report that acupuncture restores energy, improves vestibular functioning, and enhances feelings of well-being. While its mechanism of action is not fully understood, acupuncture is believed to stimulate the body's production of enkephalin (beta endorphin) and serotonin, creating changes in mood and sleep. Although many in the West view it as a radical or new treatment, acupuncture has been practiced for centuries and may become a standard component of integrated medical treatment in the future. Acupressure is similar to acupuncture, but instead of needles, a trained practitioner applies pressure to certain trigger points on the body's surface.

Chinese medicine takes a long-term preventive approach that is also helpful for chronic illness. Western medicine is acknowledged by practitioners of Chinese medicine to be more appropriate for trauma and acute illness. A combination of Eastern and Western medicine may be the accepted treatment modality of the twenty-first century.

• **Ayurvedic medicine.** One of the holistic approaches to medicine, ayurvedic philosophy and medical practice originates in India. It focuses on a wholesome lifestyle, incorporating diet, herbal preparations, massage, meditation, and behavior. The whole person rather than the disease label is the focus of treatment. Treatment is aimed at producing feelings of well-being and is claimed to be helpful for health maintenance and for minor disorders.

• **Other types of "physical" healing.** Many other healing approaches, including chiropractic and nutritional therapy, are eyed with suspicion by the medical community and society in general. Despite considerable controversy, many patients claim to have been helped by "unorthodox" methods. Each treatment has its advantages and limitations, and the patient's belief system plays a large part in determining the success of any treatment. The availability and growing popularity of alternative approaches indicate that there is no one correct approach to medical treatment. The role of nutrient supplementation and diet as an adjunct to a treatment program is discussed further in Chapter 11.

Mental and Spiritual Approaches to Healing

• **Positive thinking, faith healing, and other alternatives.** In the growing movement of patient empowerment and the belief in the healing properties of the human body, positive motivation toward healing and wellness is respected and considered potent. This discussion includes such diverse healing systems as shamanism, Christian Science, and folk healing, since in all these cases intervention is believed to be a supernatural, or at least superhuman, phenomenon. Generally regarded with disfavor as being superstitious and ritualistic, such approaches are oriented toward the intervention of forces beyond the usual range of human understanding and the limitations of our technological and cultural beliefs.

The individual's faith in the method is the basis of its success. Skeptics abound, especially in our culture, in which science and logic are highly valued. By contrast, in these healing systems illness may be seen as the result of inappropriate or negative thinking on the part of the individual, or as the result of some external supernatural force. The key ingredient is faith—in the method, in the healer, in some sort of divine intervention. Healing rituals in communities that accept and believe in them produce positive results. The group or community support and the individual's spiritual beliefs are thought to be the potent ingredients in such healing practices.

In choosing treatment for a ruptured appendix, the need for surgical intervention is clearly demonstrable. However, an interaction between an intangible illness and an unobservable intervention encourages skepticism even when successful results are obtained. The practices of prayer, imagery, belief in supernatural or invisible, innate healing sources, or any type of spiritual medicine is alien to our culture. Although we tend to believe in the "power of positive thinking," we have difficulty believing that it can truly help healing to take place. Can faith and belief transcend and overcome physical symptoms? If not, how can we explain the apparent success of these methods in many cases? We are skeptical of such procedures as hypnosis and guided imagery, but less so when technology such as biofeedback equipment is introduced to demonstrate scientifically that something measurable is happening.

"We must be receptive to possibilities that science has not yet grasped, or we will miss them," writes Bernie Siegel in *Love,*

Medicine and Miracles. "It's absurd not to use treatments that work, just because we don't understand them." Joan Borysenko, in *Minding the Body, Mending the Mind,* is open to such alternative approaches. "We are entering a new level in the scientific understanding of mechanisms by which faith, belief, and imagination can actually unlock the mysteries of healing." Emotions and beliefs exert a direct influence on the brain and thus on the immune system, thereby facilitating healing.

• **Psychology and psychiatry.** Although these fields are attaining more realistic and legitimate status in our society, the need for therapy is often as suspect as its practice. Mental health or behavioral health practitioners vary in approach, education, training, and personal style. The general goals of therapy include personal growth, insight, behavior change, enhancement of self-esteem, problem solving, and emotional support. Such issues may require only short-term therapy, while more complex, deep-seated issues may require long-term treatment. In many cases, the family of the PWC should be involved in therapy. Families have great difficulty accepting change, especially when former roles can no longer be filled by the PWC.

In my experience as a psychologist working with PWCs, I find that in most cases brief intervention is sufficient. Those who have difficulty accepting the diagnosis and limitations and those who resist modifying their activity levels and lifestyles are cause for particular concern. Denial of the illness is a natural stage in working toward acceptance, but those who become stuck in this stage may require intense therapeutic intervention to move beyond it. A PWC may have longstanding issues that are compounded and magnified by chronic illness. Such issues may involve loss of former roles (especially for those who have been overly responsible for others and neglected self-care), family of origin, financial concerns and attitudes, relationship problems, and low self-esteem. Working through these while coping with CFIDS-related concerns can be a lengthy but helpful process.

Psychological counseling helps in the treatment of primarily physiological illnesses by addressing adjustment issues and mobilizing innate healing potential. Physical and psychological treatments should be integrated.

Healthy Suspicion

Quacks and charlatans exist in all types of medical practice—physical, mental, and spiritual. A certain level of suspicion is healthy—we must not accept all new therapies blindly—but we should also guard against total rigidity and immediate rejection of anything new or unusual. Any tool that minimizes helplessness and maximizes hopefulness is doing something helpful, even if we cannot demonstrate how or why.

Alternative treatment approaches vary widely in success rates, and some of their claims are unfounded. Additionally, many systems lack credentialing organizations and accredited or recognized training institutions. Often there are considerable variations in practice. Individual practitioners of the same type of medicine often differ radically, not only in personality but in theory, approach, and cost. Medical insurance companies do not usually pay for any treatments considered by them to be "experimental." Unfortunately, with CFIDS there is no standard treatment program and so all interventions can be considered experimental.

Treatment modalities range from beneficial to harmless to dangerous—and many are quite expensive. An outbreak of a new illness or increased attention to an existing one invites the development and aggressive marketing of various new substances and treatments. Such a flurry of new miracle approaches is cause for careful consideration. Safety claims may be fabricated, especially when products are touted as "natural." (I can think of many natural substances, like cow dung and arsenic, that I would not care to ingest.) Any claims that a particular treatment program cures CFIDS or helps all PWCs is bogus; so far no treatment has been found to do either.

TOWARD A NEW CONCEPT OF HEALTH AND HEALING

We have oversold the benefits of technology and external
manipulations; we have undersold the importance of human
relationships and the complexity of nature.

M. Ferguson, *The Aquarian Conspiracy*

One flaw in medical training is the lack of education in communication skills. Doctors are confronted daily with the fears and insecurities of their patients. The doctor's manner can increase or de-crease this fear and confusion. Too often the communication is abrupt and cursory, leaving the patient with unanswered questions, assumptions, and new fears that may negatively affect the treat-ment outcome. Many doctors tend to give orders rather than offer explanations. For them, "difficult patients" are often those who ask questions, ask to participate in their health care, and expect that the physician will work with them toward a mutually satisfying outcome. Those doctors who demand patient compliance, ignore input from their patients, and act too busy to care are "difficult doctors." Patients and doctors should ask each other more ques-tions, both for a more accurate assessment of the case and to help the patient become a better-informed, more cooperative (rather than compliant) participant.

We want doctors to be something more than mechanics. We demand that they pay attention to our concerns and treat us with compassion as well as competence—a lot to ask, but the only path to successful treatment. We appreciate new technology but abhor its overuse. Treatment of the whole patient is essential—not just test results, or an isolated symptom or body part, but the whole human being. Such progress requires a team approach and the education of doctors in such areas as communication skills, alter-native approaches to healing and medicine, exercise, and nutri-tion. All healing is scientific, according to Bernie Siegel, M.D., even when we cannot explain how the healing occurs.

It is time to discard permanently the antiquated concept of mind-body duality and to use the term "psychosomatic" in its *true* sense, an acknowledgment that the integrated system called the mindbody experiences the illness. "The placebo is proof that there is no real separation between mind and body," wrote Norman Cousins:

> Illness is always an interaction among both. It can begin in the mind and affect the body, or it can begin in the body and affect the mind, both of which are served by the same blood-stream. Attempts to treat most mental diseases as though they were completely free of physical causes and attempts to treat most bodily diseases as though the mind were in no way involved must be considered archaic in the light of new evi-dence about the way the human body functions. (1979)

Empathizing with patients is said to present risk for the physician. We do not ask physicians to ignore their own needs for objectivity and distance but simply to meet us halfway. Bernie Siegel, M.D., believes that doctors are destined to fail as mechanics but have much to offer as empathetic counselors, teachers, and healers.

The power of touch should not be underestimated in the practice of medicine. Human touch brings healer and patient closer, counteracts some of the "cold" effects of modern medical technology, and conveys warmth and caring. Massage, acupuncture, and acupressure are healing modalities that involve touch. Some physicians make it a practice to touch each patient during an examination or consultation.

Effective verbal communication, too, helps to bridge the gap. Patients fare better when procedures are explained, when they feel they are listened to, when they work together with the doctor in choosing the course of medical treatment. In my experience as a mediator I have found that people who participate in a decision-making process are more likely to comply with terms they have helped to develop. The same principle applies to consumers of health care, who are more likely to follow a treatment regimen they have played a part in selecting.

Patients and doctors each have responsibilities in their relationship. A true partnership between doctor and patient combines the perceptions and strengths of both based on a foundation of communication, trust, and mutual participation.

Developing a Positive Doctor-Patient Relationship

Physicians are experts in the field of medicine but are human beings first. Arthur Schimelfenig, Ph.D., said at a monthly meeting of the CFS Association of Arizona, "If you expect your physician to pull you out of this, forget it. You're the best treatment you've got. Use your doctors to help you."

As a patient it is your responsibility to:

1. Identify and state your needs. If you have a complaint about medical care, bring it to the attention of your doctor in a straightforward, not critical or accusatory manner. Complaining isn't productive, but direct requests often are. Learn to communicate assertively.

2. Ask questions when you need information about your ill-
    ness, prognosis, medications, or other treatment options.
    Specific questions will generate clearer answers. Recognize
    that the answer to many of your questions will be, "I don't
    know." Because many doctors are uncomfortable saying
    this, you might get a circuitous answer. If you do, ask a
    more specific question or say, "Is this something you can
    look into further?" or "Do you know if any research is
    being done in this area?"

3. Become aware of the role you are playing as a patient. Are
    you playing the role of the dependent child, expecting your
    doctor to be the magic, healing parent? Most effective is an
    adult-to-adult relationship based on mutual respect and
    your need for a competent, caring medical professional—
    not a parent.

4. Differentiate between cooperation and obedience. A coopera-
    tive patient works helpfully with the physician; an obedient
    one simply does what she or he is told without questioning.
    Cooperation gets the best results in the long term.

5. Be well informed about CFIDS. Share information with
    your doctor, making it clear that your purpose is to share
    knowledge, not to tell your doctor how to practice medi-
    cine. Physicians can't keep up with every new development
    in medicine but should be willing to consider new informa-
    tion presented by patients.

6. Be a well-informed consumer of medical care. Shop care-
    fully for your experts; you're the customer. Question your
    doctor about rates for various services. Of course, your deci-
    sion to see a particular doctor should not hinge solely (or
    even primarily) on costs, but you have the right to know
    up front what the charges will be. Comparison-shop when
    filling prescriptions. Consider generic drug prescriptions
    (but be aware that in some cases generics are of lesser qual-
    ity; talk with your doctor and pharmacist about the pros
    and cons of generics).

7. Keep careful track of your appointments and give 24-hour
    notice (except in cases of emergency) if you cannot keep

an appointment. Arrive on time. If the doctor is habitually late, discuss this problem not with the staff but with the doctor, who is ultimately responsible for scheduling.

8. Be organized. Maintain lists of (a) your symptoms and concerns, (b) your questions, (c) all medications you are taking, and (d) any medications to which you have had unusual or adverse reactions in the past. If you have consulted other doctors in the past, keep copies of your medical records, including lab test results, and make them available to your new physician(s).

9. Listen attentively to what the doctor says during your discussions and take notes. Ask questions until you are sure you understand the answers. Information that makes sense at the time can be difficult to remember later. You might consider bringing someone to appointments with you to corroborate or expand on your history, offer observations, and clarify information if necessary.

10. Recognize that medicine is not a hard science, and that diagnoses and treatment plans are judgment calls based on objective and subjective information. If you still harbor the unrealistic expectation that the doctor's responsibility is to identify a single medical cure for a long-term illness, recognize that the problem is too complex for such a simple solution. The lifestyle modification that must accompany medical intervention is the responsibility of the patient.

11. Be honest. Don't fake feeling better than you do just to please the doctor. Although doctors like their patients to get well, you are doing yourself a disservice if you pretend.

12. Request extra time with the doctor when making your appointment, if you need to. Expect to be charged for the additional time. If you are a new patient, tell the receptionist so when scheduling your appointment. And make sure the doctor is someone who is experienced in diagnosing and treating CFIDS.

13. Communicate your satisfaction to the doctor if you are pleased with the medical treatment you are receiving.

Enumerate the qualities that are most valuable to you; specific praise is most helpful and gratifying to the recipient.

Your doctor has a responsibility to:

1. Jump off the pedestal. Let your patients know that you don't view yourself as omniscient.

2. Talk to your patients. Tell them what you think; tell them when you don't know or aren't sure—that you don't have all the answers. Initially you may disappoint them, but in the long run you will be doing them (and yourself) a service. Offer explanations and information and explore alternatives with the patient.

3. Listen to your patients. If you don't understand, ask questions—without preconceived notions as to what the answers will be. Their statements will be at least as informative as their lab test results, and your willingness to listen demonstrates your caring.

4. Take your patients seriously. Patients often overhear doctors talking about them or other patients in a flippant manner. This behavior is insulting, hurtful, and trivializing. Please recognize that you are dealing with human beings, not cases. No one wants to be "the appendectomy in Room 402." Avoid the labels "somatizer," "hypochondriac," "neurotic," and "crock." All symptoms have origins, and all should be taken seriously. If you don't understand what's going on, say so, but don't dispute with the patient whether a "real" illness exists.

5. Avoid assuming a parental role that creates childlike dependence and ultimately resentment on the part of your patients. This type of dependency is dangerous, making you the responsible party and the patient the passive one.

6. Patients with chronic illnesses have special needs, ongoing ones. Let patients know you cannot effect a quick cure or alleviate all of their suffering but that you are available to them as a resource and a helper. If you are unable to diagnose or threat their illnesses, tell them so and discuss options.

7. Recognize that some patients will return time after time
    without improvement. This is not your failure or theirs: it
    is characteristic of the illness. It is natural to want your
    patients' health to improve with treatment and to be disap-
    pointed if there is no change or a negative one, but avoid
    making statements that cause the patient to feel guilty for a
    lack of progress. Assume that you are both doing the best
    you can and no one is to blame for a lack of improvement.

8. Keep an open mind about newly emerging concepts regard-
    ing CFIDS treatment. Patients with CFIDS have a strong
    network and will hear of various treatments that sound "far
    out," but such options should be considered if they are not
    likely to cause harm. Sara Reynolds, M.D., adds, "Don't
    criticize any treatment which appears helpful unless it is
    known to be detrimental in some way."

9. When a referral for psychological treatment is warranted,
    explain the purpose of the referral—support, neuropsy-
    chological evaluation, or help with problem solving, adjust-
    ment issues, stress management, coping skills, etc. If you
    make the referral with an inference that the illness is "all
    in the patient's head," you are using psychology/psychiatry
    as a dumping ground and will alienate your patient.

10. Your patients have emotional needs that are not separable
    from their medical needs. Although the physician need not
    play the therapist's role, it is important that patients be
    given support and understanding. Patients need to have
    their suffering acknowledged although it can't be "fixed." A
    simple statement such as "I realize this is really rough for
    you," can be of more help than most physicians realize.
    While the doctor is conceptualizing the disease, the patient
    is experiencing difficulty, confusion, and fear.

11. Offer your patients guidance in learning to take responsibil-
    ity for their own care in terms of lifestyle modification
    (diet, exercise, etc.). Suggestions, explanation of rationale,
    and encouragement are helpful. Patients often feel "disci-
    plined" (shamed or scolded) by their doctors, which rein-
    forces dysfunctional parent-child roles. A preface such as "I

know it's really hard to give up some of the things you really like, but . . . " encourages the patient to perceive the suggestion as a source of positive motivation rather than an order. Patients are often fearful that their doctors will "yell at them" to promote compliance; empathetic guidance works better.

12. Show respect for your patients by keeping to your appointment schedule as closely as possible. It is demeaning to a patient to be kept waiting for long periods of time. In cases of emergency most patients will understand, but lateness on a regular basis is not acceptable. It may be necessary for you to discuss such chronic scheduling problems with your office staff.

13. Some of your CFIDS patients are more knowledgeable about their illness than you are. Many have read extensively, networked, and contacted support groups to obtain information. Allow patients to share this information with you.

CHOOSING A DOCTOR WISELY

The worst way to find a doctor is to consult the yellow pages for a name that sounds good or a location that is convenient.

Here are some suggestions for finding competent medical care:

- Consult your local CFIDS support group for a list of doctors who are experienced in treating CFIDS. Get referrals from other CFIDS patients or from doctors in whom you have confidence. You may need to see several types of specialists for treatment (e.g., internal medicine, allergy/ immunology, infectious disease, urology, endocrinology, and gastroenterology), but use a primary physician to consolidate and oversee treatment.

- Consult *The American Medical Directory: Physicians in the United States* in the reference section of your public library to get information about individual physicians, including type of practice, training, credentials, and board certification.

- Once you have chosen a candidate, ask if the doctor treats CFIDS and how long she or he spends with each new patient. If the answers are satisfactory, make an appointment to interview the doctor. You are in a "hiring" situation. Prepare pertinent questions in advance. Be aware of the validity of your needs.

- Use referrals and information about a doctor as a general guide, then trust your instincts to determine if you can work well with this person, if you feel a sense of trust and respect. Ask yourself these questions:
  — Do I feel comfortable with this doctor? Is this someone in whom I can confide?
  — Do I feel listened to and understood? Am I being given the doctor's full attention, free from distractions?
  — Are there likely to be power struggles? Is this person abrupt or arrogant?
  — Is this person knowledgeable about CFIDS and treatment options?
  — Does this doctor have an open, accepting, positive attitude?
  — Do we share the same treatment philosophy?
  — Is a sense of hope being communicated to me?
  — Is this person willing to admit uncertainty, to say "I don't know" when appropriate?
  — Do I have the sense that this doctor is interested in me as a person, not just a medical case?

No physician will get an A+ in every category. Decide which qualities are the most important; you won't find perfection! Don't expect inappropriate favors from the doctor, such as falsifications on insurance forms or frequent long telephone calls in place of office visits.

In some areas of the country, PWCs have been unable to find practitioners who are knowledgeable about CFIDS. As the medical community becomes better educated about CFIDS this problem will diminish. Currently these PWCs have few options: they can either educate a willing doctor or travel to a practitioner in another area.

IF YOU ARE DISSATISFIED
WITH YOUR DOCTOR . . .

Many patients complain about poor doctor-patient communication. The highly motivated patient who addresses specific problem issues directly will probably obtain better results from the health care system.

First, examine your complaints or needs to determine if they are valid. If so, discuss the problem openly with the doctor, not a member of the staff. Do not accuse, attack, or make assumptions; this will put the doctor on the defensive, making it more difficult for the two of you to solve the problem and create a mutually satisfying therapeutic relationship. Make requests for change in a considerate, positive way, focusing on each specific problem and the desired outcome or solution options, and evaluate the doctor's response. Because most patients feel more comfortable grumbling to others than discussing problems directly with their doctors, your doctor may be surprised to hear of your dissatisfaction. Your doctor may have requests of you as well; try to listen objectively to assess their validity before reacting defensively.

If you can agree on changes to be made, allow a reasonable time for them to take place. If the problem is not corrected, you can persist or switch to another doctor. Once you have chosen another practitioner, obtain previous medical records or have them transferred.

If you have switched several times and are still dissatisfied, your expectations may be unrealistic. Perhaps no doctor can provide what you're seeking. However, do not compromise your values or reasonable standards. You should expect competent, compassionate, sensitive medical care and should not tolerate arrogance or indifference.

PWCs feel considerable gratitude toward the exceptional doctors who have respected us, believed in us, and treated us with compassion. Those doctors who practice the art as well as the science of medicine and who have devoted long hours to often-unpaid CFIDS research and treatment are truly special. We respect and appreciate them beyond measure.

UNPOPULAR TRUTHS

There is no magic bullet, no universally successful form of treatment. Any treatment carries the risk of potential harm; no one has all the answers; the doctor does not necessarily know best. Marcus Welby, M.D., is a fictional character; few if any medical professionals can offer the combination of knowledge, experience, warmth, and understanding that we crave. The bottom line is that we are responsible for our own medical decisions and care. We must educate ourselves, although our physicians may be less than thrilled if we are knowledgeable and curious.

We are not to blame when a treatment fails to help; most of the time no one is to blame. There is no target for our anger and frustration, and we must resist the temptation to appoint a scapegoat (the doctor, the medical profession, or ourselves).

Finding treatments and ultimately a cure for CFIDS is no simple matter. We would like to believe that there is a single causative that we can fight and eradicate. The true picture is more complex.

We may feel rejected by our doctors, often realistically so. They are the experts regarding medical practice; we are the experts regarding the functioning of our own bodies. Doctor and patient must work together as teammates, to combine expertise. Doctors don't perform miracles, and medicine is not a perfect or exact science. The innate healing ability of our bodies is more magical than the "science" called medicine. Medical science offers a vast array of interventions that can facilitate healing, but *it is the body that heals*.

There is no such thing as "normal." What is typical of one person may be atypical for another. Each of us is unique and complex. We function differently and respond differently to treatment.

Seeking wellness is a trial-and-error process. Healing remains an art, a combination of scientific knowledge and a practitioner's skills. Our health care system is imperfect. Our task is to make use of its strengths but also to understand its weaknesses. Providers and consumers of health care together can create positive change in this system.

Chapter 11

Treatment

When diagnosed with CFIDS, many of us asked, "Okay, so what do I take to make me better?" We were naive enough to believe that every illness had a cure. Our expectations changed as the grim reality set in: there is no specific, universally successful CFIDS treatment. We then began the search for treatments that would help us to feel better rather than get better. Ideally a PWC's physician is open to exploration of treatment alternatives and prescribing on a trial-and-error basis, as well as encouraging a multifaceted healing approach that includes lifestyle management in addition to general and symptomatic treatment.

Sara Reynolds, M.D., writes:

> We have an illness for which there is (1) no positive laboratory diagnosis (according to the recent CDC criteria) (2) no usual course, and (3) no specific treatment. Hence, there are many possibilities for untried remedies. There will be the uninformed or even unscrupulous who will suggest useless and/or very expensive, certainly unproved, remedies. There is a great temptation to feel that whatever you are taking when you begin to feel better must be the magic cure. (*CFS Jigsaw,* April 1988)

But because our symptoms wax and wane unpredictably, we cannot be sure that improvement is caused by medication. Dr. Reynolds suggests several trials, going on and off a particular medication until a definite correlation between it and symptom relief can be established.

Any treatment is potentially dangerous. The current trend toward the use of "natural" products is based on the false assumption that "natural" equals "safe." Anything that enters the body can alter its functioning for better or for worse—or some of each.

Mainstream doctors typically use pharmaceutical drugs as a primary treatment modality, a good-news/bad-news proposition. Many medications ease suffering and save or prolong lives. However, medications can create new problems as they alleviate existing ones. Any substance powerful enough to affect body chemistry may cause serious side effects or severe complications. Many of today's "miracle" drugs will be deemed worthless or even harmful in the future. Thalidomide and DES are examples of pharmaceutical products once considered helpful and safe that later produced tragic results.

Also, little is really known about the complex interactions of various drugs taken simultaneously. The results of treatment with pharmaceutical drugs can be magic or tragic—or somewhere in between. A fairly conservative yet open-minded approach to treatment makes the most sense.

When we feel awful, our concern about the risks of experimental treatment seem to decrease in inverse proportion to the severity of our symptoms. We try out various medications, weighing risk, fear, and uncertainty against the degree of desperation. We keep hope alive by continuing to try new things rather than waiting helplessly for the situation to resolve itself. We can't always know for certain what the long-term effects of a drug might be, but what is the alternative? Do we wait until a cure is discovered, refusing treatment in the interim? Do we wait for the results of scientifically valid, double-blind studies to ascertain the safety and effectiveness of a drug (which can take many years) and suffer in the meantime? As one patient said, "I'm spending all this money on drugs and medical care, and I'm just being experimented on, waiting for a cure."

Most of the available information about treatment results in PWCs is anecdotal, that is, based upon nonstandardized, informal clinical trials with differing numbers of patients—sometimes only a few. Anecdotal reports provide interesting leads as to what might be helpful. We need more systematic, scientific trials, which are expensive and time-consuming, but in the meantime we need symptom relief. Physicians are placed in a bind; they want to use medications wisely but cannot wait years for results of experimentation when their patients are ill *now*. Jay Goldstein, M.D., said at the 1987 CFS Convention in Oregon:

I feel that when we are dealing with a disorder such as the chronic fatigue syndrome, you can't wait for double-blind experiments to tell you what to do. When I see a patient that has a problem for which there is no treatment anywhere in the medical literature, I feel that it is my responsibility and my obligation to use what I know as well as I can to help this person['s] suffering, even though it might be a treatment that no one has ever done before. I feel that it is a tragic failure of American medicine that they have lived in the straight jacket of the double-blind experiment. It's made doctors unnecessarily rigid, narrow, unthinking, and noncreative. That's what you don't need when you have a disease like [CFIDS].

Accepting that there is no standard treatment regimen for CFIDS is very difficult for doctor and patient. Deciding which treatments to try is confusing and frustrating. Evaluating the results of treatments is almost impossible, given the unpredictable course of CFIDS. Well-intentioned friends and family members offer advice and admonitions. ("There is a stigma now about taking drugs," said one patient. "It really bugs my mother and husband that I'm taking drugs. They think I shouldn't have to.") Our goal is to obtain as much help as possible while minimizing risks. As much as we would like to "just say no" to drugs, our need for relief is strong.

When a particular treatment seems to be effective, we are often told this is just a "placebo effect," as if the placebo response were synonymous with voodoo. It is actually the power of belief, the confidence in a treatment, that can trigger us to mobilize our own resources to obtain relief. Belief in the curative power of a treatment can be as potent as the treatment itself; neither the mind (the patient's set of beliefs) nor the body (the physiological effect of a treatment) is the sole source of a treatment's success; the interaction of the two determines the result. Although a scientific rationale for a treatment's apparent effectiveness is not always available, positive belief and hope are known to create physiological change. Paul Cheney, M.D., views the placebo response as an expectation of wellness that causes the emission of polypeptides from the central nervous system, improving immune function. He believes that a positive attitude and active imagery have a positive effect on the immune system (January 14, 1987). Other physicians concur. "I try to get the patient to understand that the *body* heals, not the therapy. . . . The most important thing is to pick a therapy you believe in and proceed with a positive attitude," writes Bernie Siegel, M.D. Norman Cousins described the placebo as "the doctor who resides within."

Instilling hope in a PWC is one of the practitioner's most valuable functions. On several occasions I saw my physician during discouraging exacerbations, and his attitude alone helped me to mobilize my will toward wellness before I even began any new treatment. Knowing that there were still options to try, that relief was possible, and that I had a good doctor on my side kept me going.

I wrote in my journal:

Sometimes I wonder what I should believe in. If I weren't so damned skeptical, something might have cured me already. If I could convince myself of the effectiveness of something, anything, I might get well . . . .

Another new medicine, and the hope that maybe this will do it. I'd sell my soul for a magic pill. And then some weird-ass reaction to the medicine; there goes all the hope . . . until I hear about the next minor miracle, which I will doubtless try. I admire people who have total faith in something—religion, herbs, whatever. . . . Hope is so important. Do I feel better because I get hopeful, or do I get hopeful when I'm feeling better? Both, I suspect.

Since then I have come to the realization that a belief system evolves—one does not simply self-impose an effective healing philosophy. Developing an understanding of the complex interactions between behavior, treatment options, and an emerging belief system is a process rather than an event.

When something—yoga, vitamins, pharmaceuticals, or acupuncture—seems to help, the properties of the treatment combined with the relief and sense of hope interact in a psychological-physiological process. Don't let anyone tell you that it's not "real," or that it's all in your head, or any other such nonsense. If you believe in it and it is helpful, the treatment is of value (as long as it does not have serious deleterious effects). If a treatment is effective initially but later loses its beneficial effects, it may be wise to discontinue it for a period of time and then restart it. If beneficial effects are not felt the second time around, eliminate the treatment and seek an alternative.

When a treatment seems to make the symptoms worse, we may be told that we are having a "healing crisis" and that our discomfort or pain results from toxins being expelled from our tissues. Although some medications cause initial temporary side effects, it is unclear whether a so-called healing crisis is a positive sign. If any form of treatment causes severe discomfort, seek competent medical advice immediately.

The spectrum of treatments undertaken by PWCs is amazingly diverse. Different physicians favor different treatment approaches, which are generally tailored to the needs of the individual and which may change over time as new discoveries are made. CFIDS practitioners have found that the results of treatment, even with the more promising drugs, are variable, producing significant alleviation of symptoms in some PWCs, modest improvement in others, and no effect or an adverse effect in the remainder.

One person's miracle treatment is another person's poison. The success of some treatments may be short-term, and symptoms may return during a course of medication or after it is discontinued. The severity of the illness in individual cases determines how aggressive treatment should be.

Consult your doctor about treatment possibilities, and get information about options from CFIDS newsletters and journals. Consider the whole picture: not only the potential side effects of medications you are considering but also their possible interactions with other medications. Also consider the cost; many available treatments are not covered by medical insurance and you may want to check with your insurance carrier before initiating more expensive treatment. Because of a lack of scientific studies, all CFIDS treatments are considered experimental, and insurance companies are erratic and unpredictable in their reimbursement.

Remember that drug combinations can be tricky. Make sure all physicians treating you have a list of all the medications you are taking, including over-the-counter remedies, vitamins and supplements, herbs, and birth control pills. Drug interactions can produce symptoms worse than those being treated and may even result in irreversible damage or death. Use of tobacco or alcohol can affect your response to medication and ideally both should be discontinued or moderated.

CFIDS treatments are of two main types: primary treatment (aimed at treating the disease in general), and symptom-specific treatment. The following discussion of treatments is presented as information rather than advice. Treatment should be initiated *only under medical supervision.* In some cases the information is technical and may be of greater relevance to the practitioner than to the PWC. Because traditional dosages may not be appropriate for PWCs, practitioners should check with informed physicians or in the CFIDS literature, or call the CFIDS 800- or 900-numbers (see Appendix C) for current treatment information, including dosages.

(*Explanation of Abbreviations:* OTC indicates those treatments that are available over the counter [without a prescription]; IM indicates administration by intramuscular injection; IV indicates intravenous administration. The trade name of the medication is given first with the generic name in parentheses.)

PRIMARY THERAPY

Included in this category are treatments that cause general improvement in CFIDS. Some of these medications are new, some are experimental, and some are controversial. Treatments vary as a result of patients' and physicians' individual philosophies and beliefs, and not all PWCs respond to the same treatments. In using immunomodulating and experimental drugs, we face certain dangers and must weigh risk against benefit.

• **Adenosine monophosphate (AMP)** is a natural cellular metabolite that has been used for the treatment of some herpesviruses. AMP has been helpful for some PWCs, who reported general improvement, including increased energy. Side effects include asthma, shortness of breath, transient flushing, palpitation, and dizziness with high doses. A popular treatment several years ago, AMP is no longer commonly used.

• **Alpha interferon (IFN),** oral or injectable, is thought to have various immune-enhancing functions including antiviral action and may be more helpful in combination with other treatments than alone. It is administered orally or sublingually. Very low doses are recommended due to toxic effects of high doses; some patients become worse with this treatment. IFN should not be given if the patient already has detectable levels of alpha interferon.

• **Ampligen** (poly(I)-poly $C_{12}U$) is a biological response modulator with antiviral and immunomodulating properties that is known to normalize the 2'–5' A synthetase/RNAse antiviral pathway in both CFIDS and HIV disease, and it may prove useful in treating other chronic diseases as well. It is manufactured for both IV and oral use and is quite expensive. When tested on severe cases of CFIDS, results have been promising: increased cognition as measured by IQ scores and memory tests, increased activity level as measured by Karnofsky performance scores, decreased fatigue, increased exercise tolerance and efficiency in oxygen uptake on treadmill testing, reduction in giant cells and reduction in virus activation, particularly HHV-6. Ampligen is generally well tolerated with few side effects. It has orphan drug status for CFIDS but is not yet FDA-approved for widespread treatment use. Financial rather than regulatory constraints seem to hinder further trials.

• **Antibiotics** are used to treat bacterial rather than viral infections. Overuse and inappropriate use of antibiotics are major criticisms of medical practice today and may play a part in candida (yeast) overgrowth. However, Vibramycin (doxycycline), an antibiotic in the tetracycline class, has been of occasional help to some PWCs.

• **Antidepressants** are often helpful in relieving not only depression but numerous other CFIDS symptoms as well. They are described later in this chapter in the section on depression.

• **Antifungals** include standard drugs such as Mycostatin (nystatin) and Nizoral (ketaconazole) and newer drugs such as Diflucan (fluconazole) and Sporanox (itraconazole), which treat systemic yeast and fungal infections. They may have immune modulating properties as well. Like other medications, they may lose their effectiveness over time and may need to be rotated or stopped and restarted to achieve beneficial effect. Some practitioners and researchers believe that candidiasis is not a problem in CFIDS and find antifungal medications and diets ineffective. Others regard fungal infection/candidiasis as playing an important role in CFIDS, as a cause or an epiphenomenon of the illness, and find antifungal treatment and dietary modifications of great benefit.

• **Antioxidant** therapy consists of using supplements to reduce the harmful effects of free radicals, molecules that can cause cell injury or death and that are believed to contribute to the development of many illnesses. Commonly used antioxidants are vitamins E, C, and beta carotene (a precursor to vitamin A); others include bioflavenoids, ginseng, ginkgo biloba, and silymarin.

• **Antivirals** are used to treat certain types of viral infections: Zovirax (acyclovir)—oral or IV—for herpes group viruses; Famvir (famciclovir)—oral—which has been shown to have action against herpesviruses; Cytovene (ganciclovir)—oral or IV—which is helpful with CMV and other viruses; and valcyclovir, aminated acyclovir which is essentially acyclovir in a more usable and effective form. Foscavir (foscarnet)—IV—inhibits all known herpesviruses and is the most expensive of the antivirals. Acyclovir is the antiviral most commonly used in CFIDS but the others may have application as well. These drugs are expensive and their use is indicated only when evidence of active viral replication is present; however, some may hold promise for treatment of CFIDS symptoms. Some antivirals are of benefit only when used intermittently, and the risk-benefit ratio of these drugs may prohibit their use unless absolutely necessary.

• **Coenzyme Q10** (OTC) is a mitochondrial coenzyme used in adenosine triphosphate (ATP) production that is believed to have antioxidant and immune-enhancing qualities and to act as a free-radical scavenger. Dr. Paul Cheney finds that large doses taken sublingually seem to be most effective. CoQ10 is often used synergistically with other medications, such as Prozac. Some patients report general improvement, cognitive improvement, and increased energy level and/or muscle strength after several weeks. CoQ10 is available at health food stores, pharmacies, and from the CFIDS Buyers' Club. Prices vary widely.

• **DHEA (dehydroepiandrosterone)** is an adrenal hormone normally present in humans, that is low in many PWCs. It has antiviral, immune modulating, and metabolic and brain enhancing properties. It can modulate T- and B-lymphocyte function, thus improving immune functioning. Those with a deficiency of DHEA may have cold hands, temperature dysregulation, dry skin, and brittle hair. Dosage is individualized, usually quite low, and must be carefully assessed. DHEA should be used only if testing reveals a deficiency. Although DHEA use in CFIDS is increasingly common, only limited research has been conducted.

• **Gamma globulin** is a blood product that contains antibodies. It is used especially for recurrent upper respiratory infections and when total IgG is low, or in the presence of IgG subclass deficiencies. IgG is one of several types of immunoglobins which are produced in the lymph cells to combat foreign substances. Although expensive and inconvenient (and not always covered by medical insurance), IV administration of gamma globulin is usually more effective than IM administration. Jay Goldstein, M.D., recommends measurement of IgA and anti-IgA antibody levels before using gamma globulin to avoid the possibility of serum sickness. Side effects at high doses include headache, nausea, malaise, phlebitis, transiently abnormal liver function tests, and an unusual excitatory response in some PWCs. Results of experimental trials have been inconsistent, in part due to the wide variability in dosages used. High-dose administration is likely to cause side effects, but if the dosage is too low, there will be no benefit. Those who do experience benefit may find this treatment losing its effectiveness over time.

• **H2 blockers** such as Zantac (ranitidine), Tagamet (cimetidine), Pepcid (famotidine), and Axid (nizatidine) suppress production of stomach acid and are often prescribed for gastric complaints. They also provide general benefit for a minority of CFIDS patients. If one of the H_2 blockers proves ineffective, another may be successful. It is wise to start with small doses, since PWCs may experience unusual side effects, such as insomnia and agitation. (Goldstein)

• **Humatrope** (somatotropin, or human growth hormone) may have application in the treatment of CFIDS. Good research studies have not yet been conducted, and treatment is quite expensive and must be continuous. Numerous side effects have been associated with its use.

• **Inosine pranobex** (Isoprinosine or Pranocin) (OTC in some countries such as Mexico) is not available in the United States. It is used to treat illnesses characterized by immune deficiencies and has received mixed reviews from PWCs. The method of action and optimum dose are unknown. Side effects are rare and include mild nausea and transient rise in serum and urinary uric acid levels.

• **Kombucha mushroom tea** is a preparation containing kombucha "mushroom" (which is actually a fungus), black tea, and sugar. Kombucha has been hailed as "the magic mushroom," but the properties of this preparation have not been studied. Only anecdotal information is available, and reports are very mixed. This one belongs in the "questionable" category.

• **Kutapressin** is a porcine liver extract of polypeptides with a long history of safety since its development in the late 1940s. It is an immunomodulator that inhibits lymphokines, has antiviral properties, and is an antiinflammatory agent. Kutapressin has been shown to suppress HHV-6, Epstein-Barr virus, and possibly herpes zoster (shingles) and human foamy virus. The SLIF test (Single Lymphocyte Immune Function) is often given before and during treatment, initially to establish immunosuppression and later to assess treatment progress. PWCs tend to improve after a series of injections (usually 30–60) and minor setbacks during therapy may occur. Those ill longer than five years are less likely to obtain benefit. Evidence of immune dysfunction and recent EBV infection predict greater treatment success. Relapse may occur upon discontinuation of treatment. The only contraindications are pork allergy and pregnancy. Side effects are minimal and are limited to local injection site reactions such as itching and bruising. A primary drawback of Kutapressin is its high cost.

• **L-Carnitine** is synthesized in the body from the amino acids lysine and methionine. It is essential for mitochondrial energy production, which is disrupted in CFIDS. It may improve fatigue and cognitive symptoms. Adverse effects are rare.

• **Lentinus edodes mycelium, or LEM,** a Shiitake mushroom extract (OTC) is believed to improve immune and liver function. It has been widely used in Japan and has become a popular treatment in the United States as well. LEM is expensive and is not usually covered by medical insurance. Reported effective by roughly half of those who have tried it, LEM may lose its benefit over time. It may increase the number of white blood cells, especially NK cells. Lentinan, an extract from another part of the same mushroom, differs from LEM and is administered by IV or injection. It is believed to have antiviral properties.

• **Magnesium** is an important supplement for many PWCs to correct intracellular deficiencies which disrupt adenosine triphosphate (ATP) functioning, leading to a vicious cycle in which even less magnesium gets into the cells. Blood levels of magnesium may be normal, which is deceiving. Magnesium may be taken in pill form, by injection, or as an elixir. Adequate calcium should be taken, since magnesium can deplete calcium. Magnesium is helpful in pain relief and cellular energy production.

• **Naphazoline** (OTC as ClearEyes or by prescription in stronger concentrations) is an ophthalmic drug (eyedrops) which directly stimulates the trigeminal nerve, allowing direct transmission to the brain. Many PWCs using naphazoline eyedrops report cognitive improvement. (See "Sympathomimetic ophthalmic solutions" later in this list.)

• **Nicotine patch** treatment has been initiated in CFIDS by Jay Goldstein, M.D., who reports that it stimulates the production of serotonin, an important neurotransmitter in CFIDS. Nicotine is a vasodilator which helps increase cerebral blood flow, thus improving cognitive function. Although the use of the patch may be helpful because nicotine is released steadily, cigarette use is not recommended because the nicotine enters the body too quickly to be of benefit, in addition to the undesirable effects of smoking.

• **Nitroglycerin,** administered sublingually at low doses, metabolizes to nitric oxide and produces beneficial effects including a reduction in pain, dyspnea (air hunger), and blurred vision as well as increased energy, improved cognition, and mood improvement. About ⅔ of those with fibromyalgia (more women than men) receive benefit, and those without fibromyalgia usually report no effect. According to Jay Goldstein, M.D., who has pioneered the use of this therapy in CFIDS, response is rapid (within three minutes) and generally persists for one to three hours after administration. Rapid tolerance is often a problem. The drug is well tolerated, with headache being an occasional side effect.

• **Omega-6 free fatty acids (evening primrose oil)** and **omega-3 fatty acids (EPA fish oil) (OTC)** are essential fatty acids (EFAs), which create metabolites (EFAMs) that have two essential functions in the body: to maintain normal membrane structure and to act as messengers which regulate aspects of cell function. EFAs cannot be made by the body. EFAs mediate cytokine effects and modulate the HPA axis. They have immunomodulating and antiviral properties. Anecdotal reports indicate substantial clinical improvement in CFIDS symptoms such as pain, fatigue, and depression.

• **Oxytocin,** a hormone and neurotransmitter that may be deficient in PWCs, is available in sublingual and nasal spray forms. It has a dramatic effect in some patients, helping with fatigue, pain, and cognition deficits (particularly short-term memory). Blood pressure should be monitored. This drug is in early experimental stages for treatment of CFIDS.

• **Peptide-T** has been known to help relieve fatigue, cognitive dysfunction, depression, pain, diarrhea, nausea, dermatitis, and frequent urination. It has undergone initial tests, but follow-up studies are needed. Dr. Candace Pert, co-inventor of this drug while working at the National Institutes of Health (NIH), reports that the government has been unwilling to continue testing peptide-T beyond the preliminary study. It is not commonly used in the treatment of CFIDS at this time but may prove beneficial, and further studies are needed.

• **Risperdal (risperidone)** is a high-affinity $5\text{-}HT_2$ antagonist and a low-affinity dopamine (D_2) agonist closely related to ritanserin. Although it is marketed as an antipsychotic, Jay Goldstein, M.D., has had success in using both this agent and ritanserin in CFIDS treatment at very low doses. Experimental; not formally studied.

• **Ritanserin** is a long-acting $5\text{-}HT_2$ receptor blocker with antidepressant and antianxiety properties which helps to increase slow-wave sleep. PWCs have varied greatly in their responsiveness to the drug, although all tolerated it well. In those who were helped, symptoms quickly returned when the drug was discontinued. Experimental; not formally studied.

• **Sympathomimetic ophthalmic solutions** include naphazoline HCl, epinephrine, dipivefrin HCl, apraclonidine, and phenylephrine to treat various symptoms. According to Dr. Jay Goldstein, these substances administered as eye drops have different effects than they would with other forms of administration, and these effects are achieved more quickly.

• **Transfer factor (TF)** is a blood product containing cells from the blood of an individual who is intimate with the PWC but not ill (e.g., a spouse or other household member). The blood is processed according to an elaborate procedure and then TF is administered by injection. Results have been spotty. Although a few practitioners claim great success with TF, most have not found it effective. It is considered highly experimental and should be used as a last resort if at all.

• **Vitamin and mineral supplements** (most OTC) should be good quality and preferably free of yeast and sugar. Multivitamins should be high in B, C, E, and beta-carotene. Supplementation with the minerals zinc, potassium, and magnesium is often recommended. Supplements are especially important because vitamins and minerals in PWCs may be easily depleted and/or poorly absorbed. See also: Vitamins C and B-12, listed separately.

• **Vitamin B12** (oral OTC; nasal gel OTC; injectable by prescription) has been very helpful in treating CFIDS, and most patients receive benefit in terms of increased energy and overall improvement. It is generally agreed that injection is the most effective route of administration, usually 1 to 2 times per week. When taking B_{12}, one should take a multivitamin or B-complex supplement that will supply large amounts of the other B vitamins. The effectiveness of B_{12} may decrease in time; if so, it should be discontinued for a few weeks and restarted.

• **Vitamin C** (oral OTC; IV by prescription) is found to be beneficial in treating CFIDS and other immune disorders. The administration of ultra high-dose vitamin C (oral or IV) is controversial; some practitioners report dramatic positive results and others find this treatment ineffective and potentially dangerous. Taken orally, large doses of vitamin C may produce gastric problems; if so, the dose should be decreased and then increased gradually.

NUTRITION, SUPPLEMENTS,
AND ENVIRONMENTAL TOXINS

Ours is a nutrition-conscious age in which "natural" products are widely advertised and self-proclaimed nutrition experts abound. Health food stores and bookstores offer a wealth of information and misinformation about nutritional programs and products, often loaded with contradictory and inflated claims. Medical schools have typically paid little attention to nutrition, yet we often turn to our physicians for nutritional advice. Fortunately, many medical schools are now requiring courses in nutrition, and research in this area is flourishing.

As we become aware of the effects of pollution on our environment, we worry about contaminated water, or foods grown in depleted soil and loaded with pesticides and antibiotics. We are bombarded with media-borne proclamations that we need fiber, complex carbohydrates, lean meat or none at all, fresh veggies . . . and yet our convenience stores and restaurants carry few or none of these products. We become suspicious that any food we enjoy is likely to contribute to an early demise. And when we develop CFIDS, one "expert" tells us to load up on protein; another tells us to eat small amounts. One expert tells us to eat a diet high in complex carbohydrates, another tells us that all carbohydrates can contribute to yeast overgrowth. When energy is low, we may crave sugar and carbohydrates ("junk food syndrome")— the very things we know must be bad for us. What to do? Who is right? There are no simple answers.

Numerous substances and treatment procedures have been suggested for treating CFIDS—prescription medications, vitamins, minerals, nutritional supplements, and various "immune boosting" products. Obtaining accurate information about all treatments under consideration and using basic common sense are imperative. Certain products seem to enhance well-being and improve immune functioning, but often we don't understand their long-term effects, their synergistic (combined) effects, or what they do outside the lab and inside the body. It is not safe to assume that natural products are harmless; anything taken in large enough quantities can be toxic. We should not seek information from self-proclaimed noncredentialed "health experts," such as the clerks in health food stores, whose knowledge is limited and whose primary interest is in selling their products. The same caution applies to fad "wonder" products and products sold in multilevel sales programs with numerous personal testimonials and little or no scientific basis or verification. Beware of those who claim that their products cure CFIDS. If a cure were available, we'd all have heard about it by now. (The CFIDS "grapevine" is remarkably efficient!) Consult a well-trained nutritionist before embarking on a program of supplementation. Be a curious, cautious, well-informed consumer. Don't count on anyone else to do this for you.

Many so-called alternative therapies are quite useful in the treatment of CFIDS even though their mechanisms of action may not be fully understood. (We still don't know how aspirin works.) When considering treatment options, ask a lot of questions: the cost of treatment and likelihood of medical insurance reimbursement; alternatives to be considered; references to well-designed scientific studies about the product or service including its success rate; the practitioner's credentials, training, and prior experience treating CFIDS with that product; side effects; expected length of treatment; and expected outcome. You are entitled to receive satisfactory answers to these questions.

• **Craniosacral manipulation** involves all the bones in the body, including those in the head. Cerebrospinal fluid and the cranial bones move in a rhythmic pattern at the rate of 10–12 times per minute. The rate in PWCs, however, is abnormal. Many osteopathic physicians are trained in this treatment modality, which is helpful in restoring normal rhythms. Treatment is gentle and noninvasive. No formal studies have been conducted, but this technique has helped many PWCs.

• **Diet** is a controversial topic in this disease, but there is general consensus about certain recommendations:

> Use certain vitamins and supplements judiciously.
> Maintain a diet high in vegetables and complex carbohydrates and moderate in protein.
> Keep your diet low in fats, especially saturated fats.
> Avoid the "Big 5": caffeine, nicotine, sugar, aspartame (Nutrasweet), and alcohol.

Use fresh rather than processed foods whenever possible.
Avoid foods that are not well tolerated (due to allergies or sensitivities); these are often dairy products, gluten, and foods with certain food additives.
Eat foods in variety so that sensitivities do not develop.
Wash fresh produce in water containing a teaspoon of Clorox; remove outer leaves or peel skins to remove pesticide residues and reduce danger of ingesting parasites.
Eat small, frequent meals.

Individual experimentation is the most accurate method of determining which foods are well-tolerated and which are not. PWCs may be sensitive to food additives, dyes, and antibiotics; dairy products; gluten products; MSG; certain spices; sulfites; nitrates; and some hard-to-digest vegetables. An elimination diet combined with careful record-keeping under medical supervision may help to uncover food allergies and sensitivites. Symptoms of food intolerance include malaise, mood alteration, digestive disturbances, food cravings, and repetitive eating patterns. Skin and blood tests are generally considered unreliable in diagnosing food allergies.

Some PWCs report carbohydrate cravings, especially during exacerbations. Although a psychological basis for these cravings has been suggested, there is evidence that the source is a largely physiological, possibly a chemical problem related to levels of serotonin and/or other neurotransmitters, to biochemical and metabolic abnormalities, or to systemic yeast overgrowth. Consumption of simple carbohydrates may increase fatigue, causing a "boost-and-crash" cycle (in which the blood sugar level rises and then plummets quickly and dramatically) and perhaps compounding candida-related problems and other symptoms. The problem can be dealt with by limiting the consumption of simple carbohydrates. Complex carbohydrates are metabolized more slowly and so don't cause the "boost and crash" effect.

• **Entero-hepatic resuscitation** is most effective for those with mild to moderate symptoms who have been ill for less than 2.5 years. The basis of this treatment is that chronic toxicity, resulting from overloaded detoxification mechanisms (liver detoxification pathways), is the basis for many CFIDS symptoms, including extreme environmental sensitivities. Leaky gut syndrome, in which toxic substances seep through the intestinal lining into the gut and ultimately to the liver and other organs, has been found in a group of PWCs. Antibodies to these substances may be produced, thereby activating the immune system inappropriately. This excess burden on the liver compromises its detoxifying ability. Thus, even minor toxic exposure then generates symptoms in PWCs who are already overloaded with toxins they cannot process adequately. Additionally, specific amino acid abnormalities are often found in nonresponders, indicating metabolic toxicity and inability to assimilate amino acids. Entero-hepatic resuscitation is achieved with a nutritional detoxification plan including supplements (UltraClear and UltraClear Sustain) and specified diet and supplementation, including magnesium and antioxidants (vitamins C, E, beta carotene, and CoQ10). These measures have been helpful in a large portion of subjects tested, resulting in significant symptom reduction. Like other CFIDS treatments, this one is not effective in all cases and requires strict attention to supplementation, diet, and expense, which is generally not reimbursable by medical insurance.

• **Herbal remedies** have been used for centuries to treat various illnesses. The scientific basis for their action is not usually known, but many of our pharmaceuticals are based on the active ingredients in botanicals. Use herbs judiciously; some offer tremendous benefit, some do little or nothing, and others are harmful. Dosages must be appropriate to the individual. Examples of herbs used in the treatment of CFIDS are:

> **aloe vera:** externally for various skin conditions; internally for digestive problems (but interferes with iron absorption)
>
> **astragalus:** increases white blood cell production; strengthens the immune response; antibacterial, energy tonic
>
> **bitter melon (mormordica charlantia):** increases NK function and numbers; regulates sugar metabolism (in enteric-coated capsules)
>
> **bromelain:** for leg pain
>
> **cayenne:** for the circulatory and digestive systems
>
> **dong quai:** analgesic; muscle relaxant; antiallergenic

echinacea (purple cone flower): respiratory and urinary tract infections; blood "purifier"; helps heal wounds; possible antitumor activity

flax seed oil: contains essential fatty acids; can help eczema, menstrual disorders, rheumatoid arthritis, and atherosclerosis; decreases inflammation of the mucous membranes

fo-ti: sedative; antitumor; blood fortification

garlic: antibacterial, antifungal, and antiviral properties; for colds and coughs; cardiovascular conditions; may increase natural killer (NK) cell activity

ginkgo biloba: improvement in neurologic/cognitive functioning and blood circulation by decreasing blood viscosity; decreases tissue damage during inflammation; antioxidant properties

ginseng: central nervous system stimulant; improves circulation and glandular functioning; stimulates heart and blood vessels; increases secretion of histamine and decreases eosinophils in blood; increases corticosteroid content of blood

goldenseal: digestive problems; antibacterial and anticandida; decreases nasal mucous; liver tonic; improves eczema; treats mouth ulcers, and gastric and respiratory infections

licorice root: to improve blood circulation, digestion, and adrenal insufficiency

lomatium tincture: for exacerbations; antiviral, immune stimulant that helps chronic fatigue and congestion; respiratory problems

ma huang or ephedra: for allergy, asthma, and cough

milk thistle or silybum: improved liver function

osha root: for congestion; antiviral; immune stimulating properties

peppermint: digestive problems

shou wu pian: Chinese herb used for treatment of alopecia (hair loss); lassitude of legs and inability to stand; dizziness; headache; memory problems

valerian: for anxiety and insomnia; often used in combination with passiflora as a sedative, hypnotic, and anodyne; calms nervous system and promotes sleep

This list is by no means complete; it is intended to provide a sample of herbal remedies that may be helpful to PWCs. Since herbs are contraindicated in certain conditions and may cause harmful effects if used inappropriately, they should be used only with the guidance of an expert who has proper training and experience.

Where the herb is grown and how it is processed affects its properties, as does the form in which it is taken (tincture, tea, powder). Few scientific studies have been conducted, so the effects of herbs are not well established. Herbs are usually used synergistically (i.e., in certain combinations). Herbal treatment can be expensive and it is not covered by medical insurance, but many have found it quite effective.

• **Avoiding environmental toxins.** Many CFIDS patients are especially sensitive to environmental pollutants and chemicals. Immune dysfunction is thought to be related to the immune system's difficulty coping with numerous substances with which we come into contact and to disruption of the body's own detoxification systems. Avoiding all toxic substances is not possible, but we need to exercise caution whenever possible to minimize adding to the total body load. Many CFIDS patients find they are sensitive to some or all of the following: hairsprays, perfumes, pesticides, chemicals, cleaning products, fuels and exhaust fumes, and tung oil (found in varnish, shellac, and some furniture oils and paint products).

• **"Sick home" improvement** is necessary for those with environmental sensitivities. One's home can be modified to minimize toxic exposure, but the process of making these modifications may aggravate existing sensitivities and it is best for the PWC to be away for a few weeks during any remodeling. Helpful changes include adequate ventilation using sophisticated air-handling systems with activated carbon filters; HEPA (high efficiency particulate air filter) room air purifiers; frequent dusting and vacuuming (preferably done by someone other than the PWC, and with a HEPA vacuum cleaner or central vacuum system); avoiding cleaning products to which one is sensitive; keeping knickknacks and "dust-catchers" to a minimum—including old books; replacement of carpeting (breeding grounds for dust mites) with ceramic tile or wood flooring; use of low-toxicity paint; a nonattached garage or a well-sealed door between garage and house; elimination of pesticide use in the house and yard; use of chemically inert building materials— stainless steel, stone, and solid wood in place of particle board; elimination of room-freshening sprays and other scented household products; and sealing off any materials that contain formaldehyde. Although most people are not in a financial position to build a new low-toxicity house, many modifications can be made in existing homes to create a less toxic environment.

SYMPTOMATIC TREATMENT

Anxiety

In addition to relaxation techniques and meditation, which must be practiced regularly in order to be effective, minor tranquilizers are helpful. Those most commonly prescribed are Xanax (alprazolam), BuSpar (buspirone), and Valium (diazepam), although Klonopin (clonazepam) may also be helpful in treating anxiety disorders. Xanax is a popularly prescribed medication that alleviates anxiety and seems to have antidepressant properties as well. Because it produces drowsiness, many PWCs with sleep disorders use Xanax to help them to fall asleep. It may be addictive, however, and sudden withdrawal is accompanied by withdrawal symptoms. Valium is less commonly used; it is addictive and causes depressions in some individuals. BuSpar is an antianxiety agent that is not related to the benzodiazepines; it is nonaddictive and does not cause the same severe withdrawal effects as Valium and Xanax. BuSpar does not cause sedation or the mild sense of euphoria associated with Xanax and Valium, and may be used along with Klonopin, which is sedating. Klonopin, a long-acting benzodiazepine, improves sleep at low doses. It also has the properties of blocking the effects of circulating cytokines and helping to normalize brain functioning.

For the treatment of occasional anxiety these medications can be taken as needed. Certain antidepressants, taken on a regular basis, are helpful in the treatment of panic disorder.

Cognitive Dysfunction

The following medications have been used to treat cognitive dysfunction with varying degrees of success:

> Acetylcarnitine
> Benzodiazepines: low-dose Klonopin (clonazepam) or Xanax (alprazolam)
> Calcium channel blockers: listed under "Headache" in this section
> Cognex (tacrine or tetrahydroaminoacridine)
> Diamox (acetazolamide)
> Dynagen: not available in the United States
> Hydergine (ergoloid mesylates)
> Ionamin (phentermine)
> Mestinon (pyridostigmine)
> Nootropics (piracetam, oxiracetam, aniracetam): not available in the United States
> Prozac (fluoxetine) and, to a lesser extent, Zoloft (sertraline) and Paxil (paroxetine)
> Stimulants: Cylert (pemoline), Ritalin (methylphenidate), Dexedrine (dextroamphetamine): should be used with caution
> Symmetrel (amantadine HCl)
> Tegretol (carbamazepine), Depakene (valproic acid), Depakote (divalproex sodium)
> Trexan (naltrexone); low dose
> Vasopressin (desmopressin acetate, DDAVP)

Some of these medications are quick-acting and others must be taken for several weeks before effects are felt. Vitamin B_{12} and CoQ10 may help as well.

Cognitive restructuring, a technique used by some neuropsychologists, helps compensate for cognitive dysfunction. A special issue of *The CFIDS Chronicle* (August 1991) focused exclusively on the work of Linda Iger, Ph.D., Tarras Onischenko, Ph.D., and Curt Sandman, Ph.D., who work extensively with PWCs experiencing cognitive difficulties. Tools and techniques, some of which may be self-implemented, are presented in this issue. Learning to cope with and compensate for cognitive deficits is often a primary focus of psychotherapy.

Neurofeedback may have application in correcting abnormal brain waves as seen in EEGs to create symptom improvement. Computerized EEGs have revealed that PWCs are in delta (slow-wave) brain activity at times when they are awake and supposed to be alert. Sensors are placed on the patient's head and linked to a system which offers feedback (e.g., changes in images on a computer screen or in the volume of music being played) as they produce the desired change in brainwave activity. The patient thus learns to increase brainwave activity over time. This form of treatment is in its early stages and has not been formally tested, but it may hold promise in normalizing brainwaves and creating symptom improvement.

Depression

Antidepressants fall into several categories according to which neurotransmitters (brain chemicals) they affect. They are nonaddictive and must be taken regularly to be effective. One is usually started on low doses of a medication, which is then increased as necessary and as tolerated. It may take several weeks for the full antidepressant effect of these medications to be felt. Sometimes different types of antidepressants are combined or used with other medications; some of these include low-dose lithium, low-dose thyroid medication, Cylert (pemoline) and BuSpar (buspirone).

• **Tricyclic antidepressants (TCAs)** are among those most widely used in CFIDS. Certain TCAs, notably Sinequan (doxepin), have antihistaminic and anti-inflammatory properties. TCAs administered in low doses often produce better sleep, decreased pain, and global improvement. Common anticholinergic side effects of TCAs include dry mouth, constipation, and weight gain. Because of drug sensitivities, TCAs are initially administered in tiny doses and increased to the patient's optimal dose. TCAs are usually administered just before bedtime because they promote sleep. If a PWC does not respond well to one drug in this class, there are many others that can be tried. Low-dose thyroid medication may enhance the antidepressant action of these medications.

• **Selective serotonin reuptake inhibitors (SSRIs)** include Prozac (fluoxetine), Zoloft (sertraline) and Paxil (paroxetine). They are less sedating than the TCAs, in fact they may give an energy boost and are therefore most often administered in the morning. In addition to their antidepressant properties, these medications decrease irritability and mood swings and may offer pain relief. They may improve energy level and cognition and usually cause fewer side effects than the TCAs. The most common side effects of the SSRIs, especially Prozac, are anxiety and a wired feeling (which often subside over time) and sexual dysfunction. Less commonly they may cause either insomnia or drowsiness. Prozac may be effective in increasing energy (at least temporarily), reducing pain, and increasing natural killer cell function. Zoloft and Paxil cause fewer of the side effects associated with Prozac and may be better tolerated.

• **Newer antidepressants.** Wellbutrin (bupropion) may help fatigue, emotional swings, and depression and does not cause the side effects associated with many of the other antidepressants. An occasional side effect in predisposed individuals is seizures. Wellbutrin is not as helpful as most other antidepressants for most PWCs. Newer medications include Effexor (venlafaxine), which is unrelated to any other antidepressants and has a shorter half-life than the SSRIs. Its side effects include nausea and increased blood pressure. Serzone (nefazodone) reportedly improves sleep pattern and produces substantial abatement of symptoms (increased alertness, decreased fatigue, and improved memory and immune parameters) without causing sedation, insomnia, or sexual dysfunction associated with the SSRIs. Luvox (fluvoxamine) is a newer antidepressant which may prove helpful in treating CFIDS.

• **Monoamine oxidase inhibitors (MAOIs)** have reportedly been somewhat effective for some PWCs, but due to strict dietary restrictions and frequent side effects they are used less often than TCAs and SSRIs.

• **Lithium,** commonly used to treat bipolar (manic-depressive) disorder, has not proven helpful in CFIDS treatment.

Finding the right antidepressant or combination of antidepressants at the most effective doses is a trial-and-error process. Even if numerous medications must be tried before the right one is found, almost all cases of depression are treatment-responsive.

• **Cognitive behavioral therapy** is a type of psychotherapy based on behavior and thought modifications, including realistic self-talk (as opposed to irrational and distorted self-messages involving misinterpretation of events or stimuli), goal setting, increased pleasurable activities or events, education about the illness, relaxation training, and other practical techniques. A combination of antidepressant medication and cognitive behavioral therapy are often most effective in treating depression.

Digestive Problems and Irritable Bowel Syndrome

Diarrhea can be treated with many OTC preparations, including Metamucil, Kaopectate, Donnagel, charcoal capsules, or Imodium (loperamide HCl). Drinking adequate amounts of fluid is important. Prescription medication, such as Lomotil, may be necessary for more severe cases.

Heartburn, or reflux of stomach acid, can be helped by H_2 blockers, antacids, and sometimes by avoiding spicy foods and not eating within a few hours of bedtime.

Intestinal gas and bloating can be relieved by charcoal capsules and other OTC products containing simethicone. Avoid offensive foods, such as dairy products, certain raw vegetables, beans and sugars, including fructose and sorbitol. Soaking beans overnight in cold water will make them less gas-producing. Beano drops (digestive enzymes) will decrease the gassiness associated with beans and other gas-producing foods. A teaspoon of Angostura bitters can also decrease gassiness.

Nausea can be relieved by such medications as Tigan (trimethobenzamide HCl) and Phenergan (promethazine), although the latter causes drowsiness. Antivert (meclizine HCl) is helpful for those who experience nausea as well as dizziness or balance problems. Spasms of the smooth muscles, such as those in the intestinal tract, may be improved by antispasmodics such as Librax, Bentyl, Donnatal, and Isordil.

General suggestions: Eliminate stress and anxiety as much as possible and do not rush meals. Chew food thoroughly. Avoid alcohol, caffeine, and nicotine and eat plenty of fiber. Avoid excessive use of laxatives and enemas. Using enzyme products or switching to reduced-lactose dairy products may help the lactose-intolerant.

Identify food intolerance by eliminating a food for 10–14 days, then reintroduce the food heavily and note any reactions. Offending foods should then be completely eliminated from the diet— these often include dairy products, gluten, corn, citrus, and food additives such as monosodium glutamate (MSG). Varying the diet (food rotation) can help avoid the development of new sensitivities. If candidiasis or systemic yeast infection is suspected, an anticandida diet will help with digestive problems, especially bloating and gas. Testing for more severe gastrointestinal illnesses, including parasites, is recommended if symptoms are persistent.

The following medications have also been of some benefit in digestive problems: Klonopin, calcium channel blockers, tricyclic antidepressants, and in severe, resistant cases, Lupron (leuprolide acetate).

Note: Do not take charcoal capsules with other medications, as they may bind to the medication and render it inactive.

Edema (Swelling)

This symptom may be reduced by using diuretics, although extended use is not advised. Many physicians are unwilling to prescribe diuretics even for short-term use. Decreasing sodium intake while increasing fluid intake is an effective nondrug treatment for swelling.

Endometriosis

Endometriosis seems to affect PWCs in higher percentages than the general population, for reasons that are not understood. Treatments include medications such as progestational agents, and surgery in severe cases.

Energy Improvement

Various general treatments discussed earlier may be helpful for boosting energy according to many physicians, including Drs. Cheney and Goldstein.

> Alpha interferon (low dose)
> Doxycycline or low-dose tetracycline

Kutapressin
Vitamin B_{12}, alone or in combination with Coenzyme Q10
Vitamin B_6 (taken with other B vitamins)
Adenosine monophosphate
Antidepressants
MAOIs, especially Parnate
Symmetrel (amantadine) for flu-like symptoms
Acupuncture, acupressure

Fever

Anti-inflammatory medicines such as aspirin, ibuprofen, and acetaminophen are often used to bring down fevers. Some doctors caution against this practice except with extremely high fevers, since an elevated temperature is one of the body's natural ways of fighting infection. In fact, a slightly elevated body temperature may be detrimental to viral reproduction and thus be beneficial to the patient.

Headache

Acetaminophen (e.g., Tylenol) and NSAID (nonsteroidal anti-inflammatory medicines) including aspirin, ibuprofen (Advil) and naproxen (Aleve, now available over the counter) may help with headaches and other pain. Some researchers have cautioned against the use of these medications on a regular basis. Taking medication at the first sign of a headache and lying in a darkened room with the head packed in ice for about 20 minutes may eliminate a heavy-duty headache before it takes hold.

Nondrug treatment of headache includes acupuncture, acupressure, relaxation and meditation, massage, osteopathic or chiropractic manipulation, herbal preparations, and avoiding headache-producing foods in some cases.

Prescription medications may be necessary for more severe headaches:

Calcium channel blockers: Calan-SR (verapamil), Nimotop (nimodipine), Procardia-SR (nifedipine), Cardene (nicardipine), DynaCirc (isradipine), Norvasc (amlodipine)
Diamox LA (acetazolamide),

Imitrex (sumatriptan)

Midrin (isometheptene, dichloralphenazone, and acetaminophen)

Nitroglycerin: low-dose, sublingual

Sandostatin (somatostatin octreotide)

Tegretol (carbamazepine)

Vicodin or Anexsia (hydrocodone)

Xanax (alprazolam) or Klonopin (clonazepam): low-dose

Nasal Congestion and Sinus Pain

Nasal congestion, sinus problems, and allergies are common complaints among PWCs. Many report increased allergic symptoms
that are not relieved by allergy injections. Antihistamines are
available OTC and by prescription. Most cause drowsiness but certain newer prescription antihistamines such as Claritin (lorata-
dine), Seldane (terfenadine), and Hismanal (astemizole) do not.

Decongestants, available OTC or by prescription, reduce nasal and sinus congestion. They may cause a feeling of being "wired"
and may interfere with sleep.

Entex LA (guaifenesin and phenylpropanolamine) is less
likely to cause insomnia or a wired feeling. Nasalcrom, nasal steroids, and seasonal injections of long-acting steroids (such as Depo-
Medrol) may be helpful.

Nasal douching is an excellent, inexpensive treatment for
sinus problems and allergic rhinitis. A mixture of 8 ounces of warm
water, $\frac{1}{2}$ teaspoon salt, and a pinch of baking soda is squirted
gently several times into each nostril using a rubber bulb syringe,
with the head tilted to the side and slightly back. The water will
exit the other nostril or pass down the throat and out through the
mouth. Afterwards, the nose should be blown gently. This procedure is initially messy, uncomfortable, and awkward but can be
easily mastered with practice. It relieves nasal irritation, eliminates
allergens from the nasal passages, and drains the sinuses.

Muscle and Joint Pain

A comprehensive approach to pain management includes sleep
improvement, medications, relaxation techniques, biofeedback,
passive stretching exercises, myotherapy, relaxation exercises,

meditation, trigger point therapy and/or injections, acupuncture, acupressure, and massage. A regimen should be developed that is appropriate for the individual without undue reliance on pain medications.

However, pain is often severe enough to warrant the judicious use of medications including:

Acetaminophen (e.g., Tylenol)
Capoten (captopril)
Felbatol (felbamate): analgesic which may be helpful in mood disorders
Feldene (piroxicam)
Imitrex (sumatriptan)
Muscle relaxants and muscle pain reducers: Flexeril (cyclobenzaprine—a tricyclic antidepressant and muscle relaxant that also promotes sleep), Lioresal (baclofen), Norflex (orphenadrine), Parafon Forte (chlorzoxazone), Robaxin (methocarbamol), and Soma (carisoprodol) for muscle pain and spasm
NSAIDS (described under "Headache")
Phenergan (promethazine HCl): available with codeine
Sandostatin (somatostatin octreotide) by injection
Sinequan (doxepin): low-dose
Tegretol (carbamazepine)
Toradol (ketorolac)
Ultram (tramadol): a newer non-narcotic, non-NSAID pain reliever
Vistaril (hydroxyzine pamoate)
Xanax (alprazolam) or Klonopin (clonazepam): low-dose, often in combination with other medications

Steroids are not recommended because of serious long-term effects. CoQ10 and Alka-Seltzer Gold (or baking soda) may be helpful, according to anecdotal reports.

Sleep Disorders

Treatment of sleep disorders in CFIDS is crucial in that other symptoms usually improve when sleep is improved. Medications for improving sleep include:

Benadryl (diphenhydramine hydrochloride): OTC

Benzodiazepines: low-dose Klonopin (clonazepam), which
   increases REM sleep, or other benzodiazepines (often
   used in combination with low-dose doxepin)

Flexeril (cyclobenzaprine)

Melatonin: OTC

Sleeping medications such as Halcion, Restoril (temaze-
   pam), or Serax (oxazepam); for short-term use

Tricyclic antidepressants, low-dose: Sinequan (doxepin),
   often used in elixir form, is the most commonly used
   TCA

Unisom (doxylamine succinate): OTC

Valerian root: OTC

Other helpful interventions include creating a pleasant sleeping environment, avoiding caffeine and alcohol, exercising early in
the day (if tolerated), developing a sleep schedule, warm baths at
bedtime, meditation, using relaxation tapes, and decreasing or dis-
continuing daytime naps if they interfere with sleep at night.

Thyroid Problems

Although thyroid tests usually fall within the normal range, some
PWCs may be hypothyroid. Symptoms of low thyroid include
modest weight gain, dry skin, hair loss, brittle hair and nails, low
body temperature, fatigue, constipation, irritability, and increased
PMS. One way of monitoring thyroid function is taking axillary
(armpit) temperature in the early morning and late afternoon daily
for a few weeks and reviewing the results with your physician.

Treatment often consists of supplementing both T3 (liothy-
ronine) and T4 (levothyroxine) on a very strict schedule, while
continuing to monitor body temperature. As symptoms improve
and temperature normalizes, maintenance on T4 alone may be
prescribed. It is essential not to suppress TSH beyond its normal
levels.

This diagnosis and treatments are controversial but have created symptom improvement in many PWCs.

Urinary Tract Symptoms

Interstitial cystitis (IC), a common problem in CFIDS, is an inflammation (not an infection) of the lining of the bladder which causes frequent and painful urination. Antibiotics are not helpful for this condition. Helpful treatments are described by Dr. Larrian Gillespie in *You Don't Have to Live with Cystitis!* Some physicians who treat IC with a solution of DMSO held in the bladder for about 90 minutes report beneficial results.

Antibiotics should be used only when a urine culture shows the presence of abnormal bacteria counts. Minipress (prazosin HCl) is often helpful in the treatment of urinary tract disorders, especially prostate problems in men.

Vestibular (Balance) Disorders

Medications helpful in treating balance disorders include:

Motion sickness medications (e.g., Dramamine, meclizine, scopolamine)
Various B-vitamin preparations (orally or by injection)
Antihistamines
Stimulants (e.g., Cylert, Ritalin)
Tranquilizers, antidepressants (used as "secondary" medications to treat persistent anxiety which often accompanies vestibular disorders)

(Reynolds, *CFS Bulletin* May 1988; Levinson 1986)

Lifestyle modification, diet, and surgery are other treatments used for various types of balance disorders. In *Phobia Free*, Harold Levinson discusses the connections between anxiety, phobias, certain learning disabilities, and inner ear disorders. This book also contains suggestions regarding specific medications.

In *Balancing Act*, Mary Ann Watson, M.A., and Helen Sinclair, R.N., M.S., offer many suggestions, including:

For acute vertigo: immobilize the head; fix the eyes on something stable; don't move until the nausea subsides and then do so gradually.
Minimize stress.
Explain your limitations to your family.

Drink adequate fluids; avoid alcohol; limit sodium, caffeine, and sugar.

Exercise if possible.

Avoid fatigue.

Take safety precautions to avoid injury.

Become aware of triggers of balance problems (e.g., competing sensory input, fluorescent lights, bright lights, certain foods, activities, or body movements) and avoid or minimize them.

Some doctors attribute the "spacey feeling" (as opposed to dizziness or vertigo) to candidiasis and report that their patients are helped by an anticandida diet and medication.

If you are seeking treatment for a vestibular disorder and your family practitioner has not been able to help, ask for a referral to an otorhinolaryngologist or neuro-otologist.

Weight Gain

The weight gain experienced by most PWCs is distressing, and the mechanism by which it occurs is unknown. There is at present no known method of reversing this problem. Crash dieting, over-the-counter diet medications, and strenuous exercise are strongly discouraged for PWCs, who are likely to become sicker on such programs. Because certain medications can cause weight gain, it is wise to become familiar with the literature on all medications and supplements being used.

DHEA, a steroid secreted by the adrenal cortex, may be low in some PWCs and is claimed to be an anti-obesity, anti-AIDS, anti-aging, and anti-stress hormone. The risk-benefit ratio of treatment with DHEA is questionable and it is not available in the United States. When we are better able to understand the reason for the CFIDS-related weight gain in the absence of dietary change, we may find new solutions to this problem.

Yeast/Fungal Overgrowth: Candidiasis

The phenomenon of generalized yeast infections or overgrowth of *candida albicans* is a controversial issue. Some doctors believe that most CFIDS patients have this problem and others believe that the condition is rare or nonexistent. Existing laboratory tests for candidiasis are expensive and unreliable, and there are no clear diagnostic criteria. Much of the literature about candidiasis and treatment approaches is anecdotal and unscientific, and is therefore regarded with skepticism by the medical community.

Some of the popular books about candidiasis list almost every symptom in the world as being related to yeast infection, including most of the CFIDS symptoms we experience. It is unclear whether there is a causal connection between CFIDS and candidiasis or whether a weakened immune system is responsible for both conditions when they exist simultaneously.

Those who have taken large amounts of antibiotics, birth control pills, or corticosteroids, and those with immune dysfunction, are thought to be more susceptible to yeast overgrowth. Treatment consists of dietary modification and medication. (See the Antifungals in the "Primary Therapy" section of this chapter.) Over-the-counter antiyeast/antifungals are available but their efficacy is uncertain. Although some doctors treat many or all of their CFIDS patients with these remedies, others have not found them to be helpful.

WHEN A PWC NEEDS SURGERY

The following excerpt regarding anesthesia is taken from a letter dated February 11, 1992, which appeared in *The CFS Dyspatch* (Summer 1992) and was written by Paul R. Cheney, M.D., Ph.D.

> I would recommend that potentially hepatotoxic anesthetic gases not be used, including Halothane. Patients with Chronic Fatigue Syndrome are known to have reactivated herpes group viruses, which can produce mild and usually subclinical hepatitis. Hepatotoxic anesthetic gases may then provoke fulminate hepatitis. Finally, patients with this syndrome are known to have intracellular magnesium and potassium depletion by electron beam x-ray spectroscopy techniques. For this reason I would recommend the patient be given Micro-K using 10 mEq tablets, 1 tablet BID and magnesium sulfate 50% solution, 2 cc IM 24 hours prior to surgery. The intracellular magnesium and potassium depletion

can result in untoward cardiac arrhythmias during anesthesia. For local anesthesia, I would recommend using Lidocaine sparingly and *without epinephrine*.

PREDICTIONS

Although a cure is not known and may never be discovered, treatment of CFIDS is available and new medications are undergoing therapeutic trials in informal and formal scientific studies. All PWCs are guinea pigs in the sense that each treatment tried successfully or unsuccessfully adds to the fund of knowledge for treating CFIDS.

Treatment efforts in the future will be enhanced by our growing understanding of the neuroimmune system and ways in which we can influence immune system and neurological functioning. New drugs known as biological response modifiers, and lymphokine therapy in particular, treat immune system and neurological abnormalities and offer exciting treatment possibilities for CFIDS and other immune disorders.

Chapter 12

Coping with CFIDS

No matter how fragile the human body,
the human spirit can take just about anything.

Cheri Register, *Living with Chronic Illness*

In *The Healing Heart*, Norman Cousins discussed the distinction between treatment and healing processes. The treatment process consists of various interventions of which the body is not capable, the use of "outside" resources. Healing is the patient's realm—using the body's own capabilities, since healing is a natural drive of the body.

"I know there's no magic bullet," I wrote in my journal,

> I really want this problem to be solved by finding and eradicating the "culprit." But I know there's more in me that needs to be taken care of. In general, I need to learn self-care, in all ways. My goal is integration of the physical, emotional, and spiritual. What I believe, my lifestyle, diet, friends . . . and the big questions. How do I choose to live? How can I best take care of myself? How can I find balance in my life? I never knew illness would raise such fundamental, difficult issues. The hunt for the magic bullet was simpler. I want life to be easy and simple, but it's complex and difficult.

I resisted the concept of "myself" as the most important resource. This notion placed too much responsibility on me for something I felt was beyond my control. I wanted the answers to come from "out there," but at the same time I didn't want to be a passive victim waiting for a gallant rescue. In time I have come to view this proposition as a cooperative one. The role of researchers and pharmaceutical companies is to keep searching for causes, effective remedies and, ultimately, cures. Simultaneously, I can maximize my internal resources both for coping with this illness and helping my body to rest and heal.

The complex interaction of factors that contribute to the development of illness (genetics, environmental influences, emotional factors, and lifestyle) suggests that the healing process is equally complex. Obviously we cannot change our genetic makeup, and most of us are not in a position to engage in scientific research, but we do have choices to make regarding belief systems, lifestyle, and the ways in which we deal with our emotions. Those of us who play an active part in our quest for coping skills will be more successful.

In a questionnaire I asked PWCs to list the treatments and healing modalities that they found helpful and not helpful. In assessing such treatments as medications, herbs, vitamins, and other "externals," the response to each was divided; some found these treatments helpful and some did not. However, such interventions as rest, positive attitude, relaxation/imaging tapes, religious faith, and stress reduction techniques were listed as helpful by all who mentioned them.

In a lecture given in October 1987, in Mesa, Arizona, Bernie Siegel, M.D., described characteristics of long-term AIDS survivors:

> Acceptance of the diagnosis, but not as a death sentence
> Personal coping system
> Altered lifestyle for coping
> Cooperation with their physicians
> Commitment to life
> Sense of meaningfulness and purpose in life
> Supportive contact with other patients
> Assertiveness
> Self-nurturance
> Open communication regarding their needs
> Open communication regarding their feelings about their
>   illness.

We can learn from patients with other illnesses to mobilize our own resources, especially our belief systems. We can remain self-reliant to whatever degree possible, maintaining a sense of adequacy and self-esteem. Rather than resign ourselves to illness, we can learn to accommodate it as best we can while striving toward improved health.

HOPE AND POSITIVE EXPECTATION

Hope is a strength-enhancing quality that is important to our overall coping effort. Unrealistic hope creates disappointment and lessens our chances of developing realistic hope—the belief that we can endure and improve, and that the way we feel now need not be forever.

Paula says:

> Mentally, I think I can affect my health by working at it, thinking more positive things, using positive visualization. Who knows how it works, but I think we can .... People with the will to live can overcome things that other people just give up on. People come back from near death to become marathon bicyclists. The rest of us just lead lives of quiet desperation.

"I have learned never to underestimate the capacity of the human mind and body to regenerate—even when the prospects seem most wretched. The life-force may be the least understood force on earth," wrote Norman Cousins in 1979, emphasizing the importance of expanding our self-imposed limits and striving toward regeneration. By 1989, Cousins' belief in the positive role of hope and positive expectations had expanded. In *Head First* he emphasized the need for a positive patient-doctor relationship, reassurance ("the human apothecary"), a sense of purpose, hope, faith, love, determination, and playfulness—which he considered "powerful biochemical prescriptions."

Other physicians, including Drs. Hans Selye, Bernie Siegel, Andrew Weil, Norman Shealy, and Stuart Berger, have written about the role of the positive emotions in determining our psychophysiological responses to illness—the powers of hope and positive expectations versus remaining stuck in anger, prolonged depression, despair, blame, hatred, and bitterness. Clinging to burdensome grievances becomes self-destructive; the negative emotions, like other forms of stress, rapidly cause an exacerbation of CFIDS symptoms, as PWCs have learned from experience.

Why are all these doctors writing about hope rather than microbes and medication? In ways that seem mysterious, love, positive beliefs, and spirituality mobilize the immune system and reinforce the notion that healing is indeed a remarkably complex process.

Psychoneuroimmunology (PNI), a relatively new branch of science with ancient roots, is likely to be the medical wonder-child of the twenty-first century. All body systems are inextricably connected; the brain, psyche, immune system, respiratory system and other systems are in constant interaction; a change in any one part will affect the entire organism. Chemical messengers dash around madly inside us influenced no less by emotions than by medications and other so-called physiological events. Imagine a delicately balanced mobile: a tap on any part will affect all other parts as the mobile is set in motion and seeks to restore equilibrium. Once balance has been restored, the mobile once again comes to rest. Each part has played a role in restoring balance.

Still, many (probably most) doctors remain skeptical because they have been trained to believe that intervention at the physiological level holds the answers. Acknowledging the need to reduce stress and to eat and exercise sensibly, they are nonetheless guilty of underrating the innate healing potential of the human body, the role of the mind and emotions in so-called physical processes. Body parts are tangible; thoughts and beliefs are not. The ways in which the two interact are not yet well understood, making it easy to underestimate the power and significance of mind-body interaction.

In our personal exploration it is important to examine our belief systems to determine if they are working for or against us. Hopelessness is a harmful medicine; hope, although not a cure-all, enables our bodies to mobilize toward healing.

In The Mile-High Staircase, Toni Jeffreys described alternating hope and despair, her unwillingness to be a passive victim, her need to fight, and her determination to remain optimistic despite discouraging setbacks. "We can be logical only up to the point where optimism and hope take over," she wrote. "That is both the limitation and the saving grace of the human condition."

Illness is a catastrophe and a challenge in which hope and despair battle like archenemies. It's a juggling act. Hope takes over only to be replaced periodically by desperation and panic as exacerbations occur. How can we maintain faith that all will be well when symptoms rage and emotions run wild? Hope flees in the face of isolation, depression, anxiety, and an inability to feel "normal," as defined by past characteristics and behavior. The loss of control and our inability to trust our body to respond predictably or productively cause doubt—in ourselves, in others, and in the concept that things can ever be made right again. How can we dare to be hopeful when everything seems to be going wrong?

I wrote in my journal:

People say, "Things could be worse." We know they're right, but what good does it do? It's hard for me to be joyous because I don't have leprosy or cancer, but I still resent what I *do* have. Is it a crime to feel sorry for myself? I feel sorry for others who have CFIDS—why not me? People talk about "pity parties," an expression that makes me shudder. The concept heaps guilt on top of self-pity on top of pain. Why shouldn't I feel sorry for myself? This is a shitty illness. Why shouldn't I complain? It's a cheap hobby. People say, "Keep your chin up." I can't always do that. I feel better when I am able to be optimistic, and I'm that way about 80% of the time, maybe . . . but when I'm at my worst, hope goes to hell, along with everything else that feels good. But I know I will feel better again, that the world will appear different . . . and I look forward to that time. I know it's not possible to feel hopeful all the time, but it helps to know hopefulness will return.

So how do we "get" hope? How can we develop and maximize it? Anything that might work is worth trying. For some, part of the answer is spiritual belief, which does not necessarily mean organized religion, but rather our way of regarding life, the world, our purpose, and our ability to find peace and happiness. We examine our beliefs about life through reading, discussion, meditation, and self-exploration. We may not find ultimate conclusions or discover any earth-shattering cosmic truths but we can discover inner sources of positive belief.

Although a Pollyanna approach is not always possible or desirable, we can search for the measure of good in all people, events, and circumstances. I'm not talking about "faking it," putting on a happy face and pretending that everything is fine, but instead about embarking upon an exploratory process that can reveal various facets of our experiences. The black-and-white "all good or all bad" approach blocks the open, creative perceptions of which we are all capable.

The following suggestions have been used successfully by PWCs:

- Focus on "right now." The Alcoholics Anonymous approach of "one day at a time" can be remarkably helpful. Rather than view CFIDS as a state of total, irrevocable deprivation, we may view it as imposing limitations *right now*, and there is every possibility of improvement with self-care and the passage of time. Now isn't forever. Most things are temporary; life's only constant is its unpredictability.

- Plan something to look forward to, an event that is not likely to be jeopardized by a downward health swing. Have short-term goals that are simple and achievable in order to create a feeling of accomplishment. Break down large tasks into smaller components and take them one step at a time.

- When we focus on our deprivations, which is natural, we need to be aware of our blessings as well—not either/or but a balance of both. Is the glass half empty or half full? We can learn to appreciate the small stuff—the beauty of sunlight captured in a prism, a child's smile, a funny movie.

- We have moment-by-moment decisions to make that affect our health. Deciding to rest when necessary rather than foolishly pushing can help avoid a "crash." We don't choose feelings but we do choose behaviors.

- Continuing to explore healing and treatment alternatives leads us to those that seem most promising. If one fails, there are many others to consider.

- The advice "Learn to love yourself" sounds trite and selfish. Despite its negative connotations, selfishness really means caring for ourselves and is a positive step in personal growth, unless carried to an extreme. Rather than criticize ourselves for our frailties (remember how we hated it when our parents did that?) let's focus on our strengths and individual worth. Our self-care will pay a bonus, allowing us to care more for others in turn. As the sum total of all of our individual ideas, feelings, values, likes, dislikes, characteristics, and traits, we are in some ways like all others and in some ways unique. We can and will endure this illness and deserve credit for making it as far as we have!

The biology of hope is powerful. One's belief system has a direct influence on the healing system. Working toward peace of mind rather than perfect wellness ensures having an attainable goal. Hope cannot heal us but it can help the healing process. A determined attitude of confidence and letting go of blame will help us to move along the paths created by our positive expectations.

LIFESTYLE MODIFICATION

Activity Level

Illness often tears a smoothly-functioning lifestyle to shreds. We go from one extreme to the other: from fully functioning to crashed, broken. When we begin to feel better, we try to do it all again, and then another crash. This cycle can continue indefinitely. I continued it long after I knew it was dysfunctional because of my denial that some lousy little virus (or whatever) had the power to devastate my chosen way of life. My tendency toward extremes compounded the problem and finally led me to seek a system that was more functional and less self-defeating: moderation—the "M" word. The concept of doing only what I was capable of in my compromised, limited state meant I could no longer pretend I could do anything and everything. It meant accomplishing less, resting more, and learning to balance priorities. I have hated this process, just as I dislike many things that are good for me; it's been a difficult yet valuable lesson in adaptation. I still don't like moderation too well, but I'm better at it, and it's helpful. I've decided not to stop living but to start living smarter and more flexibly.

Many of us are accustomed to being "on call" at all times: available to meet others' needs, to take care of things, to excel, to be busy. We're not used to considering our own needs and priorities first. We've built our identities around taking care of others; we pride ourselves on constantly achieving, giving. We don't recognize the imbalance inherent in this way of life until we get sick. Then we realize how much we've allowed others to depend on us and how we've come to expect unrealistic things of ourselves, allowing ourselves to be "enablers" by trying to be all things to all people. High expectations, self-pressure to do more and do it better, to push, to conquer and overcome obstacles, to work hard, never to disappoint ourselves or others, never to say "No"—this was normal! Anything less was unacceptable!

The opposite extreme, complete inactivity, can also be harmful. Having nothing to do and no reason to wake up in the morning is to have no meaning in one's life, no sense of purpose or value. It is devastating to one's self-esteem. Kyle reports that she feels better when she is able to work even part time, "which didn't make any sense to me, except when I stayed home I just got weaker and weaker and more depressed, and my symptoms grew larger." Many PWCs are unable to work, but some can continue full time or part time. Work can offer a sense of purpose and validity. It may not be possible to continue a prior job or career, but finding meaningful activity is essential.

We need to find flexible ways of continuing to function in accordance with our abilities, which can change weekly, daily, or hourly. It is difficult, but as long as we continue to abuse our bodies by pushing too hard, it is likely that any sort of treatment or healing efforts will fail. "Lifestyle adjustment [means] getting hold of the rheostat of your life and winding it down to 60% from what it was set at before, which was sometimes at 120%," said Paul Cheney, M.D., at the CFS Convention in Oregon (November 1987). "As you wind it down to 60%, your functional capacity goes way up."

"I've learned to stop instead of pushing," says Paula:

> When I first came down with it, I kept pushing....I've learned to back off. So the dishes don't get done. So the vacuuming doesn't get done this week. So the house isn't spotless. So what? So what? And I've never done that [before]. I've always been very hard-driving; I'm a perfectionist. Whatever I do, I had to be the best: the best mother, the best teacher, the best wife, the best whatever...the super-

woman syndrome. I had it all, but I lost it. Maybe if I moderate, I can gain back some of what I lost. I'm working part time as a substitute teacher. I don't have to make an inspirational effort because I'm not the regular teacher; I have no preplanning and my days are short. While I'm working I usually feel better; I'm up; I'm doing something I enjoy doing. As long as I stick to my routine and I make sure I get the sleep I need and eat the proper foods and take care of myself, I do better. When I stop, it's real easy to get depressed.

Paula found that if she deviated substantially from her routine, she tended to overdo, under-rest, and crash:

My energy is like a basket. I have a basketful of energy; that's all the energy I have in the world. If I waste my energy on anger, then I don't have the energy to do something else. I try to control my temper, try to mellow out. I'm learning to use moderation in all facets of my life. I don't go to the extremes that I used to go to. It probably makes me an easier person to live with.

"My personal style won't change. I can't go from Type A to being totally mellow," says Bill. "I've had a lot of trouble with relaxation . . . I really need to sit down and reschedule my life." Bill created a system in which he could continue to work when he felt able, and he learned to delegate. He felt fortunate to have this degree of flexibility in his work—flexibility that he had never allowed himself in the past.

Betty described learning to rest:

I make out schedules for the course of a day. I make sure I rest—I mean bedrest. I know how to rest now. I watch TV sometimes and go to staff meetings every now and then, but not too often. [My boss] told me I could always be rehired, but I'm going to give myself a year. I need that break. I want to make sure that I don't get too overtired or sick. I want to keep a positive attitude. I want to lick this thing. I'm not pushing myself at all.

We need to regard energy as a checking account. If we keep writing checks without making any deposits, we go into credit reserve. We tend to deplete the energy balance without giving thought to replenishing it and then are astonished when it's gone and we've crashed again. ("What do you mean I'm overdrawn? I still have checks left!") Balancing work and rest is difficult because our physical and emotional status keeps changing. Some days we can do a few things; other days, nothing at all. Sometimes we require frequent rest periods between activities and then feel rejuvenated. At other times we don't feel rejuvenated if we've rested for a week! Pushing harder won't help; it makes things worse. Adaptation is difficult but possible. Adapting doesn't mean giving in, being a wimp or a coward, but learning to be sensible, learning what to give up and what to continue—and to what degree.

CFIDS comes with a warning: adjust your life to this illness, or it will overcome you. That means sensible, flexible scheduling: often saying "no" and "maybe" in response to requests; reduced work load; increased rest and leisure. Rather than viewing CFIDS as an adversary against which to wage a futile war, learning to adapt (to choose activities wisely and to set limits) is more functional in the long run.

I used to carry a full patient load as a psychologist, teach college classes, and present frequent seminars and workshops. All that time I wished I had more time to complete further graduate studies and to write. After the onset of CFIDS I continued to work as I had before for as long as I could, becoming sicker and sicker. I didn't want to give up anything, but I finally realized I had painted myself into a corner and would need to either apply for disability benefits or cut way back on my activity level, neither of which was my style. Finally, I settled with myself: no teaching, two or three workshops a year, fewer lectures, and a decreased counseling load. It was difficult to give up so much of the work I love to do but I didn't have to give it all up. I am increasingly able to add to my load but ever cautious. In the meantime I use my "feeling good" times to write and my "down times" to rest. I still resent the down times, but I have learned to live with them. For me this has been a dramatic transformation. I have decided I never want to be as busy with "have-to's" as I was back then. I enjoy the flexibility and the time to write when I am able. I still hate this illness, but I have made positive changes in my outlook and lifestyle.

Sleep and Rest

Although some PWCs are confined to bed on a daily basis, most are able to be active to some extent. There is no formula for determining the optimum rest/activity ratio, which varies over time. Resting must be a priority. Some doctors speculate that insufficient rest will prolong the course of the illness as well as increase symptom severity.

Many of us have not learned how to rest, to turn off all outside stimuli and relax fully. We equate rest with sitting or lying down, but have not learned the relaxation skills to provide quality rest. Frequent rest periods throughout the day, or at least one rest between morning and afternoon activities, are usually beneficial, as is the use of relaxation tapes and meditation.

Although some people report that they are unable to get through the day without at least one nap, others find themselves unable to sleep at night if they have napped during the day. We must each establish our own sleep rhythms and learn what our patterns are, noting that they change over time. Sleep disturbances are common among PWCs. Getting to sleep may be facilitated by light reading or watching television at bedtime, hot baths shortly before bedtime, the use of relaxation tapes (see Chapter 14), and medications as discussed in Chapter 11.

Stress Reduction

People boast of their achievements and conquests, but not about setting limits on their activity levels. Our society awards medals for accomplishing the most, the best, the fastest. We scorn those who take it easy—while we secretly envy them. A high-stress lifestyle is trendy; we are supposed to do it all, handle the pressure, juggle the roles. Our bodies aren't built to withstand such constant wear and tear. Just as cars that are driven constantly without stopping for maintenance or refueling will conk out, so will our bodies. It's time for a different, more sensible approach. Most of us weren't going to win a Nobel Prize anyway.

We need to be selective in our activities and issues, separating events within our control from those beyond it. We need to decide on a case-by-case basis whether to take an active or passive approach, determining what to fight against and what to accept. And when we can't change events, we still have the power to alter our responses to them. Stress cannot be avoided, but its effects can be minimized. It's a matter of degree. For a CFIDS patient to work full time, to be an involved parent, and then expect to have energy left over for volunteer work and a busy social life is clearly unrealistic. It is probably unwise for a healthy person to set up such a demanding schedule. Priorities must be set. In order to lower stress levels we need to examine and modify our unrealistic notions of what "normal" is for us *now*.

The following are suggestions for minimizing stress levels:

• **Establish realistic priorities and goals.** You don't have to do it all; you don't *have to* do anything. Allow the way you are feeling to decide how much you can handle. Dump the "shoulds." No one's keeping score, and martyrs aren't awarded medals.

• **Manage time effectively.** Develop a sense of your endurance level and times when you function best, and build your schedule accordingly. Don't take on more than you can reasonably handle. If anything, take on too little; you can always add more to a minimal schedule if you are able. It is easier than eliminating things from a schedule that is too full.

• **Delegate** tasks others can do.

• **Say "no"** to inappropriate requests or to anything that isn't in your best interests. Recognize that saying "no" is not the rejection of another person but simply the refusal of a request. Too often we equate being a people pleaser with being a "good person." You can be a good person by taking care of yourself—by setting limits and doing for others only what you are reasonably able to do.

• **Make requests.** Ask others to do specific things that would be helpful to you. Remember, they, too, have the right to say "no," so allow them to assume responsibility for their responses to your requests. You know it feels good to help others; grant them the same privilege by allowing them to help you. Ask directly; don't hint or complain ("I'd appreciate your picking the kids up this afternoon," rather than "I'm so tired; I don't know how I'll ever be able to pick up the kids"). When we drop hints and others don't get the messages or act on them, we become needlessly hurt and resentful. Avoid this type of manipulative behavior by making specific requests.

- **Avoid total inactivity.** Don't give up everything; total inactivity is stressful, too. Find a balance, a reasonable load. This may take some exploration. Try to remain flexible, using energy as available.

- **Reprogram your thinking.** If you're "doing a number" on yourself, being internally critical and blaming yourself for your imperfections, examine the self-messages with which you beat yourself up. You shouldn't say anything to yourself that you wouldn't say to a close friend. Such statements as "I should be perfect," "I should accomplish more," "I shouldn't rely upon others," "I should have gotten over this by now," and "I'm just giving in to this; I'm not fighting hard enough," are just a few examples of negative messages that flourish with low self-esteem.

Such messages are irrational and damaging. They can, however, be reformulated. Many contain a grain of truth that has become terribly distorted. "I'm too lazy" can be modified into the more rational message "I feel fatigued." "I should accomplish more" can be restated as "I wish I could accomplish more, but that isn't realistic right now." "I can't handle anything" can become "It's very hard for me to cope with events when I'm feeling ill."

"Before, the house had to smell like Pine-Sol; everything had to be clean. I used to have beautiful rose bushes. Everything looked perfect," says Betty. She talked over her "laziness" with her husband, her guilt that she no longer provided a showcase home for her family. "My husband said, 'So what?' My kids didn't care. It didn't bother me like it had before." Betty received her family's permission, and finally her own, to take better care of herself than she did of the house. Realize that the worst that can happen if a particular job goes undone is usually not too terrible after all.

Another bonus: our feelings are based not on external events but on our interpretation of those events, which are our self-messages. Reformulating irrational self-messages into rational ones causes the negative feelings to change and self-esteem to soar.

"I've worked real hard on not judging myself," says Paula. "I read about 'shoulds' and 'musts' and my whole life passed before me. So I worked hard on those shoulds and am learning not to put myself down. Any time you come across a should, it's usually from the outside. 'You should do this for your mother.'" Realizing how many of her self-expectations and messages stemmed from the manipulative and demanding behavior of others helped Paula to talk less judgmentally to herself and learn to set realistic limits. "When my mother says, 'If you were a good daughter, you would...,' I say, 'Then I'm not a good daughter,' which brings her up short. Then she'll realize what she's done. It took me a long time to learn to do it." Talking rationally to ourselves gives us permission to appreciate our value and to behave more appropriately by freeing us from distorted, hurtful messages.

• **Problem solve.** Identify personal problems and seek solutions. Reading self-help books, keeping a journal, and talking with others can be helpful. If you tend to blow things out of proportion, to turn minor events into catastrophes and then live in fear of dire consequences, seek the two things that will help you to feel better: information and reassurance. For example, if your fears are illness-related, read information about CFIDS and ask others for the reassurance you need. Also become aware of the irrationality of some of your fears; again, examining self-messages can help.

• **Give up the "rescuer role."** If you habitually attempt to rescue or control others (a trait called codependency), recognize the futility of this behavior. Too often we work at "fixing" others, spending lots of energy attempting to understand them, getting them to understand themselves, and causing them to change. The result is that others do not change and we waste valuable energy. The only person you can effectively take care of is yourself. Direct your efforts toward self-care. You will continue to care *about* others, but stop trying to take care *of* them (which is taking over their job). Allow others to assume responsibility for self-care, just as you are doing.

In taking this approach you may feel as if you are abandoning others, but you are really doing them and yourself a favor. Give others credit for having the ability and the responsibility to take care of themselves. A good rule of thumb (but one difficult to follow) is never to do for others what they could and should do for themselves.

• **Find Support.** Share with others—those who have CFIDS and those who don't. PWCs can provide valuable understanding and support; they can relate directly to your situation. Those without CFIDS cannot understand in the same way but can add a valuable outside perspective and keep you from getting totally caught up in the illness. To internalize your feelings seems heroic, but it is foolish. Reach out.

- **Pamper Yourself.** Do things that make you feel good. Don't deny yourself what you want and need because you're ill. It is not your fault you are ill and you certainly don't deserve to be punished. Take a bubble bath or cuddle up with your pet. Watch television. Read a good book if your brain is working or a trashy one if it isn't. One former ice skater watches videotapes of ice skaters to keep in touch with her favorite activity. Another PWC loves to cook. She spends most of the day in bed and gets up in time to cook dinner for her family, an enjoyable activity for her. Another gave up bike riding because it was too strenuous but discovered her long-neglected guitar in the garage and began to play it again.

- **Avoid what is bad for you.** Avoid situations that tend to be stressful to avoid relapses. Drastic changes of any kind should be avoided or minimized. Air travel is problematic for many PWCs, so some avoid air travel entirely, and some continue, allowing a few days after a trip to rest. Discover your exacerbation "triggers" and avoid them.

- **Laugh!** Humor is a restorative, healing force with beneficial physiological effects. Laughter can help one to let go of negative emotions and reduce anxiety levels. It is believed to have beneficial effects on the immune system as well. Norman Cousins used laughter to help diminish pain, induce sleep, and promote healing during a serious illness, and extolled the benefits of laughter in his books *Anatomy of an Illness* and *Head First.* "Illness is not a laughing matter," he wrote. "Maybe it ought to be" (1989).

My ability to laugh is a health barometer and an important coping mechanism. My sense of humor hibernates when I am feeling ill; I worry about myself when I take life too seriously. When I am very ill my sense of humor seems irretrievably lost, but it always returns. Sometimes the right person or situation brings it out of hiding. Then I feel like me again.

Seek out the people you enjoy. Put yourself in the company of those who are funny and uplifting. Avoid the "downers" and the "needies"—especially at times when you are down and needy.

- **Holidays:** Go easy. Don't build up unrealistic expectations (Waltons' Syndrome). Perfect families exist only on TV, not in real life. Don't knock yourself out—let others pitch in; tell them what you need. If you have a rule that you must cook everything from scratch, forget it—use a mix or don't cook at all. A postholiday crash is a horror to be avoided at all costs. It's just not worth it. Others should be understanding, but if they're not, it isn't your problem. Self-care must be a priority. Enjoy the holidays as much as you can; sing "I'm dreaming of a dead virus" and "All I want for Christmas is some en-er-gy." If you lack energy to sing, then hum.

• **Learn to relax.** Many people don't know how. There are many ways to practice relaxation; experiment with techniques to determine what is most effective for you. Relaxation is a skill to be learned and practiced like any other. Its beneficial effects are felt both immediately and over time, at the emotional, spiritual, and physiological levels. Individual responses vary, and there is no one correct method or technique that is superior to others. Read about various techniques and try them on your own, purchase a prerecorded audiocassette (see Appendix C), or consult a stress management clinic, a psychotherapist, or a physician specializing in stress management.

In most relaxation exercises the individual assumes a comfortable position in an environment free of distractions. Muscle relaxation and deep breathing are employed; affirmations or certain phrases are repeated internally; and images of healing, relaxing settings, and personal enhancement are developed. The individual returns slowly to the environment. Relaxation exercises are generally practiced once or twice a day for about twenty minutes.

The use of guided imagery is based on the theory that an individual's ability to imagine and feel a positive outcome can help to create it. Imagery clearly has application in the treatment of CFIDS. It provides a time-out period during which one can clear the mind and look inward to develop insights, create peaceful feelings, and encourage self-healing, producing emotional changes that in turn create internal change in neurochemistry and physiology. Form images that are compatible with your belief system. The more appropriate and well-defined the image, the more effective the imagery will be.

• **Biofeedback** is a training process that takes place over a period of weeks or months. It employs equipment that monitors bodily functions (such as muscle tension and hand temperature) to indicate one's level of relaxation, and offers feedback in the form of noises or flashing lights to signal progress toward the desired response. Relaxation techniques are used along with biofeedback instruments, which simply monitor functioning while the individual learns to relax. The patient develops a sense of control over bodily functions that are usually beyond conscious control. Biofeedback is also helpful for treating certain symptoms such as headache and body pain.

• **Meditation** is the process of focusing one's attention on a bland stimulus in order to clear the mind and produce a sense of inward calm. Tuning out distractions and lowering body arousal brings a sense of quietness and peace, which feels good and brings about positive psychological/physiological changes. Several types of meditation are taught. Some use a mantra or a meaningless phrase for focus; others use a one-syllable word such as "one," or words related to the desired outcome, such as "calm and relaxed." Deep breathing and turning off the mind are the common denominators among all types, which may be learned from a trainer, a psychotherapist, books, or audiotapes. Benefits include relaxation, stress reduction, spiritual development, expansion of the mind, and heightened creativity.

• **Autogenic Training** is a form of relaxation that relies on passive concentration accompanied by certain phrases related to a series of specific exercises. These are aimed toward the creation of bodily sensations, such as feelings of warmth and heaviness and slowed breathing. Mastering these highly structured exercises requires continual practice. As with meditation, individual instruction, group instruction, or materials used on one's own can teach this skill.

• **Hypnosis** may be frightening to those whose only exposure has been watching people on television acting like ridiculous barnyard animals. Such simplistic, entertainment-oriented notions about the powers of hypnosis are misleading. Hypnosis is the achievement of an altered state of consciousness in which the unconscious mind plays a central role. It taps the neural links between mind and body—the psyche and the soma. In this context we attempt to convert words, ideas, sensations, beliefs, and expectations into the physiological healing process.

A hypnotized individual is in full control at all times and will refuse to do anything objectionable or harmful. Work with a reputable hypnotherapist who has training credentials, experience, and an approach with which you are comfortable. Self-hypnosis can be learned by working with a hypnotherapist, using commercially marketed cassette tapes, or practicing exercises from reputable self-help books.

• **Massage** may provide benefits such as increased relaxation, decreased pain, improved circulation, and other positive physiological and emotional effects. Massages may be given by professionals (use a reliable referral source), or someone you know may be willing to learn massage techniques.

• **Exercise** promotes cardiovascular fitness, strengthens muscles, burns calories, and fights depression. Some PWCs report that mild exercise gives them increased energy and mental alertness, which may be caused by the production of energizing hormones called catecholamines. Exercise has been speculated to enhance immune functioning. It also provides a temporary escape from problems and creates a sense of accomplishment, a self-esteem boost. One PWC reports that he walks "just to be out in public. It makes me feel like I'm part of life again."

However, exercise is not appropriate for all PWCs. Medical advice, common sense, and a trial-and-error process help determine its advisability. If you have not exercised in some time, start slowly, perhaps with only a brief warm-up routine or stretching exercises. Yoga, t'ai chi, or water aerobics may be tolerable and helpful. Stop exercising when you *begin* to feel fatigued; don't wait for exhaustion to set in. If exercise makes you feel worse over the course of 24–48 hours, discontinue or modify it.

CREATING A NEW LIFE PHILOSOPHY

Illness offers us new opportunities whether we want them or not, and forces us to examine issues that would otherwise be left unexplored. No longer able to view the world in accustomed ways, we question the meaning of life—specifically, our own lives.

If we perceived ourselves as passive victims before becoming ill, this perception may be significantly heightened when faced with CFIDS. Learning to view ourselves as active, influential forces in the course of our lives creates the opportunity to identify options and make positive choices.

Our value systems undergo change; we may become less materialistic and more in touch with health issues, the importance of relationships with family and friends, and spiritual beliefs. We come to place greater value on self-care. We become more human, loving, aware of people and things around us, and fully alive—ironically, at a time when we feel half-dead.

Spirituality, whether in the sense of organized religion or development of one's own belief system through reading, talking with others, and meditating is helpful to many PWCs. Some have stated that their religious/spiritual beliefs allowed them to get through the CFIDS ordeal. As prior beliefs are questioned, involvement with a traditional or nontraditional belief system is a source of great comfort.

We learn to rely less on the opinions and beliefs of others as a result of their misunderstanding of CFIDS and our ensuing lifestyle changes. Thus we come to rely more fully on ourselves and to respect the resources that have enabled us to learn, cope, and survive. We learn that our own approval has the most value.

No longer able to rely on former goals and life expectations, we learn to value and live in the moment, to take advantage of "right now." It is too late for yesterday, although we remain nostalgic for the way things used to be, and too soon for tomorrow, which is made especially unpredictable by radical fluctuations in health. Today is all we have to work with.

Illness offers an opportunity to develop a new sense of purpose. A retired college professor who had always wanted to learn charcoal drawing now enjoys his new-found talent. Some PWCs have adopted CFIDS as their primary cause, writing for newsletters, facilitating support groups, or becoming politically involved.

As our ability to function vacillates, our lives gain and lose meaning. Everything is up for grabs; life becomes chaotic. But from the chaos can emerge transformative insights and understandings. As we meet the major challenge of leading meaningful lives despite severe limitations, our perceptions are permanently altered. We learn to identify and rid ourselves of extraneous baggage and focus on what really matters. The process of learning to live and love more fully is necessary to our individual and collective survival.

FEELINGS

What are feelings anyway? You can't see them or find the right words for them; they defy logic. And yet they're undeniably there. Our feelings vary unpredictably, interspersed with denial or numbness born of a need to push difficult emotions away.

We are taught that hiding emotions, or better still, not having them in the first place, is a sign of maturity and strength. ("Bi-ig girls, they don't cry-iy-iy," went the song.) If we can't deny feelings, we attempt to justify them with elaborate explanations or apologies. The majority of my patients cry in counseling sessions at one time or another and most of them apologize. People are *supposed* to express feelings in a psychologist's office and yet many of them need permission because of our cultural taboo.

I am not advocating that we announce our current emotional status every thirty minutes. It is natural to have feelings and it's normal to express them. Rules to the contrary don't make any sense. We have no choices about what feelings to have; as human beings, we are going to have all of them and often unpredictably. Our rational minds will say, "No need to feel upset about *that*," while our emotions have other plans. We do have a choice, though, about how to deal with those emotions behaviorally—how we express them.

Emotions don't have to be justified. They are not to be judged. Sometimes we choose to conceal them, at least temporarily, but any strong feeling will ultimately need to be expressed in some way. However uncomfortable, feelings are a manifestation of being human. We might as well accept them and learn to handle them as best we can.

PWCs experience fear regarding the illness and its possible implications and complications. The procedures we have undergone, the new treatments we have tried, and the strange symptoms we have experienced are all frightening. There is so much that remains unknown, and the unknown is always scary. Expressing the fear and seeking both information and reassurance is enormously helpful. Talk with family, friends, and health care professionals about your fears. Sometimes we use humor to mask fear, which is healthy to a degree. It is a relief to be able to laugh at ourselves.

Anger is considered the most unacceptable emotion. We tend to equate it with shouting, belligerence, loss of control, and hurtful exchanges. It need be none of these. Anger is a natural emotion and can be expressed constructively, although many of us have never had role models for the healthy expression of anger. We are used to seeing anger displaced and have probably done so ourselves, blowing up at a child or spouse when we are really angry because of something else. We often make the mistake of allowing angry feelings to control us because we don't realize the options we have for dealing with them. Anger means there is a problem that needs to be addressed and solved. It begins with hurt or some other unexpressed feeling. When we are emotionally sensitive, as we are during CFIDS exacerbations, anger is close to the surface and can be easily triggered by minor events. Limbic system dysfunction also causes angry outbursts.

Why are we angry? We are angry that we're sick. That we are deprived. That we don't have energy. That we can't do what others can do, or what we used to do. We are angry that we have been singled out to be sick while other people are well. We are angry because we feel misunderstood by health care professionals, the media, and those close to us. We are angry because there is no cure. We are angry because we can't will CFIDS away, no matter how good we are. We are angry because we've lost so much. We are angry because we don't know if we can get back what we have lost. We are angry when others don't really listen to us or hear what we are trying to say. We are angry because we often can't express ourselves as we would like to. We are angry because we are scared, lonely, and miserable. We are angry because our income is limited and our medical bills are huge. We are angry at ourselves because we don't know what to do to make ourselves well again. We are angry because our responsibilities and expectations continue although our energy does not. We are angry because we often don't like ourselves or accept our situation very well.

We have good cause to be angry, and need to find safe outlets for our anger. Some suggestions: express it, verbally or in writing, but not in an accusatory manner. Identify the problems and feelings that may have triggered the anger; when these are dealt with, the anger may dissipate. If you feel you may explode at someone (an act that you could later regret), take a time out. Get away temporarily and return when you are capable of a more reasonable discussion. Physical activity can be helpful, if possible. Try throwing darts, pounding a pillow, throwing unbreakable things, or yelling out loud when you are alone.

Allow your anger to help you identify problem issues and work through them. Don't allow it to jeopardize your relationships with others; don't attempt to "punish" them or yourself. If you try to repress anger, it will turn to bitter resentment or to depression, both undesirable outcomes. So express it carefully, in a way that isn't belittling or damaging to others. Simply let them know how you feel. Warn your spouse or significant other when you are feeling anger in order to help them interpret your comments and actions.

Having watched a talk show about AIDS, Paula said:

> [The AIDS patients] were talking about forgiving yourself; forgiving the people around you all the hurts and the angers, to allow you to love yourself. And if you let go of the anger and the fear, your body will start to heal itself. I sat there stunned . . . . It is going to take a lot of work to let go. I hadn't thought that much about loving myself . . . . I resent my body for having failed me. To forgive that and love myself [is] something foreign . . . . Releasing suppressed anger would give me energy.

Later, Paula noted that her difficulty in asking others to do things for her caused her to become "very demanding, very resentful, very angry, which caused [them] a lot of anger in response to me. What I was giving out was what was coming back."

Depression usually waxes and wanes; for some it remains constant. Depression is a result of being ill, suffering limitations and losses, and of distorted thinking which results in irrational self-messages. It is quite painful but natural to be depressed. Sometimes the depression occurs in reaction to an event, at other times it seems to sweep in unexpectedly and is more difficult to accept because it's impossible to understand. Abnormalities in neurotransmitter levels in the brain also account for or contribute to bouts of depression. Treatment with antidepressants can correct this bio-chemical problem.

What to do? Some hot tips: allow yourself to feel, to experi-ence the depression. Allow it to run its course. Denying it and faking happiness can prolong the depression. Cry and feel sorry for yourself for a while. Tears are cathartic. One PWC described times when she was profoundly depressed but unable to cry. When the tears finally came, the depression lifted. We discussed "crying trig-gers," for example, certain songs or sad movies that would invoke tears to complete the cycle for her. You will emerge from depres-sion once you have gone through it. As difficult as it is to believe during a depressive episode, depression is not forever. You really will feel good again. Identify other issues (problems, repressed emo-tions) that have triggered the depression and deal with them when you are able.

Plan things to look forward to whenever possible. Enlist the support of others, or if you need to be alone, try to communicate this so others won't feel rejected. (When you withdraw, people often think you are angry at them.) Learn what you can from the depression; for some reason, the most meaningful learning experi-ences are painful. Physical touch may help, as can some type of meaningful activity if you are up to it.

Talking about feelings can help, even about feelings that have been talked about before. You can talk to yourself or talk with others. Let others know that your intent is only to express feelings and sort them out, that you are not expecting to be res-cued or fixed. Let them know whether or not you want feedback; sometimes we just need to talk, and other times we want to hear reactions in order to develop new perspectives.

Keeping a journal serves several functions. Writing thoughts and feelings is cathartic; it allows us to experience and clarify them in a new way and to find new meaning in them. As we write, we learn about ourselves. We should write only for ourselves but may later choose to share with others parts of what we have written. Blocked emotions will often surface; old baggage ("unfinished busi-ness") can be explored and laid to rest. A journal of events, reac-tions, thoughts, and feelings allows not only self-expression but also an opportunity to review the past by rereading. You will prob-ably surprise yourself with newly developed insights and progress.

A shy psychotherapy patient said very little during her early sessions although she was experiencing deep conflicts and insecurities. She began to keep a journal. Each week she would shyly present her recent entries for me to read. Once she had communicated in writing about events, thoughts, and feelings she could not verbalize, she became able to talk about them.

Unexpressed feelings will fester, later popping out unexpectedly and often inappropriately. Repressed emotions may be damaging psychologically and physiologically to individuals and relationships. The constructive expression of feelings can enhance relationships, but the feelings themselves (not the other person, or the other person's behaviors) must be the focus. Constructive emotional expression does not involve placing blame, labeling, or criticizing others.

GRIEVING: HANDLING LOSS

The process of grieving is a difficult, painful, but necessary reaction to any significant loss. Healing cannot take place until the loss is mourned. CFIDS-related losses include: energy, vitality and enthusiasm, good health, ability to perform responsibilities and activities, certain roles, pleasure, motivation, predictability and control, income, self-esteem, relationships, others' former perceptions of us, jobs and/or careers, educational or training plans, leisure activities, plans, and dreams. We have literally lost vital parts of our lives and of ourselves.

There are several stages in the grieving process: denial, bargaining, anger, sadness/depression, and acceptance/adaptation. We may experience the stages in order, skip around, omit certain stages entirely or return to one stage repeatedly. There is no right way to grieve, nor an easy one.

The **denial** stage is often experienced as a general numbness, reflecting our inability to absorb and deal with a painful experience all at once. We are unable to accept the possibility or the enormity of the loss. "This illness just can't be real." To protect ourselves from being overwhelmed by the sudden impact, we numb out, allowing the hurt to be absorbed gradually. During this stage we may tend to overdo in terms of activity level and then crash, often repeatedly, as we alternately deny and are reminded of our illness. Using humor or intellectualizing the problem may serve as a buffer at this stage and can be helpful if used to help us survive this stage rather than keeping us stuck there.

During the **bargaining** phase we try to make deals with ourselves, our doctors, or with God. We promise to "be good" in exchange for restoration of what we have lost. "If I eat vegetables, deny myself junk food, if I listen to 'doctor's orders,' maybe I'll get back my good health in return." And there are the retrospective "if onlys" . . . if only I had taken better care of myself, not gone on that long trip, not tried to do so much, not taken those antibiotics, not eaten junk food. We can get stuck in this stage or return to it periodically, but generally the bargaining stage is brief, if we experience it at all.

Anger! Much of the anger lies in the unfairness of a situation that is beyond our control. There is no responsible party, no single causative event, and no direct revenge to be taken. CFIDS shouldn't happen to us or to anyone. There should be a cure. Our suffering should be better understood by others. There should be more research. That all these things are true doesn't change anything. We are angry because we have been hurt and deprived. The anger stage is guilt-producing: not only are we more dependent on others, but sometimes we are not even *nice* to them. Others will tolerate and excuse some of our anger, but we need to channel it in nondestructive ways. Getting to and through the anger stage is a significant step toward recovery from emotional wounds.

Sadness and depression is the period of hurt that accompanies the full realization that what has happened is real and devastating. Hopelessness, helplessness, disappointment, isolation, and self-pity dominate the emotional scene. During this stage we may feel that our lives are over, we will never feel good again, we are totally useless, everything has been taken away, no one understands, and there is nothing left to live for. As depression lifts, anger may resurface as the feelings are directed outward instead of inward.

Acceptance and adaptation. "Ultimately chronic fatigue syndrome becomes a background fact of life, not a foreground obsession," wrote Karyn Feiden. Our losses become integrated into our lives. We give up trying to manipulate reality and accept the situation. We make peace instead of war. We adapt to a difficult situation and focus on what we can do, remaining painfully aware of what we cannot do. New strengths emerge. We stop living in the "if onlys," with what should be, and learn to live with what is. We begin to restructure our lives. CFIDS, we realize, is not the sole factor that defines us. We can live within its limitations and go on. We are able to focus outward again, to become aware of others and their needs. We are less afraid, more able to accept ourselves and others. We have learned to be flexible, for our very survival depends upon our ability to bend, to go with the flow. Rather than remain passive and stuck, we move forward, taking responsibility for the management of our lives. But our fears and doubts continue; acceptance is a matter of degree.

The grieving process is lengthy and bumpy; there are no shortcuts. We bounce back and forth between stages, sometimes feeling we have arrived at the adaptation stage, only to find ourselves back in anger, denial, or depression. Having been there before makes it a little easier the second, third, or fourth time around. Knowing we have survived these stages before, we feel less trapped and overwhelmed by them.

COUNSELING

Remember the old movies in which the psychiatrist (a bearded man on the other side of the desk or couch) remained detached, aloof, stroking his beard and saying "uh huh" occasionally? And only crazy people went to see him, right? Since then there have been movies like *Ordinary People*, in which therapists are depicted as human beings who are trained to help people sort out issues and problem-solve. There used to be a great stigma attached to therapy, but seeking help has become more acceptable—even trendy in some circles. It is not a sign of weakness to seek professional help for coping with the devastating effects of CFIDS: life adjustment issues, depression, and anxiety. Therapy is a safe place to express feelings. It can feel good to have time for yourself, focusing solely on your needs without guilt about not meeting the needs of others. As Stephanie Simonton pointed out in *The Healing Family*, "It is not a sign of failure to seek a therapist but a willingness to grow."

Local and national support groups, physicians, and other PWCs can provide names of CFIDS-educated therapists. Many qualified therapists are only vaguely familiar with CFIDS and will need to become educated by PWCs. A therapist who is experienced in treating those with chronic illnesses will generally appreciate receiving CFIDS literature.

Other people may not understand or approve of your seeking psychological help. Their opinions are not your problem, but you may be negatively affected by their attitudes. If so, explain to them the basis for your decision but don't feel you must justify it.

A good fit between therapist and client is essential. If you feel understood and taken seriously and the therapist is supportive and growth-oriented, you have probably found someone with whom you will work well. If you have reservations, discuss them with the therapist to see if the problems can be solved. If not, you are the consumer; find another therapist with whom you feel more comfortable. If this process occurs repeatedly, examine your expectations; if they are unrealistic, you will never find someone who can meet them.

SUPPORT GROUPS

There are two main types of CFIDS support groups: larger, information-oriented groups at the state- or large city-level, and smaller emotional support groups. Larger organizations often operate CFIDS hotlines and distribute newsletters to members. Smaller therapy groups, where the group's goal is to meet individual needs by sharing and interacting, may be led by professionals or by PWCs. Many PWCs participate in both types of groups.

In the group setting we are reminded that we do not suffer alone, that other PWCs share our struggle. Comfort, support, shared feelings, coping suggestions, exchange of information about treatment, and the opportunity to help others can be invaluable. As one CFIDS group participant said, "Joining this group is the best thing I ever did. Now I know I'm not crazy."

I conducted a CFIDS support group that met regularly for about eighteen months. Group size varied unpredictably because of health fluctuations. We discussed such topics as practical problem solving; life disruption and changes; dealing with the medical community; dropping the "I'm fine" facade; self-care; feelings regarding CFIDS, our lifestyles and limitations; coping and adaptation skills;

communicating with family, friends, employers, and coworkers; seeking new meaning and opportunities; learning moderation; relaxation and healing techniques; identifying and changing irrational self-messages; and exchange of individual experiences and concerns.

Some patients report that although some group interaction is helpful, too much contact or negative contact causes further preoccupation with CFIDS. Bill says, "I have decided for the time being to divorce myself, where possible, from . . . support groups and reading the literature. I found that, after a while, these contacts were making me more obsessed with the illness." Such is often the case when complaining becomes the main focus of a group—a pitfall to be avoided. Talking to people who are sicker than we are or who have been sick for a longer time can fuel our pessimism. Conversely, talking with those who are doing really well can make us feel like failures, like losers in a competition. Supportive contact with other CFIDS patients needs to be balanced with people and things in the "well world."

COPING TECHNIQUES

The following summary list of suggestions has been compiled from patient reports, personal experience, books, and articles.

> Learn moderation and self-pacing.
> Get adequate rest.
> Make self-expectations more realistic, reasonable, and
>   do-able.
> Learn to "Go with the flow." Do what you can, and let the
>   rest go.
> Talk positively to yourself.
> Focus more on taking care of yourself and less on "fixing"
>   others.
> Delegate responsibility.
> Ask for what you need (support, help, reassurance).
> Seek to build and maintain healthy relationships.
> Let go of the need to accomplish constantly.
> Recognize and express emotions constructively: deal with
>   depression and the grieving process. Don't repress
>   feelings.

Recognize and seek to eliminate self-defeating behaviors.

Develop a sensible nutrition/exercise program; exercise moderately if you can; don't force anything that doesn't feel good or right; don't push; take it very slowly.

Learn to listen to your body; understand and respect its signals.

Seek meaning and purpose in your life through activities and goals.

Become aware of the things for which you are grateful.

Learn to appreciate small pleasures.

Learn to cope with an unpredictable future.

Retain your sense of humor as much as possible.

Examine your perspectives and life philosophy—determine what really matters to you.

Learn to slow down and live in the moment—stop and smell the roses.

Accept that life is not fair and that we must learn to do the best we can with what we have.

Learn to be more patient, more flexible, less driven, less perfectionistic.

Try to communicate frequently and productively with others.

Communicate with yourself: keep a journal in which you can write all the things you aren't willing or able to communicate with others.

Identify and develop new resources.

Give yourself credit for coping with a very difficult situation.

Recognize that your primary job right now is getting well.

Learn to put away the past (hurts, angers, resentments).

Use "now" as a standard, not how you used to be.

Learn to reduce stress.

Seek positive relationships with physicians and other health care professionals.

Respect your body's innate self-healing potential and attend to your body's needs.

Learn about illness and wellness; ask questions, seek answers and new ideas.

Educate those you love about your illness.

Prioritize. As one PWC said, "If I can't do it, screw it!"

Don't define yourself solely in terms of the illness.

Keep a calendar of symptoms, activities, life changes, and medications, and try to find correlations or patterns to identify helpful and harmful factors.

Take one step at a time.

Do the things that make you feel good.

Let go of as many "shoulds" as possible.

Identify and deal with other life problems, which can compound the effects of illness.

Don't compare your progress to that of others.

Practice self-affirmations and healing imagery.

Don't apologize for being ill or having limitations.

Treat yourself with dignity and respect.

Forgive yourself and others when you can. Throw guilt and blame out the window.

Laugh!

Reach out to others: talk, hug, touch, love.

Chapter 13

CFIDS and Relationships

When CFIDS disrupts our lives, it affects those with whom we are close as well. Relationships are altered by changes in individuals. We experience the dual pull of wanting to share our pain with others and wanting to pull away from them into our cocoons. Others have the dual reaction of wanting to be understanding and helpful and wanting to escape from the pain and helplessness of watching a loved one suffer.

We ask ourselves how much it is appropriate and safe to confide in others and how to help them understand. We wonder how they can live with us and how much of our illness and our ill behaviors they will tolerate before they leave us. We wonder if caring will crumble in the face of adversity.

And as much as we try to share the experience with others, we realize that this illness is ours alone. Others may be victims of the fallout, but we bear the direct brunt. CFIDS changes us. We need to understand our changes in order to cope productively with changes in our relationships. We need the cooperation of others in order to adapt and cope with our relationships.

Important people in our lives need to be educated regarding the illness and its effects so they can better understand what is happening. In deciding how much information to give them, we should consider their roles in our lives and how much interest they have in CFIDS. Sources of information include medical literature, popular literature, books about CFIDS, discussions, and support group meetings. Some partners want to read everything available, but most will be satisfied with a few articles. It is best to select those that present a lot of general information concisely and are at an appropriate reading level. Most people will probably not want to read detailed medical information but would like to know about the possible causes, effects and symptoms, the duration of the illness, and any theories regarding contagion (see Chapter 1).

We should also help others to understand that we have greater needs than in the past. It is the responsibility of the PWC to identify these personal needs and ask others for appropriate help in meeting them. Others should act as supportive helpers rather than rescuers. The role of rescuer involves mind reading and inappropriate assistance, that is, doing for others what they should do for themselves. Rescuing may seem helpful and even heroic but it is neither. It is usually harmful to the PWC's self-esteem and puts both parties at risk of developing resentments. Giving advice is a form of rescuing and is generally not well received unless it is requested or clearly needed; otherwise it is likely to be viewed as an intrusion and disregarded. In general, caregivers are most helpful when they offer help without pushing.

Clear communication is extremely important. Often, we want to be open but also feel we should say what the other person wants to hear, which can create barriers between people. We tend to "clean up" our statements to make them seem acceptable; in the process we censor our true feelings. Acknowledging these feelings can be scary and difficult, but relationships are enhanced by the freedom to express feelings openly. The notion that good people don't have "bad" feelings is a myth. We are not saints; we are real people with real feelings.

Learning to communicate assertively is a good idea regardless of health status. Assertiveness means expressing one's ideas, feelings, and needs appropriately, not aggressively: asking for what we need, refusing inappropriate requests or demands, and making direct statements rather than hints. It allows people to communicate honestly without covering up or protecting one another. It enhances self-esteem and feelings of self-control, thus helping to combat depression.

Sexual relationships are affected by CFIDS. Many PWCs experience decreased sex drive, and men may experience difficulty having or maintaining an erection. Certain medications as well as the illness itself may cause delayed orgasm, another source of frustration for PWCs. Lack of energy contributes to these sexual difficulties. Couples should communicate about the change in sexual frequency and other issues. Less frequent sex and less vigorous or satisfying sex is disappointing; individuals and couples feel deprived of intimacy. Adaptive measures, including cuddling without pressure for sex and less vigorous sexual activities, help to make up for the losses. If discussion and problem-solving attempts are unsuccessful, a sex therapist can help with CFIDS-related sexual issues.

GRIEF AND MOURNING

Couples and families, as well as PWCs, may feel a need to grieve. The losses they experience are many: financial changes, familiar patterns and activities, ways of sharing responsibilities. In addition, those who care about the PWC will be affected personally by her or his losses as an individual. You may be able to grieve together, going through the process at the same pace, or you may arrive at different stages independently. Emotional sharing keeps loved ones in touch with each others' feelings and experiences. If emotional expression has been repressed or denied in the relationship in the past, this sharing will be doubly difficult but necessary so that people don't grow apart.

Grieving and rebuilding allow new strengths and interests to emerge. Just as we need to grieve with those we care about, we need to share laughter when we can. Seeing the humor in a situation relieves tension and provides a break from the pain. Laughing and crying are not that different from one another; each allows a letting go of feelings, expressions of the comic and tragic aspects of life.

IMPACT OF CFIDS ON FAMILIES

Chronic illness disrupts a family's usual patterns and dynamics. All families develop ways of coping with stress over time, but chronic illness is an unexpected and unusual type of stress that lingers and causes continuing disruption. Families that are cohesive, flexible, resourceful, and adaptable will be more successful at coping with CFIDS. The following suggestions can help:

Talk about what's happening. Pretending it's not there won't make it go away. Discuss the illness and its effects on the family as a whole and on individual family members. Don't assign blame;

discuss the illness as a shared problem. Make sure all family members have an understanding of the illness, even young children.

Open communication requires that all family members should be allowed to speak for themselves, not for one another, and that each accepts the others' feelings as valid. This means not trying to talk others out of how they feel or expecting them to become optimistic when they are concerned or depressed. Empathize with the others' feelings, even when you wish they didn't feel that way. When the PWC says, "I'm scared that I'll never recover," instead of saying, "That's ridiculous—of course you will!", a more empathetic statement would be, "I know this is frightening for you. Not knowing can be very hard." This allows the PWC to feel understood and supported, rather than told how to feel.

Develop as much flexibility as possible in the way the family functions. Brainstorm to seek solutions to new problems. If responsibilities have to be reassigned, make sure each family member is clear about what is expected.

In many families one person is unofficially regarded as the caretaker. This may be the person who now has CFIDS. All family members should assume some of the caretaking responsibilities, rather than regarding them as the responsibility of only one person. This lessens the burden on any one individual and teaches valuable skills to the others.

The PWC should be open in discussing his or her limitations and problems rather than covering them up in an attempt to shield the family from difficulty and pain. However, the PWC should avoid becoming overly dependent on other family members, especially young children. Taking on primary support of a parent is an inappropriate burden for a child.

The family should avoid attempts to overprotect the PWC, and avoid making assumptions about what the PWC can do or would like to do. The PWC should be involved whenever possible in making family plans and given the option of participating.

If extended family members, neighbors, or others in the community are available, they can provide additional support and perhaps help with the additional responsibilities created by the illness.

The needs of all family members, not just the PWC, must be understood and respected. In addition to showing caring for the ill family member, each must consider personal well-being a priority.

Children of PWCs often resent the limitations imposed on their lives by the illness. They may react by becoming demanding or depressed, by blaming themselves for the illness or family problems, or by developing behavior problems at school or at home. They may be unaware of the connection between their behavior and their parent's illness and the consequent disruption of stability in their lives. Their reactions and behaviors should be discussed openly and reassurance offered. Help in the form of individual or family therapy should be sought if the problems increase or do not resolve over time. In any case, it is neither helpful nor healthy to condone or ignore a child's inappropriate behavior because the parent feels guilty or incapable of discipline.

Express caring for one another openly through words and gestures. Touch; hug. Don't assume that the others know you love them—let them know! Acknowledge their feelings. Express hope. Let all family members know that they are valuable and helpful to the family. Sharing these feelings can create new strength, growth, and closeness.

FOR SINGLE PWCS

Enduring CFIDS as a single person is a mixed bag. You have the privacy and freedom to make your own schedule without taking someone else's needs into account. However, you may also lack the comfort of a primary support person. There is no one else to take up the financial slack, to complain to, to bring you tea and toast. (Remember, however, that some partners of PWCs are unwilling to do these things.) You may be forced to live with parents or grown children, and feel dependent and perhaps guilty.

If you are dating or seeking a permanent relationship, the issue of what to tell the other person inevitably comes up. It is usually best not to disclose detailed information too soon—but don't keep your illness a secret either. Look for a middle ground between these extremes and you will find the level of disclosure that works best for you. CFIDS adds a difficult dimension to new relationships; some thrive anyway and others don't last. Some people will distance themselves at the mention of CFIDS, usually because of their own fears and prejudices or their unwillingness to become involved with someone who is ill.

Even if a primary relationship is not feasible for you right now, don't isolate yourself. Plan at least minimal activities that involve contact with the outside world, such as trips to the library, a class, or a movie. Interact with others, stay in touch with friends and relatives, as well as other PWCs. It's vital that you have a support system.

Tamara Lewis, a single PWC living in Seattle, Washington, has written a sensitive piece called "Living Alone with CFIDS" and has generously allowed its inclusion in this book:

Shockingly, the world has shrunk down to the size of my apartment. And my body is no longer the vehicle with which I move through life. Rather, it *is* my life. Occasionally, after hours alone, aching and ill, a strange collapse of boundaries occurs. I cease to feel separate from the walls of my apartment. It is as if what happens in my apartment happens inside my mind; a knock on the door startles me as if someone just rapped on my skull. What happens on the television is happening to me. I feel the tragedy of the evening news in my body.

I am no longer expected anywhere by two o'clock or even by Tuesday. And I live alone, so no one's coming home for dinner—and I don't bump into anyone on the way to the bathroom. So, I can go days without seeing anyone. And I begin to feel unreal. I look out my window just to be sure—to be sure I'm still in relation to something, even if it's just the street I live on. I live on a street, therefore I live.

No one sees me staring lifelessly at the walls. No one sees me toss through another sleepless night. No one sees me lying on the floor crying. My illness and I are like an unsolved crime—no eyewitnesses.

When the relentlessness of the illness has finally gotten to me, I am without good judgment. I can't tell what's wrong and I can't tell what I need. It is at those moments that I most need someone to walk into the room and state the obvious: "Turn on the lights. Eat something. Call your doctor." It is those moments when living alone is most painful.

It may seem obvious that the solution is to reach out and call a friend. And many have said, "If you ever need anything, call." But that would require rational thought and the problem is, I've lost my brain. I can't figure out who to call. And I can't figure out what to say. And if at long last I regain my clarity and realize what I need, it is so very difficult to call someone and say: "I need to know someone cares. I need to know that I'm still me. I need to think of reasons to live. I need to be held." These are not calls people are accustomed to receiving as they're on their way to a Mariner's game. And it puts me at great risk to ask. I think this illness should be renamed Chronic Vulnerability Syndrome.

WHEN THE PWC IS A CHILD

Children generally require more attention than adults. They should be given information about CFIDS that is appropriate for their age and should be encouraged to ask questions. Don't be afraid to say, "I don't know" if you cannot answer their questions. Try to be reassuring but don't withhold the truth, as this may jeopardize their trust. Ask them about their feelings: Do they feel left out of important activities? Ignored by their peers? Burdensome to the family? Different, not okay? Unable to do "normal" things? They may be able to express their feelings and needs quite clearly, or might require your help to clarify them.

Adjust your expectations of the child in accordance with a realistic, objective assessment of strengths and impairments in cognitive and physical functioning. Unrealistically high expectations will make the child feel misunderstood or a constant failure. Expectations which are too low do not offer credit for abilities and may allow the child to escape appropriate responsibilities and standards of acceptable behavior. Sometimes the input of a third party (professional, family member, or personal acquaintance) who is familiar with CFIDS and with the child can help make this assessment. Expectations should be kept somewhat flexible since symptom severity varies.

If the child's attendance at school is a problem, look into resources for home instruction. Educate the child's teacher about CFIDS (especially its cognitive effects) and work cooperatively to develop a flexible and appropriate learning plan. If you encounter resistance from the school administration, pursue the matter assertively with the help of your health care providers and a local support group if necessary.

CFIDS may prolong a child's dependence on the family, an especially difficult issue with adolescents. Discuss this problem openly. Allow for as much autonomy in decision-making by the child as possible.

Consider the use of guided imagery (as described in Chapter 12) for self-expression and healing. Children are often more responsive to imagery than adults because they haven't yet acquired adult constraints and are usually open to playing an active role.

Don't neglect other children in the family. If they are resentful about the "privileged" status of the child with CFIDS (fewer responsibilities, more attention), allow them to express their feelings openly but not in a way that is demeaning or blaming of their ill sibling.

Treat the child with CFIDS as normally as possible. Try not to make too many special exceptions. Illness, although genuine, can be used manipulatively. Continue discipline, routines, and family structure as before to whatever degree possible. Be aware of any tendency to "baby" or rescue the child, or to "make up" for the illness with inappropriate favors or privileges. You cannot compensate for the child's losses.

Children, especially teenagers, may attempt to deny health problems, theirs or anyone else's. Let them know gently that denial won't work, that facing illness is painful but they are strong enough to do so and will have the family's support. Then allow them to express their feelings (don't "correct" them) and to grieve. Don't expect their feelings to make sense or to match yours; allow them to experience and accept illness in their own way.

Try to plan fun activities and allow the child to interact with friends as much as possible. Peer relationships are extremely important to kids; don't be insulted if peer activities take precedence over family ones.

Children are very adaptable and are capable of handling hardships and illnesses such as CFIDS amazingly well. Like all of us, they need frequent signs of support and encouragement.

RELATIONSHIPS IN THE WORKPLACE

If you are able to continue working, there have probably been changes in your attendance record, work hours, and relationships with employer and coemployees. PWCs often wonder what to tell employers and prospective employers about the illness. It is not wise to hide or lie about your illness. In the long run the cover-up may be difficult to sustain, and greater problems may ensue if your health status is discovered later on. If CFIDS does not interfere with your ability to work productively, however, there may be no reason to volunteer health information. There is no universally correct way to handle this situation; it is a matter of your own preference and judgment.

Many employers are quite understanding of the special needs created by CFIDS and even request information about the illness. Others are less tolerant. The work setting and your responsibilities might not offer the flexibility you need right now. If you are unable to meet the requirements of your present job, consider alternatives: switch to a less demanding job, cut back on work hours, do your work at home, or explore disability benefits if necessary. If you are able to perform the basic duties of your job but require assistance with special needs, the Americans with Disabilities Act (ADA) requires that your employer make reasonable accommodations so that you may continue working. If areas of difficulty arise, seek the assistance of an attorney who specializes in labor law.

If you work closely with others, some of your symptoms are likely to become apparent to coworkers. Again, you must decide what and how much to disclose. You may want to give them general information about your illness, especially those with whom you work closely. Explain how CFIDS affects you, including the unpredictable changes in mood and behavior, so they won't misunderstand you. Encourage them to ask questions. Be honest about how you feel. Expect that some coworkers will be understanding and supportive, and some will not.

RELATIONSHIPS WITH FRIENDS

Relationships change in different ways in response to the stresses of CFIDS. Some continue relatively unchanged, some become closer, and some dissolve. New friendships may be sought with both PWCs and "civilians." A mixture provides a balance between the support only other PWCs can provide, and the contact with the outside world and perspectives offered by healthier friends. Different types of friendships have varying characteristics. Some revolve around shared interests or activities; others are based on common traits or professions. Some are just for fun—humor, movies, leisure activities. Deeper relationships involve more intimate sharing. Having a variety of friends reduces boredom and loneliness.

Most PWCs feel a strong, ongoing need to talk with others about their illness and its impact on their lives. Relationships will tolerate different amounts of focus on your illness. With close friends you can discuss the impact of your present needs on the relationship. In more distant relationships the talk about CFIDS will be more superficial; in-depth discussions could strain relationship boundaries. Even though CFIDS is a main event in your life, you will need to make decisions about how much discussion of the illness is appropriate in each of your relationships.

Your friends will not always know how to respond to your statements about CFIDS. They may think you are exaggerating, and respond with disbelief. Talk about it, tell them what it's like. If their reactions are consistently disappointing, you may need to confront them, or even end the relationship.

The energy crunch and isolative tendencies that often accompany CFIDS make friendships difficult. Not everyone can understand or tolerate our alternating needs for distance and closeness. If you are fortunate, most of your friendships will last, but not all relationships can survive the toll of chronic illness.

ABOUT SUICIDE: SUGGESTIONS
FOR FRIENDS AND FAMILY

During times of desperation, most PWCs have considered suicide as the only route for escaping their great emotional pain. Although relatively few follow through with their plans, the incidence of suicide is significantly higher among PWCs than in the general population. Suicidal talk or behavior should always be taken seriously.

Discouraging relapses may lead to the irrational thinking (which seems quite real and logical at the time) that recovery will never take place, life is too painful to endure, no one cares, and no hope exists. Trying to talk a suicidal person out of being pessimistic is usually ineffective, but you can help by listening. Keep communication going. Allow the person to do most of the talking as you pay careful attention. Be supportive but not unrealistically optimistic, as this would only cause the person to feel misunderstood. Ask what you can do to help. Stay with the person until you are certain that any danger has passed. If you need to leave for a period of time, ask if the person needs anything and will feel safe being alone. Suggest resources such as counseling, group therapy, or contact with other PWCs. Once the initial feelings are expressed and you feel the timing is right, help the person identify reasons to live, to hope. If depression is severe and does not lift, hospitalization may be appropriate.

AN OPEN LETTER FROM
A CFIDS PATIENT TO A FRIEND

Dear Friend,

I know my illness is putting pressure on both of us and is straining our relationship. Don't give up on me! Please try to be patient. I have unpredictable mood swings. Sometimes I'm so depressed I want the whole world to go away and I don't want to talk to anyone. Please don't take it personally. I just need to pull back until I can interact productively again.

Let's talk together about the changes in me and the changes in our relationship. I know you've noticed them and I'd like the opportunity for us to discuss them openly. Please tell me about your life, too, even if I forget to ask. I get very self-absorbed when I feel ill and discouraged, but I still care about you. If I forget to show my caring, please let me know, gently. Your needs matter to me a lot, but sometimes mine get in the way.

I need lots of attention right now, lots of caring. I don't want my needs to overwhelm you but sometimes they overwhelm me. I don't expect you to rescue me, to make me all better, but I hope you're willing to listen while I express needs, emotions, and thoughts. Sometimes I'll need to bounce ideas off you to get some feedback. I'll try to make my needs known; tell me if I'm not being clear or if I'm expecting too much.

There are times I think I can't get through this; please remind me that I'm strong and that I've gotten through so far. Tell me you believe in me.

I feel guilty because right now I don't have much to give. Our relationship is uneven, unbalanced, and I don't feel good about being the one with greater needs. I don't expect to be babied or coddled but I often need a lot of attention and caring. I sometimes feel as if I'm a burden and you're just tolerating me to be nice. I know better; this is my insecurity I'm talking about—not you. I would like to repay you somehow, even though you probably don't expect to be repaid.

Please continue to stay in touch and invite me to do things with the understanding that I may have to respond with "maybe" or "no," wishing I could join you. Try to realize that what seems to you like a minor exertion can be a major effort for me; when I'm not doing well such an effort can deplete my energy resources and may jeopardize my health even further. I miss doing things with you but need to be very careful about my activity level.

I both love and hate it when you tell me I'm looking good. Please don't assume that means I'm feeling good. And when you ask how I am, I'll answer honestly but will try to summarize and not ramble too much or bore you.

I know you can't always be available for me, and I'll try to understand when you have conflicting needs of your own. CFIDS has helped me to realize the importance of feeling cared about. Thank you for being my friend.

AN OPEN LETTER FROM A CFIDS PATIENT TO A SPOUSE/PARTNER

Dear Significant Other,

Please understand that I am going through a horrible ordeal. I feel horrible about inflicting my illness on you. I know you're affected by my changes, and I wish it were otherwise. I don't want to be ill.

I feel guilty about not being able to shoulder my former responsibilities at work and at home, leaving you to take up the slack. I wish I could do more, or even know in advance what I will be able to do each day. Maybe sometimes you think I'm lazy or just trying to get out of doing something I don't like to do, but that's not it. Sometimes I just can't, and other times I know it would be a mistake to use up all my energy on a minor thing and then have to give up something more important.

I want to know that I can trust you, that you will be available to listen and try to understand. And I'll try to understand that you can't always be available.

At times my feelings are irrational, and I may become angry for no apparent reason. These mood swings are part of my illness. I'll try to keep them under control, but I need you to understand that even when I direct them at you, I'm not blaming you for my illness. I'll try not to use you as a scapegoat for my anger but will sometimes fail. Please don't take my mood swings personally; they're not your fault. If they become too hard to take and you feel ready to explode at me, please tell me so. Maybe one of us can leave the scene, and we can talk about it later when we're both calmer.

Sometimes I need to talk about these irrational feelings. Just listen, okay? Please don't tell me how to feel or how not to feel. You don't have to "fix" my feelings, and please don't judge them. Just accept and acknowledge them. When you say such things as, "CFIDS must be terribly frustrating for you," I feel understood and comforted. But don't tell me you know how I feel. You don't, and you can't; no one can know exactly what this is like for me. And when I cry, don't try to get me to stop. Please let me cry—I'll feel better later.

I know I complain a lot. It helps to relieve tension. If I'm complaining more than you can bear, please tell me so, gently. I probably won't handle it well, but I really do understand that you need to distance yourself from my complaints.

I need to work at making clear requests so that you'll know what I need. It's not your job to mind read—it's my responsibility to ask for what I want. This is difficult for me; it's easier for me to meet others' needs than to ask others to meet mine.

Don't try to talk me out of my symptoms or remind me that they're not as bad as they could be or not as bad as they were. I know I need to stay hopeful, but if you take an optimistic role when I feel pessimistic, it feels as if you don't understand me or validate my feelings.

I know you don't understand why I'm sick. Neither do I. It's frustrating not to have someone or something to blame, but let's acknowledge our feelings of helplessness to each other.

I don't want you to give up your whole life for me. Please continue to do the things that are important to you. I won't always be able to do them with you, so do them alone. Sometimes I resent not being able to do things and I may even resent your freedom. I'll try to keep a good perspective. If you put your life on hold because of my illness, I'll feel guilty and in time you'll come to resent me. I appreciate your invitations to do things. Your asking lets me know that you still value my company. Please don't assume what I can or can't do; ask, and I'll answer you honestly. I hope you will understand that when I say "no," it's not because I don't want to but because I can't or shouldn't.

I know I'm not the way I used to be. Let's talk about these CFIDS-related changes. I'm trying to learn from my illness, and you can help. We can't pretend that things are the way they were or that they'll ever be the same again. But as we change and grow, let's grow together rather than apart. Let's keep the lines of communication open. When I need to withdraw, I'll try to let you know so you won't take it personally. Please do the same for me. Don't just pull away; explain to me that you need to distance temporarily so I'm less inclined to feel abandoned.

Because we're both experiencing losses, we'll both need to grieve. Some of our grieving will be a solitary process, but some of it will be shared, because we've both lost so much. Let's acknowledge what we've lost by mourning together.

Please don't try to make my decisions for me. If you see me wearing down and think I should rest, please offer your observation, not advice or an order. I need to take care of myself and you can help, but don't try to take over my care. It wouldn't be good for either of us. Your encouragement helps me to do a better job of taking care of myself.

It helps me to have both my difficulties and my strengths acknowledged by you. Tell me you think I'm brave, that I'm fighting hard, that I'm weathering this calamity well. Tell me you still love me. Small tokens help—a flower, a phone call, a card. Tell me you care about me and why you value me. Please touch me; I need hugs now more than ever. Sometimes I may be unable to hear you or I may even push you away when I'm hurting, especially at times when I can't love myself. I'll try not to hurt you, but if I do, please understand that it's not you I'm rejecting, it's me and my illness.

I know our sexual relationship has changed and that we both miss the way it was. I don't know how to explain to you that my lack of energy or sexual interest is a result of my illness and not a rejection of you. I want us to continue to relate physically—to touch, hug, and cuddle. We need to remain close in every way we can.

These are rough times for us. I appreciate the efforts you've made to help me to cope and to be as comfortable as possible. I know I've been difficult to live with. At times you have been too. If we can get through these times together, our relationship will become stronger—something I want very much.

AN OPEN LETTER FROM A HEALTHY SPOUSE/PARTNER TO A PWC

Dear PWC Whom I Love,

I know you have overwhelming needs right now due to your illness. I know you have difficulty coping. Please try to see that I'm going through a hard time, too. I almost feel as if I shouldn't have needs, but your illness affects me as well, very deeply. I care about you, and when you hurt and I can't fix it then I hurt too.

I feel helpless, perhaps even more helpless than you do. I wish I knew how to make you better. Sometimes I give you too much advice. It's not always helpful but sometimes I don't know what else to give, and I want to give something. I'll try not to take over your care or tell you what's best for you. I don't want you to be dependent on me any more than you have to be.

Please tell me what you need. I won't repeat your confidences to anyone. Sometimes you hold back and I become frustrated because I don't know what you need. If you ask me to do something specific for you, I have the option of saying "yes" or "no." But you have to ask.

I take what you say seriously, even though some of it doesn't make sense to me. Please take what I say seriously as well, even when I don't make sense to you.

There are times when I just don't understand. You seem crazy, or lazy, or as if you no longer care about *my* needs. I know it isn't true but I can't help my feelings. I guess you sometimes need to feel sorry for yourself. I feel sorry for myself, too, and I'm not even the one who's sick.

Sometimes you dump on me when you're especially tired or grouchy. I understand this in my head, but I still hurt. I feel as if you're blaming me for your illness and expecting me to fix it. I'd do anything I can to help you, but I can't make it go away. Please try not to lash out. If something is really bothering you, let's try to talk about it at a good time.

When I do something that's helpful, please tell me so. I need feedback and acknowledgment from you. I'm doing an awful lot right now. I need to know that what I'm doing is noticed and appreciated.

I love you, but I need other friends and family in my life as well. I hope that my time with them won't cause you to feel left out when you're not feeling well enough to participate. I may become overly involved in work and other activities because of my need for time out. I'm trying to balance our needs, and just as you need to take care of yourself, I need to take care of myself. This is new for both of us. I still need to see friends, exercise, play, and deal with job stresses, family needs, and my own health concerns.

I agree that we should continue to make decisions together, even though I may have to carry them out alone. I'll try not to be a martyr or a dictator. If you see that I'm making too many decisions without your input and you feel left out, please tell me.

Sometimes I think you should do things differently in order to get better. When I ask you to try some special treatment, diet, or positive thinking, it's because I'm trying to help. Sometimes I even get mad at your doctor, thinking that with adequate care you'd get better.

Although I try not to burden you with the way I feel, I don't want to pretend I have no bad feelings about this. I feel afraid, hurt, vulnerable, angry, and sad at times. Sometimes I become angry at you for being sick, although rationally I know it's not your fault.

When you are depressed or stay in bed, staring into space, I feel abandoned. I *know* you're not abandoning me, but I *feel* vulnerable. Sometimes I think this illness has taken over your life, and I'm not very important anymore. Please let me know that I'm still important to you.

Let's try to do some fun things together. I know your energy is limited, but we need some time off from the gloom. Let's figure out what we can do to enjoy each other. Save some of your precious energy for *us*, even if it's just to watch a videotape together and share some popcorn.

We can get through this together. Despite the pain and the struggles, let's not forget how much we mean to each other.

Chapter 14

Conclusion

Folksinger Pete Seeger told a story many years ago about a king who wanted to have all the world's wisdom condensed into one book. He appointed a wise man to perform this awesome task but refused to read the book when it was presented to him, saying, "Now boil everything in this book down to one page." And when presented with the wisdom of the world in one page, again the king did not read it but asked that it be condensed into one paragraph. When the wise man had done this, the king asked him to condense it into one word. When he returned, the king asked for the one word that held the world's wisdom, and the wise man told the king, "The word is 'maybe.' "

After years of treating and interviewing PWCs, and researching and writing about CFIDS, I find that I really have little to offer in the way of definitive, universal conclusions or recommendations. Quite frankly, I feel inadequate writing a book based on maybes—but maybes are all we've got.

We want more. We need answers to our questions, more positive attention and treatment from the medical community, more funding for CFIDS research, more attention from government agencies, and the knowledge that our plight is being taken seriously by our government, health care providers, and loved ones.

We can provide the impetus for these changes by speaking up; by supporting our local and national support groups (of which there are more than five hundred!); by writing letters to legislators and organizations; and by educating ourselves, our health care providers, and concerned others.

Paul Cheney, M.D., testified about this "monstrous and yet subtle disease" before the Senate Appropriations Subcommittee on Labor, Health and Human Services, and Education in Washington, D.C. on May 8, 1989:

The most remarkable thing about chronic fatigue syndrome is that the impetus for its recognition as a defined clinical entity has come primarily from patients. If there was ever a grass-roots disease, this is it. What clues there are to this disorder lie *presently* in listening carefully to these patients.

The CDC now receives one hundred calls from patients and physicians each week. CFIDS-related calls to the NIAID, an AIDS-dominated institution in Bethesda, Maryland, are outnumbered only by AIDS-related calls. Thousands of social security and private disability claims list CFIDS as the principal cause of disability. Many school systems provide home-bound instruction to children with this disorder. This disorder has already or will likely cost this country billions in lost productivity and health costs, and ironically from its most productive segment, the young and middle-aged adult. It could easily dwarf the economic effects of AIDS and sap the nation of its economic vitality. (*The CFIDS Chronicle*, Spring 1989)

There are estimated millions of PWCs in the United States alone and, unfortunately, our number is growing. CFIDS is also an increasing phenomenon in other countries around the globe, where it is known by a variety of names. We are faced with individual and collective struggles. As a group, we share concerns regarding CFIDS recognition, health care, and social issues. Individually we struggle with physiological, spiritual, and emotional issues. We survive this ordeal as best we can despite dwindling checkbook balances, bizarre symptoms, and alternating hope and despair.

I have grown during the time I have been ill, and I have learned some things I would never have thought about had I remained well. I am not pretending to be glad I have CFIDS; I would just as soon be well and make do with a little less growth. But I don't have that choice, so I've decided to make the best of it in my own way. I hope you will do the same.

Susan Levine, M.D., wrote about CFIDS: "This is a silent illness which . . . robs people of their day to day sanity." Well, this illness can *borrow* my sanity, but it can't *have* it. CFIDS can spur me to examine the meaning of life in general, and of my life in particular, and it can create obstacles in everything from relationships to my ability to think coherently, but it can't take over permanently and it can't destroy my life. Tomorrow I may think differently, but my wish is to have many more hopeful and productive days like today. I can live with that.

Appendix A

CFIDS Symptom Checklist

Indicate **on a scale of 1 to 10** the severity of each symptom you experience, with 10 being the most severe.

General

___ Fatigue, usually made worse by physical exertion or stress

___ Activity level less than 50% of what it was pre-illness

___ Recurrent flu-like illness

___ Sore throat

___ Hoarseness

___ Tender or swollen lymph nodes, especially side of neck and underarm areas

___ Tender points or trigger points

___ Headache

___ Eye pain

___ Chest pain

___ Night sweats

___ Low-grade fevers

___ Feeling cold often

___ Feeling hot often

___ Cold extremities (hands and feet)

___ Subnormal body temperature (below 97.5°)

___ Low blood pressure (below 110/70)

___ Severe nasal allergies (new onset or worsened existing allergies)

___ Cough

___ Heart palpitations

___ Shortness of breath with little or no exertion

___ Frequent sighing

___ Rashes

___ Eczema or psoriasis

___ Recurrent sores

___ Hair loss

___ Dryness of eyes and/or mouth

___ Frequent thirst

Musculo-Skeletal

___ Muscle pain

___ Muscle twitching

___ Muscle weakness

___ Joint pain

___ Paralysis or severe weakness of an arm or leg

Gastrointestinal

___ Nausea

___ Vomiting

___ Esophageal reflux (heartburn)

___ Bloating, intestinal gas

___ Weight gain (_____
pounds)

___ Weight loss (_____
pounds)

___ Decreased appetite

___ Increased appetite, food
cravings

Sleep

___ Difficulty falling asleep

___ Difficulty staying asleep

___ Vivid or disturbing dreams
or nightmares

___ Unrefreshing or nonrestorative sleep

___ Altered sleep/wake schedule

___ Alertness/energy best late at
night

Cognitive

___ Word-finding difficulties

___ Memory disturbance,
short-term

___ Memory disturbance,
long-term

___ Losing the train of thought
in the middle of a sentence

___ Attention deficit

___ Concentration problems

___ Calculation difficulties

___ Difficulty speaking (slowness, stuttering)

___ Spatial disorientation (e.g.,
getting lost in familiar
locations)

___ Difficulty judging distances

___ Frequently saying the wrong
word

___ Difficulty finding the word
you want to use

___ Comprehension deficit (difficulty understanding what is
heard or read)

___ Difficulty following written
instructions

___ Difficulty following spoken
instructions

Psychological

___ Depression

___ Anxiety

___ Panic attacks

___ Phobias (irrational fears)

___ Personality changes (often
the worsening of a pre-
viously mild tendency)

___ Mood swings

___ Irritability

___ "Rage attacks" (becoming
angry or out of control for
little or no reason)

Neurological

___ Seizures; Seizure-like episodes

___ Fainting (syncope) or blackouts

___ Sensation that you might
faint

___ Numbness or tingling sensations

___ Tinnitus (ringing in one or
both ears)

___ Lightheadedness, feeling
"spaced out"

___ Disequilibrium (balance problems)

___ Staggering gait (clumsy walking, bumping into things)

___ Dizziness

___ Vertigo (feeling that the room is spinning)

___ Tremor or trembling

___ Photophobia (light sensitivity)

___ Sensitivity to noise

___ Sensitivities to odors (cleaning products, exhaust fumes, colognes, hairsprays)

___ Sensitivities to foods

___ Sensitivities to medications (inability to tolerate a "normal" dosage)

___ Alcohol intolerance

___ Alteration of taste, smell, hearing

___ Symptoms worsened by temperature extremes or changes in weather

___ Symptoms worsened by air travel

Vision

___ Changes in visual acuity (frequent changes in ability to see well)

___ Difficulty with visual accommodation (switching focus from one thing to another)

___ Blind spots in vision

Urogenital

___ Frequent urination

___ Painful urination or bladder pain

___ Prostate pain

___ Impotence, erection problems

___ Decreased libido (sex drive)

Other Disorders

___ TMJ syndrome

___ Mitral valve prolapse

___ Cancer

___ Periodontal (gum) disease

___ Worsening of PMS

___ Endometriosis

___ Aphthous ulcers (canker sores)

Appendix B

CFIDS Networking

FORMING A CFIDS SUPPORT GROUP

Having served as a facilitator, speaker, and consultant for several CFIDS support groups, I would like to share my suggestions for forming and conducting such groups. I am referring to smaller, support-oriented, self-help groups whose primary goals are sharing, mutual support, and generating ideas for managing the illness (as opposed to larger, information-oriented groups at the city or state levels).

An initial organizational meeting can bring interested parties together for the purpose of decision making. To find PWCs in your area to form a group, contact the nearest CFIDS Support/Information group in your area. Your organizational meeting date may be publicized in their newsletter, in flyers, and through a press release to the media. To send out a press release, consult the yellow pages for names of local newspapers and other periodicals, and mail them a press release following the guidelines below. Generally they will be happy to publicize your meeting at no cost and in some cases will even contact you for further information so they can write an article about CFIDS and your group. It is wise to send new press releases periodically, e.g., every few months, to keep the public informed and your group membership strong.

Press Release

Purpose of meeting: Support for persons with Chronic Fatigue Immune Dysfunction Syndrome

Date of meeting: _____

Time: _____

Location: _____

Cost: Free (Even if there will be a charge for members later on, there is usually no fee for the first meeting.)

Open to all Persons with CFIDS

For further information: Contact _____
(organizer's name and telephone number)

Give a brief description of CFIDS and the purpose of the group.

Meetings

At the initial meeting, the following issues need to be addressed:

Who will lead the group? Options: the group leader may be a PWC, may alternate among PWCs, or may be a therapist or other professional. In the latter case, there will generally be a charge.

Where and when will the group meet?

How long will each meeting last? (90-minute meetings are suggested.)

What will be the group's goals?

Will there be invited speakers or consultants? If there is a charge, how much will each member contribute?

Will there be a fee for the group? (Costs may include materials, room use, mailing, telephone, speakers, refreshments.)

Group size: maximum number of participants. (Six to twelve people is a good group size, allowing for diverse input but maintaining comfort and intimacy.)

Will significant others be included? At every meeting or at specified meetings? (e.g., every fourth meeting)

Will a telephone tree be developed to keep members informed of new information or meeting changes? (Although difficult to develop, a telephone tree saves one individual having to make all the calls; advisable if the group is large.)

Once the first meeting gets underway, the issue of confidentiality should be discussed. Those present will need to agree not to discuss the disclosures of others outside the group setting.

A Suggested Agenda

Introductions: An opportunity for the group leader and
each PWC to offer a brief time-limited biographical
sketch and medical history, as well as hopes and expectations regarding the group and specific areas of concern.
Information: It is helpful to provide members with general
CFIDS information, including data regarding larger local
groups, national organizations, and a bibliography. Community resource lists should be available.
Topics of common interest to the group.

Topics For Discussion

General information/discussion about CFIDS:
— Onset
— Symptoms (general or physical, emotional, neurological)
— Diagnosis
— The exacerbation/remission cycle
— Relapse "triggers" and techniques for minimizing them
Emotional effects of CFIDS
— Common feelings among PWCs
— Life changes brought about by CFIDS
— Changes in self-concept and self-esteem
— Individual feelings of group members
— Anxiety
— Depression
— Mood swings, irritability, "overreaction"
— Losses and stages of grieving (denial, bargaining, anger,
depression, acceptance)
— Coping with emotions
— Expression of feelings
— Learning not to judge feelings
Medical care
— Appropriate medical resources
— Dealing assertively with doctors and other medical
personnel
— Avoiding dangerous "fad" treatments
— Emotions regarding medical care (especially fears)

Lifestyle management
— Advantages of learning to manage time and cut back on activities
— Moderation and self-pacing
— Seeking a balance between self-care and responsibilities
Life philosophy
— Shifting the focus to the here and now
— Lessons learned from/during the illness
— Healthy optimism (versus false optimism and versus pessimism)
CFIDS and relationships
— Effects of CFIDS on relationships
— Coping with CFIDS in relationships
— Partners
— Friends
— Family members
— People in the workplace
— Problem-solving in relationships
Advocacy
— Letter writing to local, state, and national representatives regarding funding for CFIDS research (work with your local or national CFIDS support group)
— Fund raising for advocacy and research. Local public health agencies or support groups for other illnesses may become involved in this effort at your request (See Feiden's *Hope and Help for Chronic Fatigue Syndrome*, pp. 176–179.)
Individual CFIDS-related problems
— Brainstorming solution possibilities
— Offering support and affirmation

Some groups require attendance at all meetings regardless of how ill an individual may feel. Others operate on a "drop-in" basis: PWCs may attend as they feel the need. Some groups specify a number of sessions or months the group will meet and others keep it open-ended, continuing for as long as the demand exists. If the group does disband, referral of group members to other support groups is helpful.

Groups differ in terms of "group personality"—a product of the chemistry between its members. If you have any concerns about the group—for example, an individual who dominates most discussions, or someone presenting what you believe to be misinformation about CFIDS—it is best to address these issues immediately and diplomatically in the group session.

Keep the focus of the group open and realistically positive. Avoid getting stuck in an "ain't it awful" rut in which the tone of the group is dominated by complaints and hopelessness. If a group member seems unusually emotionally upset or is not receiving necessary medical care, make appropriate referrals.

Resource articles:

Pioneering your own support strategies: Carleen Malone, *The CFIDS Chronicle*, Summer/Fall 1989, pp. 92–97.

The view from the other side of the couch: Linda Miller Iger, same issue, pp. 102–104.

PUBLISHING A CFIDS NEWSLETTER

Many local groups publish CFIDS newsletters. Based on many I have read and reviewed, I offer the following suggestions.

Contents

General CFIDS information

Local and national events regarding CFIDS and chronic illness, including date, time, location, speaker, cost

Editorial comment and letters to the editor

Articles contributed by health professionals, editorial staff, and individual PWCs that are of general interest to those with CFIDS (e.g., emotional issues, coping, medical treatment, information for significant others, anecdotes, suggestions)

A disclaimer stating that the newsletter is intended to offer information and support but not to replace medical advice or treatment (A local attorney may be willing to help you with proper wording.)

Summaries of meetings, conventions, and symposia

Reviews and summaries of articles in medical literature and other periodicals, books, audiotapes, pamphlets—including ordering information

Referral list of local professionals (physicians, attorneys, psychologists/psychiatrists/counselors) recommended by PWCs (Contact these professionals first to see if they would like to be placed on the referral list.)

Helpline: a telephone number to call for CFIDS support and information, the hours this line is operated, and by whom (specify whether volunteers or professionals)

Encouragement of involvement in advocacy and fund-raising efforts, including letter writing (list of government officials and sample letter or outline)

PWC "ads": those looking for services, roommates, etc.

Community resources

Humorous articles and cartoons

Suggestions

A newsletter should not be dominated by the voice of any one individual. That is, the editor should not be writing all the articles, reviewing literature, etc. Ideally, staff should include an editor or coeditors, a reviewer (often a medical reviewer), and someone with a literary background who can proofread articles and make suggestions and corrections (grammar, style, punctuation).

A balance should be maintained among informational articles, editorials and letters to the editor, humor, resources for PWCs, etc. Format is important. A newsletter should be laid out carefully and be easy to read.

Sources of information should be clearly identified. Obtain permission to use material from other sources. Articles or cartoons found in other CFIDS newsletters, books, and pamphlets may be excellent for your readers and most authors are eager to have you use their material with prior permission.

Newsletters may be brief; most PWCs prefer shorter, more frequent ones. It is an unnecessary duplication of effort to cover topics already covered in national newsletters; a synopsis and suggestion for further reading should suffice.

Appendix C

Research
and Resources

The important thing is not to stop questioning.

Albert Einstein

C FIDS research is being conducted at several prestigious institutions and more informally in doctors' offices across the country. Through scientific research in combination with the serendipitous findings that often lead to breakthroughs, researchers may discover the causes, treatments, and ultimately cures for CFIDS. Andrew Lloyd pointed out that studies to date have been physician-based rather than community-based, that is, only those who have been diagnosed and treated by physicians are being studied. Those in the community who have self-diagnosed or undiagnosed CFIDS have not been included, thus potentially altering the true picture (November 1991).

Although several government agencies are now involved in conducting CFIDS research, most research to date has been funded by the private sector through donations of patients and concerned others.

NATIONAL ATTENTION TO CFIDS

Unfortunately, as a nation we have taken an ostrich-like approach to chronic viral and immune dysfunction-related illnesses. Given the magnitude of the problem, relatively little has been done to solve it.

Society's general attitude toward AIDS is a good example. Our deepest fears and prejudices about this lethal, out-of-control illness led to our avoiding the HIV problem until it was a disease of epidemic proportions. Although the problem has existed since at least the late 1970s, little attention was focused on it until two shocking events occurred: the public became aware of AIDS in the heterosexual, non-drug-using population, and Rock Hudson, a national idol, died of it. Then it got real for us. By that time it had spread dramatically and thousands of people had died, but research funding was still woefully inadequate. The disease just wasn't pleasant or convenient to deal with. We boast a huge federal budget, national research institutes, state-of-the-art health care resources, outstanding media involvement and coverage of health issues, and a humanitarian philosophy. But we turn a deaf ear to the cries of those afflicted with chronic immune-related illnesses. The bureaucracy is too busy. Politics and finances are more important than human lives.

The approach initially taken by the press to CFIDS was disappointing. All we read was about the crazy and lazy people with an imaginary new yuppie illness, an excuse to cop out. CFIDS was treated like a second-class illness seen in those unable to cope productively with life, a first cousin to hypochondria.

The government's reaction to the CFIDS problem has been as underwhelming as its response to the AIDS epidemic. It's easy to ignore an illness that's invisible, that doesn't kill people or even make them look sick. Research funding remains inadequate. They have taken a few stabs here and there, waiting for the problem to go away. It hasn't. Several government health agencies that fall under the auspices of the United States Public Health Service have played a role in the study of CFIDS: the National Institutes of Health (NIH), Centers for Disease Control and Prevention (CDC), National Institute of Allergy and Infectious Diseases (NIAID), National Cancer Institute (NCI), National Center for Research Resources (NCRR), National Institute of Neurological Disorders and Stroke (NINDS), National Institute of Child Health and Human Development (NICHD), and National Institute of Arthritis, Musculoskeletal and Skin Diseases (NIAMS). Their efforts to date have been inadequate.

Funding for CFS research has been relatively small compared to that for other chronic medical conditions such as AIDS, cardiovascular disease, and cancer," wrote Mark Loveless, Andrew Lloyd, and Rudy Perpich in "Summary of Public Policy and Chronic Fatigue Syndrome: A Perspective."(1994) "As a result, the medical literature has been characterized by a trickle of high-quality data generated by clinical, epidemiological, and basic studies of CFS." The authors recommend a general public policy for PWCs that would be sustained by the media, and efficient distribution of biomedical and epidemiological information to primary care physicians through educational programs and medical literature. A Public Health Service CFS Interagency Committee has been established to improve communication among federal health agencies and researchers in the private sector.

Extramural research centers have been established by NIAID to conduct multidisciplinary CFIDS studies and others may be added.

Research is currently addressing standardized evaluations of CFIDS patients, diagnostic markers, comparisons of CFIDS and other diseases, and abnormalities associated with CFIDS. However, extramural research remains grossly underfunded, and much of the information we have has come from informal studies conducted by dedicated health care providers at their own expense. Drs. David Bell, Paul Cheney, Jay Goldstein, Byron Hyde, Anthony Komaroff, and Daniel Peterson are among those who began studying the illness in the 1980s and continue to conduct vital research that generates new theories and information. We are endlessly grateful to these and countless other dedicated professionals who have taken a strong interest in CFIDS, which has often earned ostracism by their skeptical colleagues. These dedicated professionals have stood by us, treated us, and defended us against those who do not take CFIDS seriously.

Many studies have been funded privately by PWCs and others in the private sector through such organizations as The CFIDS Association of America, Inc., which has been active in fundraising. As one PWC wrote in a letter to The CFIDS Association, those of us who have the illness, many of whom are impoverished, should not be the primary source of funding research and other CFIDS-related projects.

A catch-22 situation results from the disease being called "chronic fatigue syndrome," a label that causes the syndrome to be taken lightly or dismissed by the public and professionals alike. We are told that once the illness is better understood, it will be granted a more appropriate name, but in the meantime it is not difficult to understand why we have trouble communicating the seriousness of this illness. The "CFS" label discourages research funding, and the lack of funding blocks potential discoveries about its pathophysiology, and thus the CFS label remains.

In addition to inadequate funding, the many obstacles to CFIDS research include lack of an adequate and consistent case definition, poorly constructed research protocols, political infighting among research centers and patient groups, the need for a stronger multidisciplinary approach, and difficulty with coordination and communication among researchers. It is not even known if everyone given this disease label has the same disease. We lack a database which would allow such comparisons to be made and patients to be followed over time.

Fortunately, progress is being made in many of these areas, but it is slow. Because of constraints involved in publishing research, many findings are not made available for several years while they are peer-reviewed and await publication in professional journals. Funding and communication among agencies have improved, but more is needed.

PWCs are impatient; we are ill now, and the answers we need are slow in coming. PWCs can help promote the cause by becoming politically active—writing to legislators, contributing to research, and educating the public. Letter writing has a significant impact on government attention to CFIDS. Letters must be written by significant numbers of PWCs to the President, federal legislators for each state, state government officials, local and national media, and to members of the House and Senate Labor, Health, and Human Services Appropriations Subcommittees. Names, addresses, and sample letters can be found in issues of The CFIDS Chronicle. Support groups must take an active role in organizing these efforts, which are often overwhelming to individual PWCs.

To date, this country has been penny-wise and pound-foolish in drastically underfunding CFIDS research because the disease is taking a huge financial toll in terms of disability benefits, medical expenses, and lost wages and productivity of PWCs. Those stricken with the disease are often in what should be their most productive years and we comprise a significant segment of our workforce. It is inhumane and financially foolish not to make this disease a strong national priority.

RESOURCES

National Organizations and Newsletters

The American Association for Chronic Fatigue Syndrome (AACFS)
P.O. Box 895
Olney, MD 20830
A nonprofit organization of research scientists, physicians, licensed medical health care professionals, and other professionally involved individuals and institutions. Its mission is to promote the stimulation, coordination, and exchange of ideas for CFS research and patient care as well as periodic reviews of current clinical, research, and treatment data on CFS for the benefit of CFS patients and others.

The CFIDS Association of America, Inc.
P.O. Box 220398
Charlotte, NC 28222-0398   800-442-3437   900-988-2343

Resource line (for educational materials, membership renewals, and donations)   704-365-2343
The Association is a charitable organization whose mission is "to conquer CFIDS and related disorders and to inform and empower those affected by these disorders until a cure is found." The Association publishes The CFIDS Chronicle, the most widely distributed source of CFIDS information, whose purpose is "advocacy, information, research,

and encouragement for the CFIDS community." The Association maintains resource/support group lists for each state. Information about various aspects of CFIDS is available at the 900 number, with a charge (stated at no cost at the beginning of the call) that covers the cost of maintaining both telephone lines.

Membership: $30/year; waived in cases of financial hardship; includes quarterly issues of *The CFIDS Chronicle*, periodic updates, and a membership packet.

CFS Crisis Center
27 West 20th Street, Suite 703
New York, NY 10011   212-691-4800

National Chronic Fatigue Syndrome and Fibromyalgia Association
   (NCFSFA)
3521 Broadway, Suite 222
Kansas City, MO 64111   816-931-4777
Publishers of *The Heart of America* newsletter and various pamphlets as well as patient resource information.

National Organization for Rare Disorders, Inc. (NORD)
P.O. Box 8923
New Fairfield, CT 06812-8923   203-746-6518

CANADA:

The Nightingale Foundation
383 Danforth Avenue
Ottawa, Ontario K2A 0E1, Canada

The ME Association of Canada
246 Queen Street, Suite 400
Ottawa, Ontario K1P 5E4, Canada 613-563-1565

Advocacy

CFIDS Activation Network (CAN)
P.O. Box 345
Larchmont, NY 10538   212-304-5631

C-ACT (CFIDS Activation Network)   800-442-3437
Leave your name in the advocacy "mailbox" to become involved in supporting The CFIDS Association of America's advocacy group. An information packet and enrollment postcard will be mailed to you. This opportunity to become involved in advocacy efforts is open to members and nonmembers and is free of charge.

San Francisco CFIDS Task Force
3543 18th Street, #20
San Francisco, CA 94110   415-525-6415

RESCIND
9812 Falls Road
Suite 114-270
Potomac, MD 20854

Minann, Inc.
P.O. Box 582
Glenview, IL 60025

Buyers Club

CFIDS Buyers' Club
1187 Coast Village Road, #1-280
Santa Barbara, CA 93108   800-366-6056
Founded by Rich Carson, the Buyers' Club offers discounted nutritional
supplements and donates a portion of profits to CFIDS research. A com-
plementary catalog is available. Publisher of *Health Watch*, a newsletter
regarding CFIDS research and treatment.

Christians

Share, Prayer and Pen-Pal Chain
919 Scott Avenue
Kansas City, KS 66105
Information packets are available; donations are appreciated.

Consumer Resources

Consumer Information Center 2A
P.O. Box 100
Pueblo, CO 81002
Consumer information catalog available at no charge.

The Food and Drug Administration (FDA)
Consumer Affairs and Information
5600 Fishers Lane, HFC-110
Rockville, MD 20857   301-443-3170
Fraudulent health products may be reported to the FDA and to your
state attorney general's office.

Consumer Health Research Institute
3521 Broadway
Kansas City, MO 64111   800-753-8850
If you have questions about specific health products, send SASE and
$1.00.

National Council Against Health Fraud
Victim Redress Taskforce
P.O. Box 33008
Kansas City, MO 64114

Write to this organization if you believe you have been harmed by a quack remedy.

The U.S. Postal Service
Chief Postal Inspector
475 L'Enfant Plaza
Washington, DC 20260
Write to the U.S. Postal Service if mail fraud was involved in the purchase of faulty or quack products.

Electronic Resources

CFS/ME Computer Networking Project
P.O. Box 11347
Washington, DC 20008-0567
Send SASE with $.55 postage. Information about CFIDS computer networks on GEnie, Internet, CompuServe, Prodigy, America Online, Fidonet, Usenet, and Free-net. To obtain a copy via Internet, send a request to cfs-me@sjuvm,stjohns.edu.

Canada: CFS/ME Computer Networking Project
3332 McCarthy Road
P.O. Box 37045
Ottawa, Ontario K1V 0W0
Send SASE. Internet CFIDS information and support: Roger Burns, Internet address: CFS-NEWS @LIST.NIH.GOV for details on how to reach Internet information services.

CompuServe CFIDS Support Area
CFS/CFIDS/FMS Section (16)
Health & Fitness Forum (GOODHEALTH)
CFIDS Info: 505-898-4635   CompuServe Info: 800-898-8199

Literature search:
Steve Clancy, M.L.S.   714-856-7996   714-846-5087
Wellspring RBBS   714-725-2700 Voice: 714-856-7309
The Wellspring BBS is a service of the Science Library of the University of California at Irvine and includes citations for current medical literature.

Emotional Support: Newsletters for PWCs

CFIDS Pathfinder
P.O. Box 2644
Kensington, MD 20891-2644   301-530-8624

The CFIDS Reality Check
12 Wildwood Estates
Plattsburgh, NY 12901

Send SASE. A personal and positive newsletter helping PWCs to share experiences, coping and recovery techniques.

Expressions
P.O. Box 16294
St. Paul, MN 55116-0294
A semiannual, nonprofit magazine for writers and artists with disabilities and/or chronic illness.

The National Link
P.O. Box 51952
Durham, NC 27717-1952
Quarterly publication that provides an opportunity for CFS patients, their families, and friends to share their thoughts, experiences, humor, and methods of coping.

Gay Men

GMWC
P.O. Box 340251
Columbus, OH 43234
Newsletter for gay men with CFS.

Government Agencies and Publications

Centers for Disease Control and Prevention (CDC)
Division of Viral Diseases
Building 6, Room 120
Atlanta, GA 30333   404-639-1388
Pamphlet: "The Facts about CFS."

National Institute of Allergy and Infectious Diseases (NIAID)
Office of Communications
Building 31, Room 7A32
9000 Rockville Pike
Bethesda, MD 20892   301-496-5717

National Institutes of Health (NIH)
Clinical Center Communications
9000 Rockville Pike
Building 10, Room 1C255
Bethesda, MD 20892   301-496-5717

CFS Interagency Coordinating Committee (CFSICC)
Dr. Philip Lee, Assistant Secretary for Health, Chair
A partnership between CFIDS advocates and the federal public health officials. Committee members represent the CDC, NIH, FDA, SSA (Social Security Administration), and patient advocates.

Disability, Social Security, and Financial Aid

Government Entitlement Services
22144 W. Nine Mile
Southfield, MI 48034   800-628-2887
Information about disability benefits.

Social Security Administration (SSA)
U.S. Department of Health and Human Services
Baltimore, MD 21235
Booklets: Understanding Social Security, Supplemental Security
Income, Disability, Benefits for Children, Working While Disabled,
The Appeals Process.

Pocket Guide to Federal Help for Individuals with Disabilities
Publication E-89 22002
U.S. Department of Education
Washington, DC 20202

Clearinghouse on Disability Information
U.S. Department of Education
Switzer Building, Room 3132
Washington, DC 20202-2524   202-732-1241
Information, resources, referrals.

National Organization of Social Security Claimants' Representatives
    (NOSSCR)
19 East Central Avenue
Pearl River, NY 10965   800-431-2804
Referrals to local attorneys for SSI and SSDI matters.

Superintendent of Documents
U.S. Government Printing Office
Washington, DC 20402
Booklet: "Summary of Existing Legislation Affecting Persons with
Disabilities."

Office on the Americans with Disability Act
Civil Rights Division
U.S. Department of Justice
P.O. Box 66118   202-514-0301
Washington, DC 20035-6118   TDD 202-514-0381
Information on ADA requirements, telecommunications, public serv-
ices, transportation, public accommodations, and employment.

Job Accommodation Network
809 Allen
P.O. Box 6122
West Virginia University, WV 26506
Help with adaptive assistance.

National Health Law Program, Inc.
2025 M Street, NW, Suite 400
Washington, DC 20036   202-887-5310

National Health Law Program, Inc.
2639 S. La Cienega Boulevard
Los Angeles, CA 90034   213-204-6010
Services to low-income persons with health care-related legal problems.

National Library Service for the Blind and Physically Handicapped
Library of Congress
1291 Taylor St., NW
Washington, DC 20542   202-287-5100
Free material loans to those unable to read standard printed items be-
cause of physical or visual problems. Linked to regional libraries.

Independent Living Centers
704-375-3977
300 centers located in all 50 states.   704-375-3977

National Council on Independent Living   312-226-1006

Senate Special Committee on Aging
Indigent Patient Programs
Dirksen Senate Office Building, Room G-31
Washington, DC 20510-6400
Information about Pharmaceutical Manufacturers' Prescription Drug
Indigent Programs: explanation of programs and a directory of pharma-
ceutical companies willing to provide medicines for those unable to
afford them.

The CFIDS Association of America, Inc., offers materials regarding
obtaining social security benefits. Call their 800 number and request a
materials list/order form.

Pen Pal Clubs

FMS/CFS Pen Pal Program
c/o Cathy Rich, Coordinator
1557 De Anza Boulevard
San Mateo, CA 94403
Donations appreciated.

PWC Pen-Pal Exchange
15865-B Gale Avenue
Box 818
City of Industry, CA 91745

Single/Adult Pen Pal Club
c/o Jane Ortiz
12412 Park Street
Sugar Creek, MO 64054

Children of PWC pen pals:
Mandee McCracken
96 Delaware Ave.
Penns Grove, NJ 08069-1318
Send SASE.

Teen Pen Pals:
Global Teen Club International
Cathryn Michael Murray
3120 Oak Road, Suite 309
Walnut Creek, CA 94569
Send SASE.

Teen CFIDS Pen Pal Connection (ages 10–19)
c/o Connie Howard
1810 Cliffwood Court
New Albany, IN 47150
Send SASE and 25¢.

Significant Others

Well Spouse Foundation
P.O. Box 801
New York, NY 10023   212-724-7209   800-838-0879

Support Group for Support Groups

The CFIDS Support Network of America (CSN)
PO Box 220398
Charlotte, NC 28222-0398
The CSN is a support group member-organization dedicated to provid-
ing information services to CFIDS support groups nationwide.

Newsletter Exchange Program
c/o Linda Commons
Indiana CFS Association
810 N. Bancroft
Indianapolis, IN 46201

Twins

Dedra Buchwald, M.D., a Seattle-based researcher, seeks sets of twins,
fraternal or identical, at least one of whom has CFS/FM for a study of
genetic factors. Contact Sandy Oung at Harborview, 206-223-3111

Youth

National Information Center for Children and Youth with Disabilities
   (NICHCY)
P.O. Box 1492
Washington, DC 20013   800-999-5599

National Parent to Parent Support & Information System, Inc.
P.O. Box 907
Blue Ridge, GA 30513   800-651-1151
Purpose: To link parents whose children have special health-care needs
and/or rare disorders.

Protection and Advocacy, Inc. (a federal agency that provides services
   for the disabled, including children).
Consult the business white pages or look under the Department of
Health and Human Services in the Federal Government section of your
telephone book.

Your State Department of Education.

RELATED DISORDERS:
SUPPORT AND INFORMATION

Allergy and Environmental Disorders

Allergy and Asthma Information Center & Hotline
P.O. Box 1766
Rochester, NY 14603   800-727-5400

American Academy of Allergy and Immunology
611 East Wells Street
Milwaukee, WI 53202   800-822-2762

American Academy for Environmental Medicine
P.O. Box 16106
Denver, CO 80216   303-622-9755

American College of Allergy and Immunology
800 East Northwest Highway, Suite 1080
Palatine, IL 60067-6516   800-842-7777

Asthma and Allergy Foundation of America
1717 Massachusetts Ave. NW, Suite 305
Washington, DC 20036   202-265-0265

Chemical Injury Information Network
P.O. Box 301
White Sulphur Springs, MT 59645-0301   406-547-2255

Environmental Health Network
P.O. Box 1155
Larkspur, CA 94977   415-541-5075

Environmental Health Association/HEAL Chapter
1800 S. Robertson Blvd., Suite 380
Los Angeles, CA 90035   301-837-2048

Food Allergy Network
4747 Holly Avenue
Fairfax, VA 22030-5647   800-929-4040

Human Ecology Action League
P.O. Box 49126
Atlanta, GA 30359   404-248-1898

Balance Disorders

Dizziness and Balance Disorders Association of America
1015 NW 22nd Avenue
Portland, OR 97210   503-229-7348 or 800-227-5726

Candidiasis

Candida Research Foundation
1638 B Street
Hayward, CA 94541   510-582-2179

Candida Research Foundation
Elizabeth Naugle, Director
P.O. Drawer J-F
College Station, TX 77840

Depression

National Organization for Seasonal Affective Disorder (SAD)
PO Box 40133
Washington, DC 20016

Endometriosis

The Endometriosis Association
8585 N. 76th Place
Milwaukee, WI 53223   414-355-2200

The Endo/CFIDS Data Project
P.O. Box 501
Hillsborough, NC 27278

Fatigue

Center for Fatigue Sciences
Dr. Ruby Simpkins, Director
28240 Agoura Road, Suite 201
Agoura Hills, CA 91301

Fibromyalgia and Chronic Pain

Fibromyalgia Network
5700 Stockdale Highway, #100
Bakersfield, CA 93309   805-631-1950
Membership: $15/year, includes quarterly newsletters.

Fibromyalgia Network
P.O. Box 31750
Tucson, AZ 85751-1750   520-290-5508

American Chronic Pain Association
PO Box 850
Rocklin, CA 95677   916-632-0922

National Chronic Pain Outreach Association
7979 Old Georgetown Road, Suite 100
Bethesda, MD 20814-2429

Arthritis Foundation
P.O. Box 19000
Atlanta, GA 30326   800-283-7800

Interstitial Cystitis

Interstitial Cystitis Association (ICA)
P.O. Box 151323
San Diego, CA 92175
Membership: $25, library of medical reprints, newsletter, support group
list, free consultation.

Interstitial Cystitis Association (ICA)
PO Box 1553   800-HELP-ICA
Madison Square Station, NY 10159   212-979-6057

Lupus

American Lupus Society, National Office
23751 Madison Street
Torrance, CA 90505

The Lupus Foundation of America, Inc.
P.O. Box 12897
St. Louis, MO 63141

Lyme Disease

The Midwestern Lyme Disease Association
3835 South 37th
Lincoln, NE 68506

Multiple Sclerosis

National M.S. Society
733 Third Avenue
New York, NY 10017   212-986-3240

Sjögren's Syndrome

Sjögren's Syndrome Foundation, Inc.
29 Gateway Drive
Great Neck, NY 11021

Thyroid Disorders

Thyroid Foundation of America, Inc.
Massachusetts General Hospital
Ruth Sleeper Hall, Room 350
Boston, MA 02114   800-832-8321

For physician referrals:
American Thyroid Association
Walter Reed Medical Center
Washington, DC 20307-5001   800-542-6687

MEDICAL INSURANCE

Resources for obtaining health insurance include the following:

• **Employer-sponsored plans.** Be sure to be familiar with your policy-covered expenses, deductible, coverage for experimental medications, and procedures. Find out if pre-certification is required and in what situations. If you are disabled, you may continue your insurance coverage for a specified period of time through a program called COBRA; you will be financially responsible for paying premiums. Information regarding coverage, including COBRA, is available from individual employers; large companies have human resource or benefit offices. If you have checked with them and believe you have been given vague or erroneous information, ask to see your policy or benefits booklet. The policy may be detailed and difficult to read but contains the most accurate information regarding coverage.

• **Individual insurance coverage.** You will need to shop around, both in terms of price and preexisting conditions. This type of coverage is expensive and difficult for PWCs to qualify for. Consider an insurer's track record, especially length of time in business, before purchasing a policy. Information is available from independent insurance agents or representatives of each insurance company.

- **Medicare.** For those not yet of retirement age, Medicare coverage is automatic 24 months after the effective date of Social Security Disability.

- **Organization group plans.** Professional and other organizations may offer insurance plans. However, such organizations may change insurance companies or make changes in the policies while they are in force. The cost is generally less than individual coverage, but individuals still have to qualify for coverage. For information, contact any organizations of which you are a member.

- **State insurance.** The availability, cost, and qualifying specifications vary from state to state. For information, call the appropriate state office listed in the government pages of the telephone book.

FURTHER READING

The list of books and resources below is not intended as an endorsement. These are sources of information for PWCs and their significant others. It is vital that the patient work with credentialed, experienced health care personnel in making decisions regarding treatment.

Most CFIDS support groups maintain libraries from which patients may borrow various materials, including books, audiotapes, videotapes, and reprints of medical journal and popular press articles. Public libraries often maintain CFIDS information files as well as CFIDS-related books. The psychology and self-help sections of bookstores are generally well stocked with books that may be helpful to CFIDS patients who wish to use "down time" as an opportunity to learn and grow. Additional resources are listed in the Bibliography.

Medical Journal Articles about CFIDS

Many CFIDS articles which have appeared in medical journals are available from The CFIDS Association, Inc., of Charlotte, North Carolina. The newsletters published by CFIDS organizations often contain summaries, excerpts, and critiques of the most important articles emerging from current research and practice.

Books about CFIDS

Ali, M. (1994). *The canary and chronic fatigue.* Bloomfield, NJ: Institute of Preventative Medicine.

Bell, D. S. (1994). *The doctor's guide to chronic fatigue syndrome: Understanding, treating, and living with CFIDS.* New York: Addison-Wesley. A somewhat technical but very helpful guide for health practitioners and patients.

Bell, D. S. (1991). *The disease of a thousand names: CFIDS.* Lyndonville, New York: Pollard Publications. A somewhat technical yet readable book with emphasis on epidemiology, symptomatology, causal hypotheses, and treatment.

Berne, K. H. (1990). *CFIDS lite: Chronic fatigue immune dysfunction syndrome with 1/3 the seriousness.* BHB Communications. 2207 East Ivy, Mesa, AZ 85213. $10.00 plus $2.00 shipping and handling. A humorous look at CFIDS: cartoons, jokes, limericks, more.

Collinge, W. (1993). *Recovering from chronic fatigue syndrome.* New York: Putnam. Techniques for helping the healing process and enhancing wellness.

Conant, S (1990). *Living with chronic fatigue.* TX: Taylor. A well-written book that addresses coping issues. Highly recommended.

Dayger, K. (Ed.) (1995). *Ft. Lauderdale notebook series (1994 AACFS Research Conference).* Rochester, NY: CFIDS Rochester Research Project.

Dayger, K. *Review of mainstream CFIDS research in the USA, 1990 through June 1992.* Rochester, NY: CFIDS Rochester Research Project. For information on both of these books, send SASE to CFIDS Rochester Research Project, 1200 Edgewood Avenue, Rochester, NY 14618.

Feiden, K. (1990). *Hope and help for chronic fatigue syndrome.* New York: Prentice Hall. A comprehensive and well-written book. Highly recommended.

Goldstein, J. A. (in press). *Treatment options in chronic fatigue syndrome and related neurosomatic disorders: A guide for physicians and patients.* Binghamton, NY: Haworth Medical Press.

Goldstein, J. A. (1993). *Chronic fatigue syndrome: The limbic hypothesis.* Binghamton, NY: Haworth Medical Press. Very technical but interesting guide to limbic system involvement in CFIDS.

Goldstein, J. A. (1990). *Chronic fatigue syndrome: The struggle for health.* Anaheim, CA: CFS Institute. Excellent guide for CFIDS diagnosis and treatment. Somewhat technical.

Hyde, B. (Ed.) (1992). *The clinical and scientific basis of myalgic encephalomyelitis/chronic fatigue syndrome.* Ottawa, Canada and Ogdensburg, New York: The Nightingale Research Foundation. A comprehensive and useful source of CFIDS/ME information.

Jeffreys, T. (1982). *The mile-high staircase.* Auckland: Hodder and Stoughton. Order from Waiake Wordsmiths, P.O. Box 35-0429, Browns Bay,

Auckland 10, New Zealand. $20 surface or $25 airmail. The author's account of her experience with ME. Interesting and well written.

Johnson, H. (in press). *Osler's web: Inside the labyrinth of the chronic fatigue syndrome epidemic.* An examination of the NIH and CDC responses to the CFIDS crisis, beginning with the investigation of the Lake Tahoe epidemic of 1984-85.

Kenny, T. (1994). *Living with chronic fatigue syndrome: A personal story of the struggle for recovery.* New York: Thunder's Mouth Press. The author's account of his experiences with CFIDS. Well-written.

Murray, M. T. (1994). *Chronic fatigue syndrome: Getting well naturally.* Rocklin, CA: Prima.

Schwartz, L. S. (1995). *The fatigue artist.* New York: Scribner. A novel in which the main character has CFIDS.

Teitelbaum, J. (1995). *From fatigued to fantastic!* Annapolis, MD: Deva Press. A treatment manual for CFIDS and fibromyalgia.

CFIDS Audiotapes and Videotapes

Audiotapes

Berne, K. (1995). *Understanding chronic fatigue syndrome.* A 60-minute discussion of what CFIDS is and is not, suspected causes, diagnosis, treatment, and coping techniques.

Berne, K. (1995). *Chronic fatigue syndrome relaxation tape.* Side A: Daytime: Relaxation and Energy Enhancement. Side B: Evening: Relaxation and Sleep Induction.

Berne, K. (1995). *CFS: For those who care.* Information and coping techniques for partners, family, and friends.

Berne, K. (1995). *CFS and self-esteem.* Sources of low self-esteem in PWCs and reassurance and practical techniques for increasing self-confidence.

Berne, K. (1995) *Neurocognitive aspects of CFS (or life on 7 brain cells a day).* A discussion about the neurologic/cognitive deficits associated with CFS: strategies for coping with these deficits and the embarrassment and frustration they cause.

For ordering information, see the back of this book.

Collinge, W. *Recovering from CFS: The home self-empowerment program.* A set of four tapes: 1. *Hope and recovery in CFS and mind/body medicine in CFS;* 2. *Deep relaxation; Breath, imagery and healing;* 3. *Understanding your immune system; Breathing and energy in CFS;* 4. *Meeting your inner healer; Supporting your inner child.* Ordering information: William Collinge, Ph.D., P.O. Box 2002, Sebastopol, CA 95473; 800-745-1837.

Chopra, D. *The mind/body solution to chronic fatigue.* Ordering information: Available from the CFIDS Buyers' Club.

Videotapes

Lapp, C., M.D. *Chronic fatigue syndrome—A real disease.*

Lapp, C., M.D. *CFS for health professionals: What we know.*

Cheney, P., M.D., Ph.D. and Lapp, C., M.D. *Chronic fatigue syndrome update*, Richmond, VA conference.

Hyde, B., M.D. *U.S. vs. British Research Comparisons.*

Goldberg, M., M.D. *Chronic fatigue syndrome in children.* Order from The CFIDS Foundation, 10 Wild Partridge Court, Greensboro, NC 27455-2715

Journal

The Journal of Chronic Fatigue Syndrome: Multidisciplinary Innovation in Research, Theory and Clinical Practice. Order from Haworth Press, Inc., 10 Alice Street, Binghamton, NY 13904-1580. Cost: $18 individuals; $24 institutions; $32.00 libraries. Free sample upon request.
This quarterly journal is the first devoted solely to CFIDS research.

Other CFIDS Resources

The CFIDS Reality Check. A newsletter dedicated to helping PWCs support one another. Send a SASE to The CFIDS Reality Check, 12 Wildwood Estates, Plattsburgh, NY 12901. Subscriptions $15.00.

Walders, V. (1993). *CFIDS Pathfinder to information: Comprehensive CFIDS citations.* Cost: $12 ($24 for institutions) plus $1.05 postage. Addenda (each) $6.00 plus $1.05 postage. Order from CFIDS Pathfinder, P.O. Box 2644, Kensington, MD 20891-2644. Telephone: 301-530-8624.

For PWCs and Their Families

Simonton, S. M. (1985). *The healing family.* New York: Bantam.

Strong, M. (1988). *Mainstay: For the well spouse of the chronically ill.* Boston: Little, Brown.

Books: Related Disorders

Arnold, C. (1986). *Pain: What is it? How do we deal with it?* New York: Morrow.

Backstrom, G. and Rubin, P. R. (1992). *When muscle pain won't go away.* Dallas, TX: Taylor.

Ballweg, M. L. and The Endometriosis Association (1987). *Overcoming endometriosis.* Chicago: Congdon and Weed.

Catalano, E. M. (1987). *The chronic pain control workbook.* Oakland, CA: New Harbinger Publications.

Chalker, R. and Whitmore, K. E. (1990). *Overcoming bladder disorders.* New York: Harper and Row.

Crook, W. G. (1992). *Chronic fatigue syndrome and the yeast connection.* Jackson, TN: Professional Books.

Information about systemic candidiasis and its relationship to CFIDS.

Ediger, B. (1991). *Coping with fibromyalgia.* Toronto: LHR Publications.

Friedman, A. M. *Treating chronic pain.* New York: Plenum.

Gillespie, L. (1986). *You don't have to live with cystitis.* New York: Rawson.

Levinson, H. L. (1986). *Phobia free.* New York: Evans.

Information about cause and treatment of balance disorders.

Marcus, N. J. (1994). *Freedom from chronic pain.* New York: Simon and Schuster.

Prudden, B. (1980). *Pain erasure, The Bonnie Prudden way.* New York: Evans.

Watson, M. A. and Sinclair, H. (1986). *Balancing act: For people with dizziness and balance disorders.* Portland, OR: Good Samaritan Hospital and Medical Center.

Disability

Massachusetts CFIDS Association. *How to apply for Social Security disability benefits if you have chronic fatigue syndrome.* 808 Main St., Waltham, MA 02154. 617-893-4415.

National Chronic Fatigue Syndrome Association. *Social Security disability benefits information* (pamphlet). 3521 Broadway, Suite 222, Kansas City, MO 64111. 816-931-4777.

National Organization of Social Security Claimants Representatives. *Social Security disability and SSI claims, your need for representation* (pamphlet) and *Preparing for your Social Security disability or SSI hearing* (pamphlet). 19 E. Central Avenue, Pearl River, NY 10965. 800-431-2804.

Ross, J. W. *Social Security disability benefits: How to get them! How to keep them!* R. D. 3, Three Forrester Road, Slippery Rock, PA 16057. 412-794-2837.

Social Security Administration. *Understanding Social Security and disability evaluation under Social Security.* Baltimore, MD 21235. 800-772-1213.

Coping with Chronic Illness

Donoghue, P. J., and Siegel, M. E. (1992). *Sick and tired of feeling sick and tired: Living with invisible chronic illness.* New York: Norton.

Kabat-Zinn, J. (1990). *Full catastrophe living: Using the wisdom of your body and mind to face stress, pain, and illness.* New York: Dell.

Lewis, K. S. (1985). *Successful living with chronic illness.* Wayne, NJ: Avery.

Pitzele, S. K. (1986). *We are not alone: learning to live with chronic illness.* New York: Workman.

Register, C. (1987). *Living with chronic illness: Days of patience and passion.* New York: Free Press.

Stearns, A. K. (1984). *Living through personal crisis.* Chicago: Thomas More Press.

Healing and Wellness

Borysenko, J. (1990). *Guilt is the teacher, love is the lesson.* New York: Warner.

Borysenko, J. (1987). *Minding the body, mending the mind.* Reading, MA: Addison-Wesley.

Chopra, D. (1993). *Ageless body, timeless mind.* New York: Harmony Books.

Chopra, D. *(1990). Perfect health.* New York: Harmony Books.

Chopra, D. (1989). *Quantum healing.* New York: Bantam.

Chopra, D. (1987). *Creating health.* Boston, MA: Houghton Mifflin.

Cousins, N. (1989). *Head first.* New York: Dutton.

Cousins, N. (1983). *The healing heart.* New York: Norton.

Cousins, N. (1979). *Anatomy of an illness as perceived by the patient.* New York: Norton.

Dion, S. (1993). *Write now: Maintaining a creative spirit while homebound and ill.* Teaneck, NJ: Puffin Foundation. May be ordered from S. Dion, 432 Ives Avenue, Carneys Point, NJ 08069. Free of charge; donations are appreciated. Send SASE (with one 32 cent and four 23 cent stamps). Also available on diskette.

Kastner, M. (1993). *Alternative healing.* La Mesa, CA: Halcyon Publishers.

Kievman, B. and Blackmun, S. (1989). *For better or for worse: A couple's guide to dealing with chronic illness.* Chicago: Contemporary Books.

Lewis, K. S. (1985). *Successful living with chronic illness.* Wayne, NJ: Avery.

Locke, S., and Colligan, D. (1986). *The healer within: The new medicine of mind and body.* New York: New American Library.

MacFarlane, E. B. and Burstein, P. (1994). *Legwork: An inspiring journey through a chronic illness* [multiple sclerosis]. New York: Scribner.

Matthews-Simonton, S., Simonton, O. C., and Creighton, J. L. (1980). *Getting well again.* New York: Bantam.

Mizel, S. B. and Jaret, P. (1986). *The human immune system: The new frontier in medicine.* New York: Simon and Schuster.

Siegel, B. S. (1986). *Love, medicine and miracles.* New York: Harper and Row.

Siegel, B. S. (1989). *Peace, love and healing.* New York: Harper and Row.

Weil, A. (1988, rev. ed.). *Health and healing.* Boston: Houghton Mifflin.

Weil, A (1990). *Natural health, natural medicine.* Boston: Houghton Mifflin.

Weil, A (1995). *Spontaneous healing.* New York: Alfred A. Knopf.

Weil, A (1990). *Natural health, natural medicine.* Boston: Houghton Mifflin.

Medical Care

Berger, S. M. (1988). *What your doctor didn't learn in medical school . . . and what you can do about it.* New York: Morrow.

Inlander, C. B., Levin, L. S., and Weiner, E. (1988). *Medicine on trial.* New York: Prentice Hall.

Robin, E. D. (1984). *Matters of life and death: Risks versus benefits of medical care.* New York: W. H. Freeman.

Weil, A. (1988, rev. ed.). *Health and healing.* Boston: Houghton Mifflin.

Bibliography

BOOKS

Achterberg, J. (1985). *Imagery in healing: Shamanism and modern medicine.* Boston: New Science Library.

Barry, D. (1988). *Dave Barry's greatest hits.* New York: Crown.

Berger, S. M. (1988). *What your doctor didn't learn in medical school . . . and what you can do about it.* New York: Morrow.

Brooks, B., and Smith, N. (1988). *CFIDS: An owner's manual.* Silver Springs, MD: BBNS.

Crook, W. G. (1986). *The yeast connection: A medical breakthrough.* New York: Random House.

Epstein, M. A., and Achong, B. G. (eds.). (1979). *The Epstein-Barr virus.* New York: Springer-Verlag.

Ferguson, M. (1980). *The Aquarian conspiracy: Personal and social transformation in the 1980s.* Los Angeles: J. P. Tarcher.

Feuerstein, M., Labbe, E., and Kuczmierczyk, A. (1986). *Health psychology: A psychobiological perspective.* New York: Plenum.

Fisher, G. C. (1987). *Waiting to live: The debilitating effects of chronic Epstein-Barr virus.* Montclair, NJ: Montco, revised and released as *Chronic fatigue syndrome: A victim's guide to understanding, treating, and coping with this debilitating illness.* New York: Warner.

Franklin, M. and Sullivan, J. (1989). *M.E.: What is it? have you got it? how to get better.* London: Century.

Gentry, W. D. (ed.). (1984). *Handbook of behavioral medicine.* New York: Guilford Press.

Goldberger, L., and Breznitz, S. (eds.). (1982). *Handbook of stress: Theoretical and clinical aspects.* New York: Free Press.

Goodnick, P. J. and Klimas, N. G. (eds.) (1993). *Chronic fatigue and related immune deficiency syndromes.* Washington, DC: American Psychiatric Press.

Halstead, L. S., Weichers, D. O., and Rossi, C. D. (1985). Late effects of poliomyelitis: A national Survey, in Halstead, L. S. and Weichers, D. O. (eds.) in *Late effects of poliomyelitis.* Miami, FL: Symposia Foundation.

Herzlich, C. (1973). *Health and illness: A social psychological analysis.* New York: Academic Press.

Inlander, C. B., Levin, L. S., and Weiner, E. (1988). *Medicine on trial: The appalling story of ineptitude, neglect, and arrogance.* New York: Prentice Hall.

Janiger, O. and Goldberg, P. (1993). *A different kind of healing*. New York: Tarcher.

Jenkins, R. and Mowbray, J. F. (eds.) (1991). *Post-viral fatigue syndrome*. New York: Wiley.

Koch-Hattem, A. (1987). Families and chronic illness. In Rosenthal, D. (ed.). *Family Stress*. Rockville, MD: Aspen.

LeMaistre, J. (1985). *Beyond rage: The emotional impact of chronic physical illness*. Oak Park, IL: Alpine Guild.

Levin, A. S. and Byers, V. S. (1987). Environmental illness: A disorder of immune regulation, in *State of the art reviews: Occupational medicine*. Philadelphia: Hanley and Belfus, 669–681.

Monette, P. (1988). *Borrowed time: An AIDS memoir*. New York: Harcourt Brace Jovanovich.

Morozov, P. V. (ed.). (1983). *Research on the viral hypothesis of mental disorders*. Basel, Switzerland: Karger.

Nash, O. (1969). *Bed riddance: A posy for the indisposed*. Boston: Little, Brown.

Pearsall, P. (1987). *Superimmunity: Master your emotions and improve your health*. New York: Fawcett.

Pelletier, K. R. (1977). *Mind as healer, mind as slayer*. New York: Dell.

Pincus, J. H. and Tucker, G. (1974). *Behavioral neurology*. New York: Oxford University.

Podell, R. N. (1987). *Doctor, Why am I so tired?* New York: Pharos.

Randolph, T. G. (1980). *An alternative approach to allergies*. New York: Lippincott and Crowell.

Restak, R. M. (1984). *The brain*. New York: Bantam.

Robin, E. D. (1984). *Matters of life and death: Risks versus benefits of medical care*. New York: W. H. Freeman.

Roessler, R., and Decker, N. (Eds.) (1986). *Emotional disorders in physically ill patients*. New York: Human Science.

Rooney, A. A. (1981). Mr. Rooney Goes to Work (orig. broadcast July 5, 1977). In *A few minutes with Andy Rooney*. New York: Warner.

Rooney, A. A. (1982). *Pieces of my mind*. New York: Avon.

Rossi, E. L. (1986). *The psychobiology of mind-body healing: New concepts of therapeutic hypnosis*. New York: Norton.

Schlossberg, D. (ed.). (1983). *Infectious mononucleosis: Praeger monographs in infectious diseases (Vol. 1)*. New York: Praeger.

Seligman, M. E. P. (1975). *Helplessness: On depression, development and death*. San Francisco: W. H. Freeman.

Selye, H. (1974). *Stress without distress*. New York: Signet.

Selye, H. (1976). *The stress of life* (rev. ed.). New York: McGraw-Hill.

Shealy, C. N. (1979). *90 days to self health*. New York: Bantam.

Shilts, R. (1987). *And the band played on: Politics, people and the AIDS epidemic*. New York: St. Martin's.

Simonton, O. C., Matthews-Simonton, S., and Creighton, J. L. (1984). *Getting well again*. New York: Bantam.

Solomon, N. (1989). *Sick and tired of being sick and tired*. New York: Wynwood.

Sontag, S. (1977). *Illness as metaphor*. New York: Farrar, Straus and Giroux.

Sontag, S. (1988). *AIDS and its metaphors*. New York: Farrar, Straus and Giroux.

Spink, W. (1978). *Infectious diseases: Prevention and treatment in the 19th and 20th centuries*. Minneapolis: University of Minnesota.

Trowbridge, J. P., and Walker, M. (1986). *The yeast syndrome*. New York: Bantam.

Viorst, J. (1986). *Necessary losses*. New York: Simon and Schuster.

Weiner, M. A. (1986). *Maximum immunity*. Boston: Houghton Mifflin.

Wood, T. M. (1989). *Life in the slow lane*. Madison, TN: Woodshed.

PERIODICALS

Ablashi, D. V. and Pearson, G. R. (1993-1994, Winter). How frequently HHV-6 is activated in CFS patients. *Heart of America News*, 1–5.

Ablashi, D. V., Berneman, Z., et al. (1994). Kutapressin inhibits in vitro infection of human herpesvirus type 6. *Clinical Infectious Diseases*, 18(Suppl.1), S113.

Ablashi, D. V. (1994). Summary: Viral studies of chronic fatigue syndrome. *Clinical Infectious Diseases*, 18(Suppl.1), S130–133.

Adler, T. (1990, July). Neurotoxics called major health threat. *The APA Monitor*, 18.

Adler, T. (1991, February). Optimists' coping skills may help beat illnesses. *The APA Monitor*, 12.

Allen, A. D. (1986, May 3). Epstein-Barr: A causative cofactor [Letter]. *Science News*, 275.

Allen, A. D., and Tilkian, S. M. (1986). Depression correlated with cellular immunity in systemic immunodeficient Epstein-Barr virus syndrome (SIDES). *Journal of Clinical Psychiatry*, 47(3), 133–135.

Altman, L. K. (1990, December 4). Chronic fatigue syndrome finally gets some respect. *The New York Times*.

Amsterdam, J. D., Henle, W., et al. (1986). Serum antibodies to Epstein-Barr virus in patients with major depressive disorder. *American Journal of Psychiatry, 143,* 1593–1596.

ANZME Society, Inc. (1991, August). *Meeting-Place 36* [Journal]. Auckland, New Zealand.

Baer, K. (1993, September). Chronic fatigue syndrome: Still puzzling after all these years. *Harvard Health Letter, 18*(11), 1–4.

Barker, E., Fujimura, S. F., et al. (1994). Immunologic abnormalities associated with chronic fatigue syndrome. *Clinical Infectious Diseases, 18*(Suppl.1), S136–141.

Behan, P. O., Haniffah, B. A. G., et al. (1994). A pilot study of sertraline for the treatment of chronic fatigue syndrome [abstract]. *Clinical Infectious Diseases, 18*(Suppl.1), S111.

Behan, P. O., Behan, W. M. H., and Bell, E. J. (1985). The postviral fatigue syndrome—an analysis of the findings in 50 cases. *Journal of Infection, 10,* 211–212.

Bell, D. S. (1992). Chronic fatigue syndrome. *Postgraduate Medicine. 91*(6), 245–252.

———. (1995). Chronic fatigue syndrome in children. *Journal of Chronic Fatigue Syndrome, 1*(1), 9–33.

Bender, C. E. (1962). Recurrent mononucleosis. *Journal of the American Medical Association, 182*(9), 954–956.

Bennett, W. I. (ed.) (1988, July). Chronic fatigue syndrome. *Harvard Medical School Health Letter,* 1–3.

Berris, B. (1986). Chronic viral diseases. *Canadian Medical Association Journal, 135,* 1260–1268.

Boffey, P. (1987, July 28). Fatigue 'virus' has experts more baffled and skeptical than ever. *New York Times.*

Boly, W. (1987, July-August) Raggedy Ann town. *Hippocrates,* 31–40.

Bothe, K., Aguzzi, A., et al. (1991, August 2). Progressive encephalopathy and myopathy in transgenic mice expressing human foamy virus genes. *Science,* as annotated and excerpted in *CACTUS September 1991 Research Update,* 16–18.

Bou-Holaigah, I., Rowe, P.C., et al. (1995, September 27). The relationship between neurally mediated hypotension and the chronic fatigue syndrome. *Journal of the American Medical Association, 247:* 961–967.

Brigham, C. R. (1988, January). Medical consultant updates: Chronic fatigue syndrome. *LTD Advisor,* Miele and Associates, 12–14.

Broadgate Consultants, Inc., Ampligen. Background on an experimental drug for the treatment of HIV infection and AIDS, chronic fatigue syndrome, several forms of cancer, chronic hepatitis B. New York: Broadgate Consultants, Inc.

Brody, J. E. (1985, June 12). An elusive herpes virus makes double misery for its victims. *The New York Times.*

———. (1988, February 16). Personal health: Coping with chronic illness can be grueling in a society that is often blind to the problems. *The New York Times.*

———. (1988, July 28). Personal health: Chronic fatigue syndrome: How to recognize it and what to do about it. *The New York Times.*

Bruno, R. L., Frick, N. M., et al. (1994, Fall). The physiology of postpolio fatigue: A model for postviral fatigue syndromes and a brain fatigue generator. *The CFIDS Chronicle,* 36–42.

Buchwald, D., Cheney, P. R., et al. (1992, January 15). A chronic illness characterized by fatigue, neurologic and immunologic disorders, and active human herpesvirus type 6 infection. *Annals of internal medicine,* 116(2), 103–113

Buchwald, D., Pascualy, R., et al. (1994). Sleep disorders in patients with chronic fatigue. *Clinical Infectious Diseases,* 18(Suppl.1), S68–72.

Buchwald, D., Sullivan, J. L., and Komaroff, A. L. (1987). Frequency of 'chronic active Epstein-Barr virus infection' in a general medical practice. *Journal of the American Medical Association,* 257, 2303–2307.

Burden, D. (1989, July/August). Caring for the caregiver. *Psychology Today,* 22.

Burns, R. (1995, Spring). Johns Hopkins research may hold promise for PWCs. *The CFIDS Chronicle,* 4–8.

Caffery, B. E., Josephson, J. E., and Samek, M. J. (1994). The ocular signs and symptoms of chronic fatigue syndrome. *Journal of the American Optometry Association,* 65(3), 187–191.

Calabrese, L., Danao, T., et al. (1992, March). Chronic fatigue syndrome. *American Family Physician,* 45(3), 1205–1213.

Calabrese, L. H., Davis, M. E., and Wilke, W. S. (1994). Chronic fatigue syndrome and a disorder resembling Sjögren's syndrome: Preliminary report. *Clinical Infectious Diseases,* 18(Suppl.1), S28–31.

Caliguiri, M., Murray, C., et al. (1987). Phenotypic and functional deficiency of natural killer cells in patients with chronic fatigue syndrome. *Journal of Immunology.* 139, 3306–3313.

Carpman, V. (1993, Fall). Chemical warfare: CFIDS, multiple chemical sensitivity and silicone implant disorder. *The CFIDS Chronicle,* 33–41.

————. (1995, Spring). CFIDS treatment: The Cheney Clinic's strategic approach. *The CFIDS Chronicle*, 38-45.

The CFIDS Association, Inc. *The CFIDS Chronicle*. 1988–1995.

Cheney, P. R. and Lapp, C. W. (1993, March/April). The diagnosis of chronic fatigue syndrome. *The CFS DysPatch*, 3(2), 1–8.

Chester, A. C., and Levine, P. H. (1994). Concurrent sick building syndrome and chronic fatigue syndrome: Epidemic neuromyasthenia revisited. *Clinical Infectious Diseases*, 18(Suppl.1), S43–48.

Chronic fatigue: all in the mind? (1990, October). *Consumer Reports*, 671–675.

Chronic Fatigue Immune Dysfunction Syndrome Foundation (1990, Summer). *CFIDS Treatment News*, 1(1).

Chronic Fatigue Syndrome Association of Arizona newsletters: *CEBV Jigsaw*, 1987–88; *CFS Bulletin* 1988–89.

'Chronic mononucleosis' puzzles clinicians. (1987, October 15). *Patient Care*, 19.

Consumers Union. (1994, August). Breathing on a jet plane, 501–506.

Coulter, P. (1988). Chronic fatigue syndrome: An old virus with a new diagnosis. *Journal of Community Health Nursing*, 5(2), 87–95.

Cowley, G. (1992, September 7). AIDS or chronic fatigue? *Newsweek*, 66, 69.

Cowley, G. with Hager, M. (1991, September 30). A clue to chronic fatigue. *Newsweek*, 66.

Cowley, G., with Hager, M. and Joseph, N. (1990, November 12). Chronic fatigue syndrome: A modern medical mystery. *Newsweek*, 62–70.

Cowley, G., with Springen, K., et al. (1990, March 26). The promise of Prozac. *Newsweek*, 38–41.

David, A. S., Wessely, S., and Pelosi, A. J. (1988, July 9). Myalgic encephalomyelitis, or what? [Letter]. *The Lancet*, 100.

————. (1988). Postviral fatigue syndrome: Time for a new approach. *British Medical Journal*, 296, 696–699.

DeFreitas, E., Hilliard, B., et al. (1991, April). Retroviral sequences related to human T-lymphotropic virus type II in patients with chronic fatigue immune dysfunction syndrome. *Proceedings of the National Academy of Sciences*, 88, 2922-2926.

DeLisi, L. E., Nurnberger, L. R., et al. (1986). Epstein-Barr virus and depression [Letter]. *Archives of General Psychiatry*, 43, 815–816.

DeLisi, L. E., Smith, S. B., et al. (1986). Herpes simplex virus, cytomegalovirus and Epstein-Barr virus antibody titres in sera from schizophrenic patients. *Psychological Medicine*, 16, 757–763.

Demitrack, M. A., Dale, J. K., et al. (1991). Evidence for impaired activation of the hypothalamic-pituitary-adrenal axis in patients with chronic fatigue syndrome. *Journal of Clinical Endocrinology and Metabolism, 7*(6), 1224–1234.

Dengler, R., Thomssen, H., et al. (1987). Chronic Epstein-Barr virus infection and human immunodeficiency virus infection [Letter]. *Annals of Internal Medicine, 106,* 775.

Dreifus, C. (1993, October-November). Prince of PBS. *Modern Maturity,* 73.

DuBois, R. E. (1986). Gamma globulin therapy for chronic mononucleosis syndrome. *AIDS Research, 2*(Suppl.1), 191–195.

DuBois, R. E., Seeley, J. K., et al. (1984). Chronic mononucleosis syndrome. *Southern Medical Journal, 77,* 1376–1382.

Edwards, D. D. (1987). Viruses in search of 'compatible' diseases. *Science News, 132,* 246.

English, T. L. (1991, February 21). Skeptical of skeptics. *Journal of the American Medical Association, 265*(8), 964.

Englund, J. A. (1988). The many faces of Epstein-Barr virus. *Postgraduate Medicine, 83*(2), 167–173, 176–180.

Findlay, S. (1988, October 31). New hope for tired people. *U.S. News and World Report, 71,* 73.

Fotheringham, C. (1987, November 18). Tests reveal new clue in fatigue illness. *North Lake Tahoe Bonanza.*

Fukuda, K., Straus, S. E., et al. (1994, December). The chronic fatigue syndrome: A comprehensive approach to its definition and study. *Annals of Internal Medicine, 121,* 953–959.

Gantz, N. M. and Holmes, G. P. (1989). Treatment of patients with chronic fatigue syndrome. *Drugs, 38* (6), 856–862.

Garlock, K, (1993, December 20). Chronic fatigue treatment patented. Charlotte, NC: *The Charlotte Observer.*

Garry, R. F. (1994, April). New evidence for involvement of retroviruses in Sjögren's Syndrome and other autoimmune diseases. *Arthritis and Rheumatism, 37,* 465–469.

Gin, W., Christiansen, F. T., and Peter, J. B. (1989). Immune function and the chronic fatigue syndrome. *Medical Journal of Australia, 151,* 117–118.

Goldenberg, D. L. (1990). Fibromyalgia and its relation to chronic fatigue syndrome, viral illness and immune abnormalities. From the Rheumatology, Arthritis-Fibrositis Center, Tufts University School of Medicine, published in *The Mass. CFIDS Update,* Summer, 1990, 27–29.

Goldenberg, D. L., Simms, R. W., et al. (1990). High frequency of fibromyalgia in patients with chronic fatigue seen in a primary care practice. *Arthritis and Rheumatism, 33*(3), 381–387.

Goldstein, J. A., Mena, I., et al. (1995). The assessment of vascular abnormalities in late life chronic fatigue syndrome by brain SPECT: Comparison with late life major depressive disorder. *Journal of Chronic Fatigue Syndrome, 1*(1), 55–79.

Goldstein, J. A. (1994, Summer). New treatments for CFS. *The CFIDS Chronicle,* 2–6.

————. (1993, Fall). The neuropharmacology of chronic fatigue syndrome. *The CFIDS Chronicle,* 24–27.

————. (1991, January). Chronic fatigue syndrome. *The Female Patient, 16*(1), 39–50.

————. (1986). Treatment of Epstein-Barr virus with H_2 blockers [Letter]. *Journal of Clinical Psychiatry, 47,* 572.

Goodnick, P. J. and Sandoval, R. (1993, January). Psychotropic treatment of chronic fatigue syndrome and related disorders. *Journal of Clinical Psychiatry, 54*(1), 13–20.

————. (1993). Psychotropic treatment of chronic fatigue syndrome and related disorders. *Journal of Clinical Psychology, 54,* 13–20.

Gow, J. W., Behan, W. M. H., et al. (1994). Studies of enterovirus in patients with chronic fatigue syndrome. *Clinical Infectious Diseases, 18*(Suppl.1), S126–129.

Greenberg, D. B. (1986). Depression, anxiety, and Epstein-Barr virus infection [Letter]. *Annals of Internal Medicine, 104,* 449.

Grierson, H., Holmes, G. P., and Straus, S. E. (1987, November 15). Coping with chronic fatigue syndrome. *Patient Care,* 79–82.

Grinspoon, L. (ed.) (1994, August and September). Sleep Disorders—Parts I and II. *The Harvard Mental Health Letter, 11*(2), 1–4, and (3), 1–5.

Hamblin, T. J., Hussain, J., et al. (1983). Immunological reasons for chronic ill health after infectious mononucleosis. *British Medical Journal, 287,* 85–88.

Heneine, W., Woods, T. C., et al. (1994). Lack of evidence for infection with known human and animal retroviruses in patients with chronic fatigue syndrome. *Clinical Infectious Diseases, 18*(Suppl.1), S121–125.

Henle, W. and Henle, G. (1981, January). Serodiagnosis of infectious mononucleosis. *Resident and Staff Physician,* 37–43.

Henle, W., Henle, G., and Lennette, E. T. (1979). The Epstein-Barr virus. *Scientific American, 241*(1), 48–59.

Hickie, I., Lloyd, A., et al. (1990). The psychiatric status of patients with the chronic fatigue syndrome. *British Journal of Psychiatry, 156,* 534–540.

Holmes, G. P., Kaplan, J. E., et al. (1988). Chronic fatigue syndrome: A working case definition. *Annals of Internal Medicine, 108,* 387–389.

Holmes, G. P., Kaplan, J. E., et al. (1987). A cluster of patients with a chronic mononucleosis-like syndrome: Is Epstein-Barr the cause? *Journal of the American Medical Association, 257,* 2297–2302.

Horrobin, D. F. (1991). Essential fatty acids and the post-viral fatigue syndrome. In Jenkins, R. and Mowbray, J. (eds.) *Postviral fatigue syndrome,* 393–404. New York: Wiley.

Ichise, M., Salit, I. E., et al. (1992). Assessment of regional cerebral perfusion by $^{99}Tc^m$-HMPAO in chronic fatigue syndrome. *Nuclear Medicine Communications, 31,* 767–772.

Jamal, G. A., and Hansen, S. (1985). Electrophysiological studies in the post-viral fatigue syndrome. *Journal of Neurology, Neurosurgery and Psychiatry, 48,* 691–694.

Jaret, P. (1986). Our immune system: The wars within. *National Geographic, 169,* 702–735.

Johnson, H. (1987, August 13). Journey into fear: The growing nightmare of Epstein-Barr virus [Part 2]. *Rolling Stone,* 42–46, 55–57.

———. (1987, July 16). Journey into fear: The growing nightmare of Epstein-Barr virus [Part 1]. *Rolling Stone,* 56–63, 139–141.

Joncas, J. H., Ghibo, F., et al. (1984, February 1). A familial syndrome of susceptibility to chronic active Epstein-Barr virus infection. *Canadian Medical Association Journal, 130,* 280–285.

Jones, J. F. (1986, October). Epstein-Barr virus: Probable cause of a broad range of infections. *Consultant,* 77–81.

Jones, J. F., Ray, C. G., et al. (1985). Evidence for active Epstein-Barr virus infection in patients with persistent, unexplained illnesses: Elevated anti-early antigen antibodies. *Annals of Internal Medicine, 102* (1), 1–7.

Jones, J. F., Shurin, S., et al. (1988). T-cell lymphomas containing Epstein-Barr viral DNA in patients with chronic Epstein-Barr virus infections. *New England Journal of Medicine, 318,* 733–741.

Kaslow, A. (1987, March). Chronic Epstein-Barr virus syndrome. *Let's Live,* 11–12, 14.

Kelly, J. (1988, August). Immunomodulators hailed as Rx. *Medical World News,* 25. (Reprinted in *CFS Bulletin,* CFS Association of Greater Phoenix, December 1988–January 1989).

Kilsheimer, J. (1994, January 8). New cures become available for those owning "sick homes." *The Arizona Republic,* AH-14.

Klimas, N. G., Salvato, F. R., et al. (1990). Immunologic abnormalities in chronic fatigue syndrome. *Journal of Clinical Microbiology, 28*(6), 1403–1410.

Kohl, R. L., and Lewis, M. R. (1987, December). Mechanisms underlying the antimotion sickness effects of psychostimulants. *Aviation, Space, and Environmental Medicine*, 1215–1218.

Kolata, G. (1990, October). Using body's controls to develop new class of immune boosters. *The New York Times*.

Komaroff, A. L. (1987, May 30). The 'chronic mononucleosis' syndromes. *Hospital Practice*, 71–75.

———. (1988). Chronic fatigue syndromes: relationship to chronic viral infections. *Journal of Virological Methods*, 21, 3–10.

Kroenke, K. (1991). Chronic fatigue syndrome: Is it real? *Postgraduate Medicine*, 89(2), 44, 46, 49, 50, 53, 55.

Kroenke, K., Wood, D. R., et al. (1988). Chronic fatigue in primary care: Prevalence, patient characteristics, and outcome. *Journal of the American Medical Association*, 270, 929–934.

Kruesi, M. J. P., Dale, J., and Straus, S. (1989, February). Psychiatric diagnoses in patients who have chronic fatigue syndrome. *Journal of Clinical Psychiatry*, 50(2), 53–56.

Landay, A. L., Jessop, C., et al. (1991, September 21). Chronic fatigue syndrome: clinical condition associated with immune activation. *The Lancet*, 338 (8769), 707–712.

Lapp, C. W. (1992, Winter). Chronic fatigue syndrome is a real disease. *North Carolina Family Physician*, 43(1).

Lever, A. M. L., Lewis, D. M., et al. (1988, July 19). Interferon production in postviral fatigue syndrome [Letter]. *The Lancet*, 101.

Levy, J. A. (1994). Introduction: Viral studies of chronic fatigue syndrome. *Clinical Infectious Diseases*, 18(Suppl.1), S117–120.

Lloyd, A., Gandevia, S., et al. (1994). Cytokine production and fatigue in patients with chronic fatigue syndrome and healthy control subjects in response to exercise. *Clinical Infectious Diseases*, 18(Suppl.1), S142–146.

Lloyd, A., Hickie, I., et al. (1990). A double-blind, placebo-controlled trial of intravenous immunoglobin therapy in patients with chronic fatigue syndrome. *The American Journal of Medicine*, 89, 561–568.

Lloyd, A. R., Hickie, I., et al. (1990, November 5). Prevalence of chronic fatigue syndrome in an Australian population. *The Medical Journal of Australia*, 153, 522–528.

Lloyd, A. R., Wakefield, D., et al. (1988, June 4). What is myalgic encephalomyelitis? [Letter]. *The Lancet*, 1286–1287.

Loveless, M. O., Lloyd, A., and Perpich, R. (1994). Summary of public policy and chronic fatigue syndrome: A perspective. *Clinical Infectious Diseases*, 18(Suppl.1), S163–65.

Mangano, J. J. (1994, Winter). Could CFIDS be a radiation-related disorder? *The CFIDS Chronicle*, 36–38.

Manu, P., Matthews, D. A., and Lane, T. J. (1988). The mental health of patients with a chief complaint of chronic fatigue. *Archives of Internal Medicine, 148*, 2313–2320.

Marchesani, R. B. (1992, November). Crimson crescents facilitate CFS diagnosis. *Infectious Disease News, 5*(11), 1, 3.

Martinovic, A. M. and Gray, J. B. (1994, Summer) EFAMs in the pathogenesis and management of CFS. *The CFIDS Chronicle*, 18–28.

Marx, J. L. (1985). The immune system 'belongs in the body.' *Science, 227*, 1190–1192.

The Mass. CFIDS Association. *The Update* (newsletter): 1990: Summer, Winter; 1991: Summer; 1992: Summer.

Masterson, M. (1989, January 29–February 3). The poison within (special series). *The Arizona Republic*.

Matthews, D. A., Manu, P. and Lane, T. J. (1991). Evaluation and management of patients with chronic fatigue syndrome. *American Journal of the Medical Sciences, 302*(5), 269–277.

Moldofsky, H. (1991, Spring) Sleep disorders in fibromyalgia and CFIDS [lecture transcript]. In *The CFIDS Chronicle*.

Murdoch, J. C. (1984). Myalgic encephalomyelitis and the general practitioner. *New Zealand Family Physician, 11*, 127–128.

National Chronic Fatigue Syndrome Association. *Heart of America News* (Newsletter). 1988: September; 1988–89: December/January; Fall/Winter; 1990: Spring/Summer, Fall/Winter; 1993: Fall; 1993–94: Winter.

National Institute of Allergy and Infectious Diseases. (1988, June; 1990, December; 1993, February). Reports: *Backgrounder* and *News from NIAID*, National Institutes of Health.

National Jewish Hospital for Immunology and Respiratory Medicine. (1984). Epstein-Barr virus. *Med Facts*.

National Jewish Hospital and Research Center; National Asthma Center. (1984). Baffling illness traced to virus. *New Directions, 14*(3).

Nelson, P. K. (Fall, 1994). Fingerprint "loss"—Is it a sign of CFIDS? *The CFIDS Chronicle*, 49–50.

Nightingale Research Foundation. *The Nightingale* (newsletter). 1989: Fall; 1990: Spring. Ottawa, Canada.

Ojo-Amaize, E. A., Conley, E. J., and Peter, J. B. (1994). Decreased natural killer cell activity is associated with severity of chronic fatigue syndrome. *Clinical Infectious Diseases, 18*(Suppl.1), S157–159.

Olson, G. B., Kanaan, M. N., et al. (1986). Correlation between allergy and persistent Epstein-Barr virus- infected patients. *Journal of Allergy and Clinical Immunology, 78*, 308–314.

Olson, G. B., Kanaan, M. N., et al. (1986). Specific allergen-induced Epstein-Barr nuclear antigen-positive B cells from patients with chronic-active Epstein-Barr virus infections. *Journal of Allergy and Clinical Immunology, 78*, 315–320.

Orbaek, P., and Lindgren, M. (1988). Prospective clinical and psychometric investigation of patients with chronic toxic encephalopathy induced by solvents. *Scandinavian Journal of Work Environment and Health, 14*, 37–44.

Osterholm, K. (1988, January/February). The 10 most hunted viruses. *American Health*, 67–78.

Ostrom, N. (1990). CFIDS: A selected chronology of events. *That New Magazine, Inc.*

Pagano, J. S., Sixbey, J. W., and Lin, J. C. (1982). Acyclovir and Epstein-Barr infection. *Journal of Antimicrobial Chemotherapy, 12*(Suppl. B), 113–121.

Peterson, P. K., et al. (1990). A controlled trial of intravenous immuno-globin G in chronic fatigue syndrome. *The American Journal of Medicine, 89*, 554–560.

Potzanick, W. and Kozol, N. (1992). Ocular manifestations of chronic fatigue and immune dysfunction syndrome. *Optometry and Vision Science, 69*(10), 811–814.

Ramsay, A. M. (1988, July 9). Myalgic encephalomyelitis or what? [Letter]. *The Lancet*, 100.

———. (1981, October 7). A baffling syndrome. *Nursing Mirror*, 40–41.

———. (1976, September). Benign myalgic encephalomyelitis or epidemic neuromyasthenia. *Update*, 539–541.

Rigden, S. (1995, Spring). Entero-hepatic resuscitation program for CFIDS. *The CFIDS Chronicle*, 46–49.

Rowe, P., Bou-Holaigah, I., et al. (1995). Is neurally mediated hypotension an unrecognized cause of chronic fatigue? *Lancet, 345*, 623–624.

Salahuddin, S. Z., Ablashi, D. V., et al. (1986). Isolation of a new virus, HBLV, in patients with lymphoproliferative disorders. *Science, 234*, 596–601.

Sandman, C. A, Barron, J. L., et al. (1993). Memory deficits associated with chronic fatigue syndrome. *Biological Psychiatry, 33*, 618-623.

Schluederberg, A., Straus, S. E., et al. (1992, August 15). Chronic fatigue syndrome research: Definition and medical outcome assessment. *Annals of Internal Medicine, 117*(4), 325–331.

Schwartz, R. B., Garada, B. M., et al. (1994). Detection of intracranial abnormalities in patients with chronic fatigue syndrome: Comparison of MR imaging and SPECT. *American Journal of Roentgenology, 162,* 935–941.

Schwartz, R. B., Komaroff, A. L., et al. (1994). SPECT imaging of the brain: Comparison of findings in patients with chronic fatigue syndrome, AIDS dementia complex, and major unipolar depression. *American Journal of Roentgenology, 162,* 943–951.

Seligman, J., with Abramson, P., et al. (1987, Spring). Epstein-Barr: A puzzling virus. *Newsweek, 7.*

Solomon, G. F. (1995). Psychoneuroimmunology and chronic fatigue syndrome: Toward new models of disease. *Journal of Chronic Fatigue Syndrome, 1*(1), 3–7.

South Sound CFIDS Support Group. (1991, April). *South Sound Newsbrief.* Orting, WA.

Spracklen, F. H. N. (1988). The chronic fatigue syndrome (myalgic encephalomyelitis)—myth or mystery? *South African Medical Journal, 74,* 448–452.

Staver, S. (1989, May 26). Meeting sheds light on chronic fatigue. *American Medical News,* 9–10

Steeper, T. A., Horwitz, C. A., et al. (1987). Selected aspects of acute and chronic infectious mononucleosis and mononucleosis-like illnesses for the practicing allergist. *Annals of Allergy, 59,* 243–250.

Steinbach, T., Hermann, W., et al. (1994). Subjective reduction in symptoms of chronic fatigue syndrome following long-term treatment with a porcine liver extract: A phase 1 trial. *Clinical Infectious Diseases, 18*(Suppl.1), S114.

Stewart, D. E. (1986). Environmental illness and patients with multiple unexplained symptoms [Letter]. *Archives of Internal Medicine, 146,* 1447.

Straus, S. E. (1988). The chronic mononucleosis syndrome. *Journal of Infectious Diseases, 157,* 405–412.

————. (1987). EB or not EB—that is the question [Editorial]. *Journal of the American Medical Association, 257,* 2335–2336.

Straus, S. E., Dale, J. K., et al. (1988). Acyclovir treatment of the chronic fatigue syndrome: Lack of efficacy in a placebo-controlled trial. *New England Journal of Medicine, 319,* 1692–1697.

Straus, S. E., Tosato, G., et al. (1985). Persisting illness and fatigue in adults with evidence of Epstein-Barr virus infection. *Annals of Internal Medicine, 102*(1), 7–16.

Strayer, D. R., Carter, W. A., et al. (1994). A controlled clinical trial with a specifically configured RNA drug, Poly(I)-Poly (C$_{12}$U), in chronic fatigue syndrome. *Clinical Infectious Diseases, 18*(Suppl.1), S88–95.

Strayer, D. R., Carter, W., et al. (1995). Long-term improvements in patients with chronic fatigue syndrome treated with Ampligen. *Journal of Chronic Fatigue Syndrome, 1*(1), 35–53.

Suhadolnik, R. J., Reichenbach, N. L., et al. (1994). Upregulation of the 2-5A Synthetase/RNase L antiviral pathway associated with chronic fatigue syndrome. *Clinical Infectious Diseases, 18*(Suppl.1), S96–104.

Sumaya, C. V. (1977). Endogenous reactivation of Epstein-Barr virus infections. *Journal of Infectious Diseases, 135*(3), 374–379.

Swartz, M. N. (1988). The chronic fatigue syndrome—One entity or many? [Letter]. *New England Journal of Medicine, 319,* 1726–1728.

Tansey, M. A. (1993, Fall). EEG neurofeedback and chronic fatigue syndrome: New findings with respect to diagnosis and treatment. *The CFIDS Chronicle,* 30–32.

Tobi, M., David, Z., and Feldman-Weiss, V., (1982, January 9). Prolonged atypical illness associated with serological evidence of persistent Epstein-Barr virus infection. *Lancet,* 61–64.

Tobi, M., and Straus, S. E.. (1985). Chronic Epstein-Barr virus disease: A workshop held by the National Institute of Allergy and Infectious Diseases. *Annals of Internal Medicine, 103,* 951–953.

Tosato, G., Straus, J., et al. (1985). Characteristic T-cell dysfunction in patients with chronic active Epstein-Barr virus infection (chronic infectious mononucleosis). *Journal of Immunology, 134,* 3082–2088.

Trubo, R. (1986, May 12). Viruses: The lurking menace. *Medical World News,* 56–58, 63–71.

Turkington, C. (1985, November). Viruses tied to mental symptoms. *Monitor,* American Psychological Association, 16(11).

Wakefield, D., Lloyd, A., et al. (1988, May). Human herpesvirus 6 and myalgic encephalomyelitis [Letter]. *The Lancet,* 1059.

Walsh, R. D., and Cunha, B. A. (1993, April). The diagnostic approach to chronic fatigue syndrome. *Journal of Infectious Medicine, 14*(4), 48–52

Weikel, W. J. (1989, May). A multimodal approach in dealing with chronic Epstein-Barr viral syndrome. *Journal of Counseling and Development, 6,* 522–524.

Wilber, K. and Wilber, T. (1988, September/October). Do we make ourselves sick? *New Age Journal.* (Reprinted in *CFS Bulletin,* CFS Association of Greater Phoenix, 1988–89, December/January).

Wilson, A., Hickie, I., et al. (1994, June). The treatment of chronic fatigue syndrome: Science and speculation. *American Journal of Medicine, 86,* 544–550.

Winslow, R. (1991, September 16). Virus may have role in causing chronic fatigue. *The Wall Street Journal*, B1, B2.

Zarski, J. J., West, J. D., et al. (1988). Chronic illness: Stressors, the adjustment process, and family-focused interventions. *Journal of Mental Health Counseling, 10,* 145–158.

Zoler, M. L. (1988, December 12). Chronic fatigue: Taking the syndrome seriously. *Medical World News,* 33–41.

OTHER RESOURCES

American Association for Chronic Fatigue Syndrome (1994, October 7–9). Proceedings: Research Conference, Fort Lauderdale, FL.

American Association for Chronic Fatigue Syndrome (1994, October 9 and 10). Proceedings: Clinical Conference, Fort Lauderdale, FL.

Archard, L. (1990, February). Molecular virology of muscle disease: Persistent virus infection of muscle in patients with post-viral fatigue [lecture]. Los Angeles: Chronic Fatigue Syndrome and Fibromyalgia: Pathogenesis and Treatment.

Bastien, S. (1991, May 19). Neuropsychological deficits in CFS [lecture]. Bel Air, CA: CFS: Current Theory and Treatment.

Behan, P. (1990, February). Recent findings in patients with post-viral fatigue syndrome [lecture]. Los Angeles: CFS and FM: Pathogenesis and Treatment.

Bell, D. (1990, February). Chronic fatigue syndrome in children: The role of symptom severity rating [lecture]: Los Angeles: CFS and FM: Pathogenesis and Treatment.

———. (1988, October). Lecture presented at the Rhode Island CFIDS Symposium [audiotape].

———. (1987, November 6). Outbreak of chronic fatigue syndrome in New York State [lecture transcript]. Wilsonville, OR: National CEBV Convention.

Blanck, R. (1994, October). Gulf War Syndrome. Proceedings: AACFS Clinical Conference, Fort Lauderdale, FL.

Buchwald, D. and Mease, P. (1990, February). Chronic fatigue syndrome and fibromyalgia: Current research findings and treatment approaches [lecture]. Los Angeles: CFS and FM: Pathogenesis and Treatment.

Caro, X. (1990, February). Is there an immunologic component to the fibrositis syndrome? [lecture]. Los Angeles: CFS and FM: Pathogenesis and Treatment.

The Centers for Disease Control (1990, January). The chronic fatigue syndrome: An information pamphlet.

The CFIDS Association, Inc. In *The CFIDS Chronicle* (1991, Spring).

Unraveling the mystery: The CFIDS Association research conference [transcript].

Cheney, P. R. (1991, May 18). CFS: A current perspective [lecture]. Bel Air, CA: CFS: Current Theory and Treatment.

————. (1990, February). Chronic fatigue syndrome: An immunological perspective [lecture]. Los Angeles: CFS and FM: Pathogenesis and Treatment.

————. (1988, October). Lecture presented at the Rhode Island CFIDS Symposium [audiotape].

————. (1987, November 7). Closing comments: Final remarks concerning chronic fatigue syndrome [lecture transcript]. Wilsonville, OR: National CEBV Association Convention.

————. (1987, November 5). Definition of chronic fatigue syndrome: Causes, health concerns. Is this a real entity? [lecture transcript]. Wilsonville, OR: National CEBV Association Convention.

————. (1987, January 14). Chronic Epstein-Barr virus syndrome [audiotaped lecture]. Incline Village, NV.

————. (1987, January 13). An outbreak of chronic fatigue illness characterized by fatigue, neurologic, and immunologic disorders: Epstein-Barr virus, cause or effect? [videotape]. Reno, NV: Washoe Medical Center.

Daly, J. (1992). The ventilatory response to exercise in chronic fatigue syndrome [lecture], Chronic Fatigue Syndrome and the Brain Symposium, Los Angeles, CA.

De Becker, P., De Meirleir, K., et al. (1994, October). Ampligen activity in chronic fatigue syndrome [in drug trials in Belgium]. Proceedings: AACFS Research Conference, Fort Lauderdale, FL, 86.

DeFreitas, E., Hiliard, B., et al. (1990, September). Evidence of retrovirus in patients with chronic fatigue immune dysfunction syndrome [presentation at 11th International Congress of Neuropathology]. Kyoto, Japan.

De Freitas, E. (1991, November 13). Chronic fatigue syndrome: Diagnosing the doubt [teleconference]. CTV World Television.

Demitrack, M. (1991, November 13). Chronic fatigue syndrome: Diagnosing the doubt [teleconference]. CTV World Television.

Fudenberg, H. H. (1990, February). Immunotherapy of chronic fatigability immune dysregulation syndrome [lecture]. Los Angeles: CFS and FM: Pathogenesis and Treatment.

Fylstra, D. H. (1995). Dr. Martin's stealth virus research: A closer look. CFS Newswire, Prodigy CFS Bulletin Board.

Goldenberg, D. (1990, February). A controlled study of tender points in patients with chronic fatigue syndrome [lecture]. Los Angeles: CFS and FM: Pathogenesis and Treatment.

Goldstein, J. A. (1991, May 19). Medical management of the CFS patient in family practice [lecture]. Bel Air, CA: CFS: Current Theory and Treatment.

———. (1991, May 18). Limbic encephalopathy in a dysregulated neuroimmune network [lecture]. Los Angeles: CFS: Current Theory and Treatment.

———. (1990, February). Presumed pathogenesis and treatment of the chronic fatigue syndrome/fibromyalgia complex [lecture]. Los Angeles: CFS and FM: Pathogenesis and Treatment.

———. (1988, October). A unified hypothesis of CFIDS: Pathophysiology, diagnosis, and treatment. [lecture audiotape]. Rhode Island CFIDS Symposium.

———. (1987, November 6). The psychoneuroimmuno- pharmacology of the chronic fatigue syndrome [lecture transcript]. Wilsonville, OR: National CEBV Association Convention.

Grufferman, S. (1987, November 5). CEBV controversy: What we need to do to gain credibility in the research world and with the general public [lecture transcript]. Wilsonville, OR: National CEBV Association Convention.

Gunn, W. (1991, November 13). Chronic Fatigue syndrome: Diagnosing the doubt [teleconference]. CTV World Television.

Hallowitz, R. (1988, October). Lecture presented at the Rhode Island CFIDS Symposium [audiotape].

Handleman, M. J. (1990, February). Neurological substrates of behavior: Brain mapping and the chronic fatigue patient [lecture]. Los Angeles: CFS and FM: Pathogenesis and Treatment.

Herberman, R. B. (1990, February). Abnormalities in immune system in patients with chronic fatigue syndrome [lecture]. Los Angeles: CFS and FM: Pathogenesis and Treatment.

Hermann, W. (1990, February). Inhibition of T-cell mitogen response in chronic fatigue syndrome [lecture]. Los Angeles: CFS and FM: Pathogenesis and Treatment.

Hyde, B. (1990, February). The definition and history of ME/CFS [lecture]. Los Angeles: CFS and FM: Pathogenesis and Treatment.

Hyde, B. (1991, May 18). A report on the NIH consensus conference redefining CFS [lecture]. Bel Air, CA: CFS: Current Theory and Treatment.

Iger, L. M. (1992, April 26). Changes on the chronic fatigue syndrome profile with the MMPI-2 [lecture]. Bel Air, CA: Chronic Fatigue Syndrome and the Brain Symposium.

————. (1991, May 19). Cognitive restructuring with the CFS patient [lecture]. Bel Air, CA: CFS: Current Theory and Treatment.

————. (1990, February). The MMPI as an aid in confirming a chronic fatigue syndrome diagnosis [lecture]. Los Angeles: CFS and FM: Pathogenesis and Treatment.

Imperati, S. (1987, November 6). Social security disability: A lawyer's view [lecture transcript]. Wilsonville, OR: National CEBV Association Convention.

Jacobson, E. (1991, May 18). Drug therapy in CFS: A psychobiologic approach [lecture]. Bel Air, CA: CFS: Current Theory and Treatment.

Johnson, A. (1987, November 6). Environmental factors and their effect on chronic fatigue syndrome [lecture transcript]. Wilsonville, OR: National CEBV Association Convention.

Jones, J. F. (1988, October). Lecture presented at the Rhode Island CFIDS Symposium [audiotape].

————. (1987, February 4). Sinequan used as treatment for symptoms of CEBV [memorandum]. Denver: National Jewish Center for Immunology and Respiratory Medicine.

Jones, J. F., and Cheney, P. (1986, June). Chronic Epstein-Barr virus [videotaped lecture]. Lake Tahoe, NV.

Jones, J. F., and Hutter, M. J. (1983). Instructional guide to chronic Epstein-Barr infection [transcript of videotaped lecture]. Tucson, AZ: Biomedical Communications.

Khalsa, G. S. S. (1987, November 6). Naturopathic medicine: Applications in chronic viral illness [lecture transcript]. Wilsonville, OR: National CEBV Association Convention.

Komaroff, A. (1991, November 13). Chronic fatigue syndrome: Diagnosing the doubt [teleconference]. CTV World Television.

Komaroff, A. (1988, October). Lecture presented at the Rhode Island CFIDS Symposium [audiotape].

Levinson, H. (1987, November 7). Cerebellar-vestibular dysfunction and phobias [lecture transcript]. Wilsonville, OR: National CEBV Association Convention.

Levinson, H. (1987, November 6). Introduction to balance disorders [lecture transcript]. Wilsonville, OR: National CEBV Association Convention.

Lloyd, A. R. (1990, February). The pathophysiology of "fatigue" in patients with chronic fatigue syndrome [lecture]. Los Angeles: CFS and FM: Pathogenesis and Treatment.

Lloyd, A. (1991, November 13). Chronic fatigue syndrome: Diagnosing the doubt [teleconference]. CTV World Television.

Lottenberg, S. (1990, February). Positron emission tomography in chronic fatigue syndrome [lecture]. Los Angeles: CFS and FM: Pathogenesis and Treatment.

Loveless, M. O. (1991, May 18). Chronic immunologic activation and CFS [lecture]. Bel Air, CA: CFS: Current Theory and Treatment.

———. (1987, November 7). Chronic fatigue syndrome: A post-viral immunologically mediated disease? [lecture transcript]. Wilsonville, OR: National CEBV Association Convention.

Martin, W. J. (1990, February). Detection of viral sequences using the polymerase chain reaction [lecture]. Los Angeles: CFS and FM: Pathogenesis and Treatment.

McGregor, H. L., Zerbes, M., et al. (1994, May). Chronic fatigue syndrome: A urinary biomarker. Proceedings: M.E. Symposium, Dunedin, New Zealand.

Mena, I. (1991, May 18). Study of cerebral perfusion by NeuroSPECT in patients with CFS [lecture]. Bel Air, CA: CFS: Current Theory and Treatment.

———. (1990, February). Study of cerebral perfusion by NeuroSPECT in patients with chronic fatigue syndrome [lecture]. Los Angeles: CFS and FM: Pathogenesis and Treatment.

Minann, Inc. Statistical data on diagnosed patients [unpublished study]. Glenview, IL.

Moldofsky, H. (1990, February). The significance of sleep-wave physiology and immune functions to chronic fatigue syndrome and fibromyalgia [lecture]. Los Angeles: CFS and FM: Pathogenesis and Treatment.

National Cancer Institute, Office of Cancer Communications. (1986, October). NCI isolates new human herpes-like virus. Cancer Facts.

National CEBV Syndrome Association, Inc. Guidelines for interpreting EBV antibody titers [report]. Prepared with the help of James F. Jones, M.D., Denver: National Jewish Center for Immunology and Respiratory Medicine.

National CFS Association. Chronic fatigue syndrome [brochure]. Kansas City, MO.

National Institute of Allergy and Infectious Disease. (1991, November 12). NIAID funds three CFS cooperative research centers. Update.

Nightingale Research Foundation (Spring, 1990). The Cambridge symposium on Myalgic Encephalomyelitis (M.E.): Summary of proceedings.

Nord Disease Database (1986, May 1). Information on CMV [report].

Peterson, D. (1991, November 13). Chronic fatigue syndrome: Diagnosing the doubt [teleconference]. CTV World Television.

————. (1991, May). Phoenix, AZ: Lecture given at monthly meeting of The CFS Association of Arizona.

————. (1991, May 18). Progress report of Ampligen 2-5A study [lecture]. Bel Air, CA: CFS: Current Theory and Treatment.

Plioplys, S. and Plioplys, A. V. (1994). Amantadine and L-carnitine therapy of chronic fatigue syndrome: preliminary results. Proceedings: AACFS Research Conference, Fort Lauderdale, FL, 92.

Reed, J. C. (1988, March). Treating CEBV [lecture]. Phoenix, AZ: monthly meeting of the CFS Association of Arizona.

Rubin, P. (1988, September 6). Phoenix, AZ: Lecture given at monthly meeting of the CFS Association of Arizona.

Russell, I. J. (1990, February). Fibrositis syndrome: Diagnosis, pathogenesis and management [lecture]. Los Angeles: CFS and FM: Pathogenesis and Treatment.

Sandman, C. (1991, May 18). How CFS affects memory [lecture]. Bel Air, CA: CFS: Current Theory and Treatment.

————. (1990, February). Is there a CFS dementia? [lecture]. Los Angeles: CFS and FM: Pathogenesis and Treatment.

Schluederberg, A. (1988, May). Information on research conducted by the National Institute of Allergy and Infectious Diseases (NIAID) on chronic Epstein-Barr (CEBV) infection and chronic fatigue syndrome (CFS). NIAID: Bacteriology and Virology Branch, Microbiology and Infectious Diseases Program.

Sleight, R. B. (1988, October). Lecture presented at the Rhode Island CFIDS Symposium [audiotape].

Steinbach, T., and Hermann, W. (1994). The diagnosis and treatment of CFIDS with Kutapressin. *The CFIDS Information Line*. Charlotte, NC: The CFIDS Association of America, Inc.

U.S. Department of Health and Human Services (1991, December 2). HHS News.

Wakefield, D. (1990, February). Immunological abnormalities and immune therapy in chronic fatigue syndrome [lecture]. Los Angeles: CFS and FM: Pathogenesis and Treatment.

Index

A

Abdominal pain, 67
Abnormalities, multisystem, 35–44
Aches. *See* Pain
Activity level, 9, 213–216
Acupuncture, 159–160
Acyclovir, 181
Adenosine monophosphate (AMP), 179
Adenoviruses, 4, 94
Age, and incidence of CFIDS, 6, 53
Agencies, government, 267–268, 273
Aid, financial, 124, 274–275
AIDS, 13, 134, 208, 255, 266–267
Allergies, 64, 89, 277–278
Allopathy, 151, 156–158
Alpha interferon (IFN), 179–180
Alternative treatments, 158–163
The American Association for
  Chronic Fatigue Syndrome
  (AACFS), 35, 269
American Medical Association
  (AMA), 159
The American Medical Dictionary: Physi-
  cians in the United States, 170
Americans with Disabilities Act, 245
Ampligen, 180
Anatomy of an Illness (Cousins), 221
Anesthesia, 205–206
Anger, 131, 227–228, 231
Annals of Internal Medicine, 27
Antibiotics, 180
Antibodies, 35, 89
Antidepressants, 51, 180, 193, 195–197
Antifungals, 180–181
Antigens, 87, 88, 91
Antioxidants, 181
Antivirals, 181
Anxiety, 76–77, 102, 193
Associations, 269–280
Attitudes, about CFIDS, 3–4, 132–135
Audiotapes and videotapes, CFIDS re-
  lated, 283–284

Autogenic training, 223
Autoimmune disorders, 5, 91
Ayurvedic medicine, 160

B

Balance disorders, 63, 73–75, 197,
  203–204, 278
Balancing Act (Watson and Sinclair),
  203–204
Barry, Dave, 24
Bastien, Sheila, 69
B-cells, 88, 89, 90
Behan, Peter, 68
Beliefs, about CFIDS, 3–4, 132–135
Bell, David, 32, 57, 96, 144–146, 268
Berger, Stuart, 26, 209
Biofeedback, 222–223
Bladder problems, 66–67
Blood cells, white, 87
Books. *See* Publications
Borysenko, Joan, 162
Brain, xiii, 11, 28, 38–39, 66, 105–106
Breastfeeding, 68
Breast implants, xiii, 48
Browning, David J., 73
Bupropion, 196
BuSpar (buspirone), 193
Buyers' Club, 271

C

Cancer, 90
Candidiasis. *See* Yeast overgrowth
L-carnitine, 183
Centers for Disease Control and Prevention (CDC), xiii, 4, 8, 14–15,
  255, 267
Central nervous system, 38–39, 44,
  68–75
Cerebellar-vestibular system, malfunction of, 74–75
CFIDS
  causes of, 4, 11, 47, 52, 87–114
  defined, 3–5, 11–15

To Order Other Books and Audiotapes by Katrina Berne

CFIDS LITE: Chronic Fatigue Immune Dysfunction Syndrome with 1/3 the Seriousness *(Paperback book — illustrated — 110 pages)*
CFIDS is no laughing matter, but humor can help us keep a healthy perspective on living with chronic illness. The jokes, riddles, limericks, and cartoons in *CFIDS Lite* help to combat the pain and isolation caused by CFIDS. Perhaps laughter *is* the best medicine.

AUDIOTAPES (All are 60 minutes long and narrated by the author)

UNDERSTANDING CHRONIC FATIGUE SYNDROME
Developed for PWCs and interested others. Basic information about symptoms, diagnosis, relapses and remissions, causal theories, treatment modalities, and resources.

CFIDS...FOR THOSE WHO CARE
For spouses, partners, family members, friends, and coworkers. **Side 1** contains information about CFIDS and its impact on relationships. **Side 2** offers techniques for helping PWCs in a way that enhances the relationship: communicating about the illness; giving and receiving emotional support, setting reasonable limits, coping with the illness, handling guilt and disappointment, affirming both partners.

CFIDS AND SELF-ESTEEM
Addresses sources of low self-esteem in PWCs (changed abilities, appearance, productivity, and self-expectations) and offers techniques for enhancing self-image and confidence; developing realistic and affirming internal messages; and improving self-care and nurturing.

NEUROCOGNITIVE ASPECTS OF CFIDS
Addresses concerns about neurological and cognitive dysfunctions such as short-term memory deficit; spatial disorientation; brain fog; difficulty using words and numbers; sensory overload; difficulty with concentration, comprehension, and sequencing. Includes strategies for coping.

RELAXATION, IMAGERY, AND HEALING EXERCISES
Side 1: Daytime. Relaxation exercise for use as an adjunct to medical treatment to promote healing, reduce stress, create positive imagery, and help to mobilize the body's healing and energy-producing potential.
Side 2: Evening. Relaxation exercise designed to reduce anxiety, bring about a sense of peace and balance, and help to achieve sound sleep.

Ordering Information ** (see note below)

CFIDS Lite	$10.00
Understanding Chronic Fatigue Syndrome	8.50
CFIDS...For Those Who Care	8.50
CFIDS and Self Esteem	8.50
Neurocognitive Aspects of CFIDS	8.50
Relaxation, Imagery and Healing Exercises	8.50

Shipping/handling: $2.50 for the first item; $.50 for each additional item.

These materials may be ordered from: BHB COMMUNICATIONS, 761 East University, Suite F, Mesa, AZ 85203

** Please send all orders for items on this page and make checks payable to BHB Communications — *not* to Hunter House